Current Topics in Pathology
81

Geraint T. Williams (Ed.)

Gastrointestinal Pathology

Contributors

D.C. Allen · A.J. Blackshaw · W.V. Bogomoletz
H.J.R. Bussey · M.F. Dixon · V. Duchatelle
C. Fenger · P.A. Hall · P.W. Hamilton · Ph.U. Heitz
P. Hermanek · J.R. Jass · P. Komminoth
D.A. Levison · M.M. Mathan · V.I. Mathan · F. Potet
A.B. Price · A.H. Qizilbash · N.A. Shepherd
P. Sipponen · J.M. Sloan · P.S. Teglbjærg
P.C.H. Watt

Springer-Verlag Berlin Heidelberg New York
London Paris Tokyo Hong Kong

G. T. Williams, B. Sc., M. D., M. R. C. P., M. R. C. Path.,
Department of Pathology,
University of Wales College of Medicine,
Cardiff CF4 4XN, United Kingdom

C. L. Berry, Professor, M. D., Ph. D., F. R. C. Path.,
Department of Morbid Anatomy, The London Hospital,
London E1 1BB, United Kingdom

E. Grundmann, Professor Dr.,
Gerhard-Domagk-Institut für Pathologie der
Universität Münster, Domagkstraße 17,
4400 Münster, Federal Republic of Germany

With 126 Figures and 28 Tables

ISBN 3-540-51016-8 Springer-Verlag Berlin Heidelberg New York
ISBN 0-387-51016-8 Springer-Verlag New York Berlin Heidelberg

Typesetting, printing and bookbinding: Druckerei Parzeller, D-6400 Fulda
2122/3130-543210 – Printed on acid-free paper

List of Contributors

Allen, D. C., Dr.	Department of Histopathology, Belfast City Hospital, Lisburn Road, Belfast, Northern Ireland, BT9 7AD
Blackshaw, A. J., Dr.	Department of Histopathology, Bedford City Hospital, Bedford, United Kingdom
Bogomoletz, W. V. Dr.	Laboratoire d'Anatomie Pathologique, Institut Jean Godinot, B.P. 171, F-51056 Reims, France
Bussey, H. J. R., Dr.	Department of Pathology and the Polyposis Registry, St. Mark's Hospital, City Road, London EC1V 2PS, United Kingdom
Dixon, M. F., Dr.	Department of Pathology, University of Leeds, Leeds, LS2 9JT, United Kingdom
Duchatelle, V., Dr.	Service d'Anatomie Pathologique, Hôpital Avicenne, F-93000 Bobigny, France
Fenger, C., Dr.	Department of Pathology, Odense University Hospital, DK-5000 Odense C, Denmark
Hall, P. A., Dr.	Keratinocyte Laboratory, Imperial Cancer Research Fund, Lincoln's Inn Fields, London, WC2A 3PX, United Kingdom
Hamilton, P. W., Dr.	Department of Pathology, Royal Victoria Hospital, Grosvenor Road, Belfast, Northern Ireland, BT12 6BA

HEITZ, PH. U., Prof. Dr.	Institute of Pathology, University of Zurich, Schmelzstraße 12, CH-8091 Zurich Switzerland
HERMANEK, P., Prof., Surg. Path.	Department of Surgical Pathology, University of Erlangen, Maximiliansplatz D-8520 Erlangen, Federal Republic of Germany
JASS, J. R., Prof. Dr.	Department of Pathology, University of Auckland, School of Medicine, Private Bag, Auckland, New Zealand
KOMMINOTH, P., Dr.	Institute of Pathology, University of Zurich, Schmelzstraße 12, CH-8091 Zurich Switzerland
LEVISON, D. A., Prof. Dr.	Department of Histopathology, Guy's Hospital, London Bridge, London SEI 9RT, United Kingdom
MATHAN, M. M., Prof. Dr.	The Wellcome Research Unit, Christian Medical College Hospital, Vellore 632004, India
MATHAN, V. I., Prof. Dr.	The Wellcome Research Unit, Christian Medical College Hospital, Vellore 632004, India
POTET, F., Prof. Dr.	Service d'Anatomie Pathologique, Hôpital Beaujon, F-92118 Clichy Cedex, France
PRICE, A. B., Dr.	Department of Pathology, Northwick Park Hospital, Harrow, Middlesex, HAI 3UJ United Kingdom
QIZILBASH, A. H., Dr.	Department of Pathology, North York General Hospital, 4001 Leslie Street at Highway 401, Willowdale, Ontario, M2K 1E1, Canada
SHEPHERD, N. A., Dr.	Department of Histopathology, Gloucestershire Royal Hospital, Great Western Road, Gloucester GL1 3NN, United Kingdom

Sipponen, P., Dr.	Department of Pathology, Jorvi Hospital, 02740 Espoo, Finland
Sloan, J. M., Dr.	Department of Pathology, Royal Victoria Hospital, Grosvenor Road, Belfast, Northern Ireland, BT12 6 BA
Teglbjærg, P. S., Prof. Dr.	Department of Pathology, Aalborg Sygehus, DK-9000 Aalborg, Denmark
Watt, P. C. H., Dr.	Department of Pathology, Royal Victoria Hospital, Grosvenor Road, Belfast, Northern Ireland, BT12 6BA

Preface

There have been many advances in the field of gastrointestinal pathology which are of considerable clinical significance during the 13 years since the last publication of a volume of *Current Topics in Pathology* devoted to this subject. Many have arisen from the application of new techniques of histochemistry, immunocytochemistry, quantitative morphometry and molecular and cell biology to gastrointestinal diseases, but some, notably the recognition of the association of *Campylobacter pylori* with the commonest type of chronic gastritis, have been achieved using such long established 'routine' histological procedures that one wonders how their significance had escaped recognition for so long. The topics covered in this volume have been selected because they present advances of relevance to the diagnostic clinical pathologist. However, they represent the personal selection of the editor, and are in no way exhaustive. Many other examples of progress in our understanding of the pathophysiology of gastrointestinal diseases have been omitted, either because of the confines of space or because they have been well reviewed recently in other publications.

Most of the workload of the practising gastrointestinal pathologist involves the diagnosis and assessment either of inflammation or of neoplasia in the alimentary tract, and this is reflected in the topics presented in this book. Thus there are expert contributions on current ideas of the pathology of gastritis and duodenitis, the biopsy diagnosis of collagenous colitis, ischaemic colitis, and intestinal spirochaetosis, and an assessment of the value of quantitative techniques in the diagnosis of chronic inflammatory bowel disease. Increasing international travel has meant that all pathologists should now have more than a passing acquaintance with conditions which have previously been regarded as tropical diseases, and a chapter by MATHAN and MATHAN, who have a vast experience in this area, is included.

In the field of gastrointestinal neoplasia, there are chapters covering the histological recognition of precancerous lesions of the oesophagus, stomach, small intestine and anus; descriptions of important advances in both the genetics and pathology of the gastrointestinal polyposis syndromes; the assessment and significance of newly recognised prognostic factors in colorectal cancer; and the role of the surgical pathologist in the clinical management of locally excised malignant polyps of the large intestine. A critical evaluation of quantitative techniques in diagnostic gastrointestinal pathology is given by the Belfast group, who have made a special contribution to this field, and valuable guidance is given on the biopsy diagnosis of disorders of intestinal neuronal innervation by HEITZ and KOMMINOTH, based on their great personal experience. Finally, the benefit of combining classical morphology with the newly available techniques of immunology and cell and molecular biology is well illustrated in a chapter on the gut-associated lymphoid tissue and gastrointestinal malignant lymphoma.

Although this book is written primarily for diagnostic histopathologists, is is hoped that it will also be of value to all practitioners of clinical and surgical gastroenterology who depend on the pathologist for their daily management of patients.

I wish to express my wholehearted gratitude and appreciation to the contributors of this volume, who have given generously of their precious time. I am also most grateful to my personal secretary, Mrs. N. J. Owen, and to the staff of Springer Verlag, notably Ms. H. Herion, Ms. U. Davis, and Mrs. D. Oelschläger, whose patient assistance has been invaluable.

Cardiff, United Kingdom GERAINT T. WILLIAMS

Contents

Indexed in ISR

Progress in the Pathology of Gastritis and Duodenitis

M. F. DIXON

1 Introduction

Although for many years a simple classification of 'non-specific' gastritis into acute, chronic superficial and chronic atrophic categories has sufficed in routine histopathological practice, the clinical significance of the latter diagnoses is uncertain. While acute gastritis has well established and consistent clinical associations (a recent history of drug ingestion or alcohol excess leading to haemorrhagic erosions), the clinical features of chronic gastritis are much more nebulous. The finding of chronic gastritis in 'healthy volunteers' (KREUNING et al. 1978) and in random population surveys (VILLAKO et al. 1976) has led some to conclude that the condition is a normal aging process of no clinical consequence. While this is a minority view, even those who believe it to be a pathological process have difficulty in recognising at what point the density of the inflammatory cell infiltration becomes 'abnormal', and the relationship between this inflammatory process, symptomatology and associated pathology.

There have been several attempts to refine the histological classification of chronic gastritis, the best known being that of WHITEHEAD et al. (1972), who advocated a system based on the type of mucosa, subdivision into superficial and atrophic forms, the 'activity' (presence of polymorph infiltration), and the presence and type of metaplasia. Thus according to their scheme a biopsy might be reported as showing 'antral active chronic superficial gastritis without metaplasia' or 'body inactive chronic atrophic gastritis with intestinal metaplasia'. These authors also endorsed the additional category of 'gastric mucosal atrophy' for biopsies showing marked glandular atrophy, widespread metaplasia and negligible inflammmatory cell infiltration. However, others, such as CHELI and GIACOSA (1983), prefer to consider this picture as simply the severe end of the spectrum found in chronic atrophic gastritis and do not feel that a separate diagnostic category is warranted. These authors also address the not infrequent problem of categorising cases where deep (transmucosal) chronic inflammatory infiltration is found without convincing glandular atrophy. Insofar as neither *superficial* nor *atrophic* gastritis is appropriate, they advocate the term 'interstitial gastritis', but the introduction of this additional diagnosis would only serve to confuse further an already confusing subject. Putting these semantic problems to one side, an expedient classification is that recently proposed by KEKKI et al. (1987), where chronic gastritis in the absence of glandular loss is termed *superficial* irrespective of the depth and intensity of the inflammatory cell infiltrate, and where there is glandular loss the varying degrees are reflected in the terms mild, moderate and severe *atrophic* gastritis. This classification has the merit of simplicity and when applied to body mucosa is closely allied to functional changes.

These attempts to classify chronic gastritis on morphological grounds have brought increased uniformity to histological reporting but have added nothing to our understanding of the pathogenetic mechanisms involved.

Classifications based on topography and clinical associations have achieved more in this regard. STRICKLAND and MACKAY (1973) recognised two major categories of chronic gastritis, one mainly affecting body mucosa and associated with marked hypochlorhydria, high gastrin levels and antiparietal cell antibodies in the serum which they designated type A, and one showing predominantly antral involvement, low gastrin levels and no parietal cell antibodies which they termed type B. This classification was expanded by GLASS and PITCHUMONI (1975) to include cases with patchy involvement of antrum and body – type AB. A more refined analysis of the three categories was provided by CORREA (1980), who, as before, distinguished an auto-immune type, but separated the remainder into *hypersecretory* and *environmental* types. Hypersecretory chronic gastritis is predominantly antral and is associated with duodenal or prepyloric gastric ulceration and excessive production of acid and pepsin. Environmental chronic gastritis is multifocal, affecting both antrum and body, and is associated with more proximal gastric ulcers and an increased tendency to develop dysplasia and carcinoma. From an aetiological point of view CORREA proposed that hypersecretory gastritis was possible triggered by psychosomatic or neurogenic mechanisms, and that environmental gastritis was related to dietary toxins and irritants.

Our views on the aetiology of chronic gastritis have undergone a dramatic reappraisal since 1983, when WARREN and MARSHALL 'rediscovered' curved bacilli, later named *Campylobacter pylori*, on the surface of gastric biopsies from patients with gastritis and peptic ulceration. The pathogenic status of this organism remains controversial, but sufficient evidence has accumulated to suggest that most non-auto-immune chronic gastritis can be considered a consequence of *Campylobacter* infection. We have therefore proposed that the designation type B, indicating bacteria-associated chronic gastritis, remains entirely appropriate (WYATT and DIXON 1988).

The ability to recognise these organisms readily in biopsy material has led to a great upsurge in interest in gastritis, and it has rapidly become apparent that there is wide variation in the prevalence of *C. pylori* in different clinicopathological settings. In turn, this has prompted an increased awareness of heterogeneity within chronic gastritis, and it is these 'new' forms of gastritis which I principally intend to explore in this chapter.

2 Type B Chronic Gastritis

The histological features of type B gastritis are well known. There is an increase in the number of lymphocytes and plasma cells within the lamina propria which is termed *superficial* in the absence of glandular atrophy and *atrophic* if the infiltrate is associated with glandular loss. Polymorph infiltration is taken as a sign of *activity*, and polymorphs are usually seen as an interstitial infiltrate between the pits and within foveolar and surface

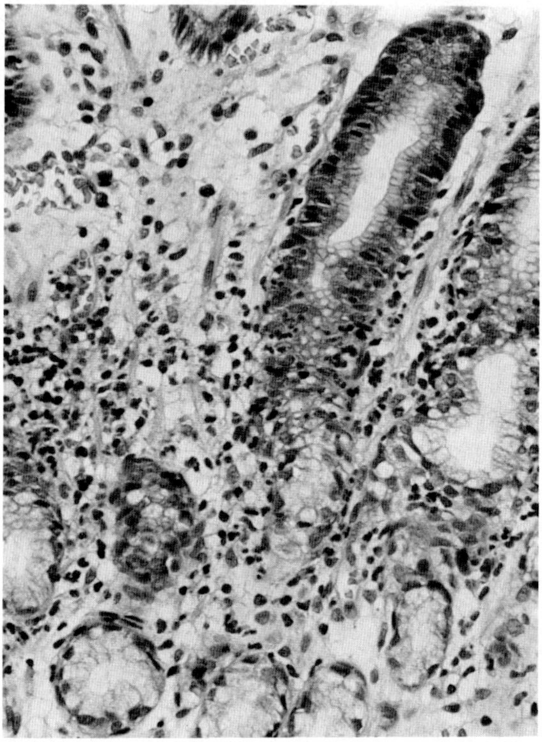

Fig. 1. Type B gastritis. Neutrophil polymorph infiltration concentrated around the isthmic region of a gastric pit

epithelium. In severe activity they collect in the pits, forming the equivalent of crypt abscesses. In many cases polymorphs appear to congregate specifically around the pit-isthmic region which corresponds to the proliferative compartment (Fig. 1), and damage to stem cells at this site may be a factor in producing glandular atrophy (HOPWOOD 1988). It is this histological picture, for so long regarded as 'non-specific', that is closely associated with *C. pylori* infection.

The long history of 'spiral organisms' in the stomach and their recent rediscovery and characterisation has been the subject of several good reviews (GOODWIN et al. 1986; MCNULTY 1986; RATHBONE et al. 1986a; BLASER 1987). The organisms were originally identified using the Warthin Starry silver stain, but this method is time consuming and capricious so that simpler techniques, such as the modified Giemsa (GRAY et al. 1986), which we favour, have been widely adopted. Some pathologists believe that the organisms are just as readily recognised in routine haematoxylin and eosin sections, but in our experience scanty organisms can be missed without a 'special' stain. Their association with type B gastritis was noted in WARREN and MARSHALL's first report, and several studies (Table 1) have since confirmed the strength of the association with active, but not inactive, chronic gastritis. *C. pylori* is equally prevalent in chronic super-

Table 1. *C. pylori* and activity in chronic gastritis

	Active			Inactive		
	n	Cp+		*n*	Cp+	
Goodwin et al. (1985) Perth, WA	51	47	(92%)	23	8	(35%)
Morris et al. (1986 a) Auckland, NZ	28	23	(82%)	7	1	(14%)
Rawles et al. (1986) Baltimore, USA	23	16	(70%)	47	7	(15%)
Wyatt et al. (1986) Leeds, UK	109	95	(87%)	35	13	(37%)
Jiang et al. (1987) Shanghai, China	49	44	(90%)	72	36	(50%)

Table 2. *C. pylori* gastritis in children

	n	Chronic gastritis	Cp+	Age range (yrs)
Czinn et al. (1986)	5	5	5	10 –16
Drumm et al. (1987)	67	10	7	8.7–15.5
Mahony et al. (1987)	38	10	9	10 –16
Thomas et al. (1988)	50	10	10	5 –16

ficial and chronic atrophic gastritis (ROLLASON et al. 1984) with the exception of gastric atrophy and intestinal metaplasia. When infection is present the organisms are widely distributed throughout the stomach and it has been claimed that the finding of the organism can be taken as a marker of active chronic gastritis within that stomach, although not necessarily at the site of detection (HAZELL et al. 1987). Examination of multiple biopsies has shown that two antral biopsies will reveal their presence in all positive cases (WYATT et al. 1988 b). The organism inhabits exclusively gastric-type epithelium, including gastric metaplasia in the duodenum (PRICE et al. 1985; ROLLASON et al. 1984; STEER 1984); it does not colonise intestinal-type epithelium either in the intestine proper or in metaplastic areas in the stomach, nor does it colonise severely dysplastic epithelium (unpublished observations) or the surface of cancer cells (JIANG et al. 1987).

Just as the prevalence of chronic gastritis rises with age (VILLAKO et al. 1986), so does the prevalence of *C. pylori* infection as detected both histologically (WYATT and RATHBONE 1988) and by serological testing for *C. pylori*-specific IgG antobodies (JONES et al. 1986; MORRIS et al. 1986 a). Where serological studies have included the investigation of children (KAL-

DOR et al. 1985; JONES et al. 1986) these have revealed uniformly low antibody titres, suggesting that, in general, infection is acquired later in life. However, *C. pylori* is an occasional cause of 'primary' chronic gastritis in children and several groups have now reported on their findings in paediatric practice (Table 2). The detection of *C. pylori*-associated gastritis in children who have recently developed dyspeptic symptoms is further evidence in support of an aetiological role. However, the question as to whether or not *C. pylori* is pathogenic still remains unresolved. Evidence in support of its pathogenetic role can be drawn from morphological observations, human and animal infection, immunological studies, biochemical mechanisms and treatment studies.

2.1 Morphological Observations

In our experience histologically detectable *C. pylori* are never found on normal antral mucosa; invariably in positive cases there is some increase in mononuclear cells. However, in patients with gastritis limited to the antrum one can find colonisation of the morphologically normal body mucosa (WYATT et al. 1986), so that inflammation is neither a prerequisite for colonisation nor an inevitable consequence of local colonisation. Failure to provoke an inflammatory response may be linked to low virulence of the particular strain of *C. pylori*; BURNIE et al. (1988) have identified nine

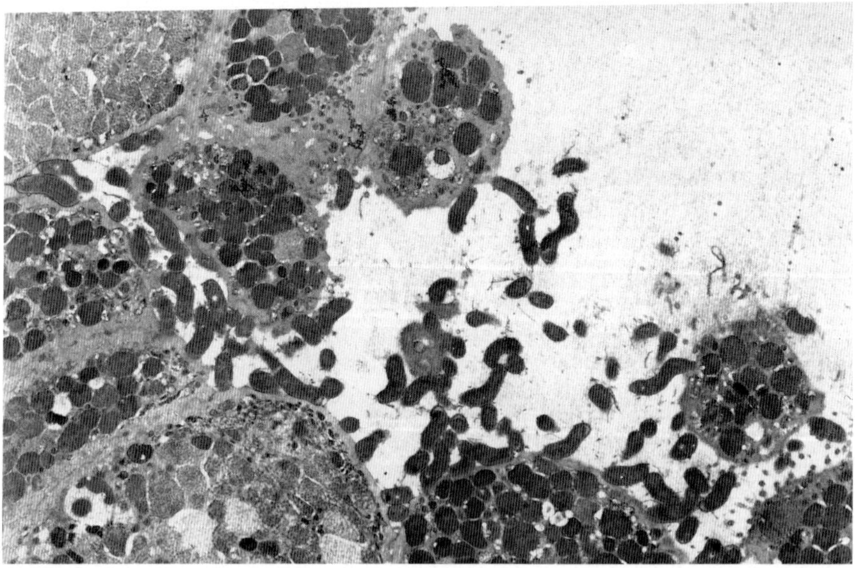

Fig. 2. Type B gastritis. Low power electron micrograph showing numerous *C. pylori* either in the mucus layer or attached to the surface epithelial cells. A few cell fragments have become detached from the epithelium

types of which type 2 was isolated from patients with normal mucosa. We have found *C. pylori* to be more numerous in active inflammation and both neutrophil and eosinophil polymorphs are significantly increased in positive cases (KARTTUNEN et al. 1987). The organisms show a close spatial relationship to polymorphs (ANDERSEN et al. 1987), and to some extent the number of bacteria present can be correlated with the number of neutrophils (STEER 1985). Although these findings are strong support for a local infection, the relationship between activity and *C. pylori* has been disputed by other workers (PRICE et al. 1985; NIEDOBITEK et al. 1987).

Ultrastructurally, the organisms are found very closely apposed to the epithelial plasma membrane (Fig. 2), where there is loss of microvilli and formation of shallow cup-like attachment sites (Fig. 3) similar to the adhesion pedicles of pathogenic *E. coli* (GOODWIN et al. 1986). However, the mere presence of these cell-bacteria interactions does not indicate pathogenicity as similar attachments are seen with some commensal or-

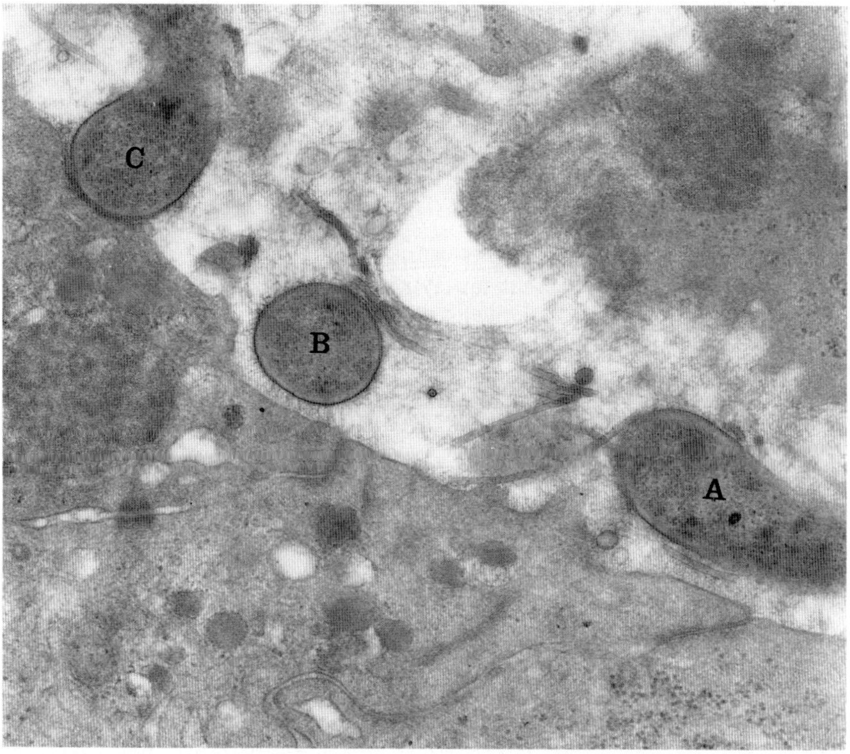

Fig. 3. Tpye B gastritis. Electron micrograph in which three *Campylobacter* organisms show aspects of the attachment process. Organism *A* is possibly attached by a flagellum; *B* shows an ill-defined 'corona' of electron-dense material around the organism, maximal towards the plasma membrane; *C*. appears to be firmly attached at one pole to a saucer-like depression in the plasma membrane, forming a so-called adhesion pedestal

ganisms in a variety of animal species (SAVAGE 1970). Nevertheless, the infected epithelium shows degenerative changes comprising intercellular oedema, detachment from the basal lamina and cell necrosis, and partly digested organisms are seen in vacuoles within epithelial cells (TRICOTTET et al. 1986). Furthermore, organisms have been identified within the canaliculi of parietal cells (CHEN et al. 1986) and in phagocytic vacuoles inside polymorphs (SHOUSHA et al. 1984).

2.2 Human and Animal Infection

Marshall's 'heroic' experiment, in which following ingestion of approximately 10^9 *C. pylori* organisms he developed a symptomatic gastritis (MARSHALL et al. 1985a), seemed to be clear evidence of the organism's pathogenicity. However, this apparently crucial experiment did not confirm a role for *C. pylori* in *chronic* gastritis as the gastritis that developed was histologically acute and proved to be self-limiting. Chronic gastritis did develop in a subsequent human volunteer study (MORRIS and NICHOLSON 1987), and it is likely that two epidemics of hypochlorhydria among volunteer subjects were caused by *C. pylori* transmitted by non-sterilised pH electrodes (RAMSEY et al. 1979; GLEDHILL et al. 1985). In both studies an initial hypochlorhydric illness progressed to histological chronic gastritis in several cases, and in one of these studies retrospective serological testing revealed that antibody titres to *C. pylori* rose in 9 of 12 gastritis patients during the convalescent phase (PETERSON et al. 1987). Sceptics could argue that even these observations do not prove a causal relationship and instead raise the possibility that the hypochlorhydria predated exposure to *C. pylori* and allowed the organisms to colonise and proliferate (HOWDEN and HUNT 1987). It is certainly recognised that the organisms are acid intolerant and do not survive below a pH of 2.5 (HAZELL and LEE 1985) so that at least a transient hypochlorhydria is required to facilitate their safe passage from the gastric lumen to their protected niche beneath the mucus-bicarbonate barrier, where the pH is near neutral. However, a sufficiently hypochlorhydric episode probably occurs with every meal, so there is no need to invoke more esoteric mechanisms.

The establishment of an animal model of *C. pylori* gastritis has proved difficult. Rodents traditionally used in peptic ulcer research have proved unsuitable, but there have been recent reports of chronic gastritis following administration of *C. pylori* to gnotobiotic piglets (LAMBERT et al. 1987; MORGAN et al. 1988) and rhesus monkeys (BASKERVILLE and NEWELL 1988). Gastric colonisation by a related *Campylobacter*-like organism accompanied by chronic gastritis has also been observed as a natural infection in aging ferrets (FOX et al. 1986).

The outcome of these human and animal studies has been to demonstrate that the establishment of *C. pylori* infection in previously normal gastric mucosa results in a chronic inflammatory response.

2.3 Immunological Studies

The fact that patients with *C. pylori* gastritis have raised levels of specific antibody in their serum has already been mentioned. The elevation is of sufficient magnitude to permit serological diagnosis (Rathbone et al. 1986b); Jones et al. 1986) and is proving useful in epidemiological studies, for example among endoscopy personnel (Rawles et al. 1987) and meat workers (Morris et al. 1986a). Specific IgA and IgM antibodies can be detected in gastric juice (Rathbone et al. 1986c) and coating of mucosal *C. pylori* has been demonstrated by immunohistological techniques

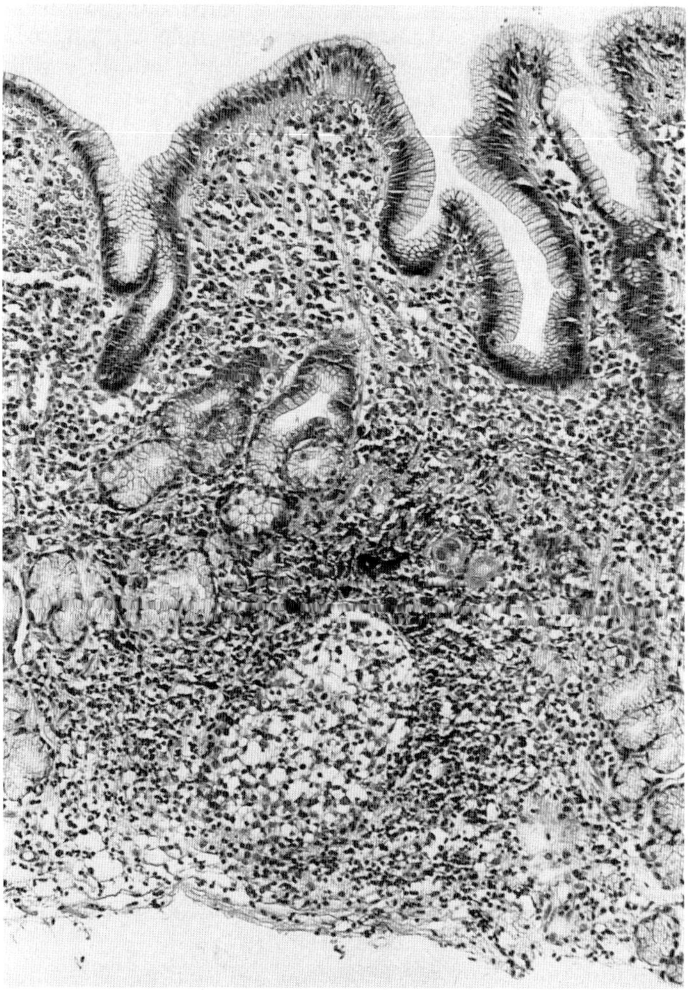

Fig. 4. Type B gastritis. *Campylobacter*-positive chronic gastritis showing a lymphoid aggregate with germinal centre formation

(WYATT et al. 1986). Local production of antibodies to *C. pylori* by plasma cells in the lamina propria has been confirmed by in vitro culture of gastric mucosal biopsies (WYATT and RATHBONE 1988). In keeping with this local specific antibody production, synthesis of secretory component is increased in antral chronic gastritis, as is production of the non-specific antibacterial substances lysozyme and lactoferrin (ISAACSON 1982; VALNES et al. 1984). It has also been shown that the number of CD-4 positive lymphocytes (helper-inducer T cells) increases relative to CD-8 suppressor cells in *C. pylori*-positive gastritis (RATHBONE et al. 1988b) and that these changes are paralleled by the acquisition of lymphoid follicles with germinal centres in about one-third of cases (Fig. 4), such follicles being almost invariably absent in normals and *C. pylori*-negative gastritis (WYATT and RATHBONE 1988). Thus the increase in mononuclear cells seen in type B gastritis is explicable in terms of a cellular and humoral immune response directed towards *C. pylori*. Secretion of IgA antibody is likely to interfere with bacterial adhesion, and coating of organisms by IgM and IgG, which have complement fixing and opsonising properties, would be likely to enhance neutrophil activity against *C. pylori* and explain the association between colonisation and polymorph activity (WYATT et al. 1986a). Enhanced production of the chemotactic factor leukotriene LTC_4 has also been demonstrated in *C. pylori*-associated gastritis compared with normal mucosa (AHMED et al. 1987).

2.4 Biochemical Mechanisms

One of the most remarkable features of *C. pylori* is its urea-splitting capacity (OWEN et al. 1985), and the generation of ammonia in its immediate microenvironment may further protect the organism against acid attack (GOODWIN et al. 1986). The organism's high urease activity has been utilised in developing rapid diagnostic tests based on incubation of gastric biopsies in urea-containing media with a pH indicator (MORRIS et al. 1986b) and in non-invasive breath tests following oral administration of ^{14}C- and ^{13}C-labelled urea (GRAHAM et al. 1987). Whether or not ammonia production is a pathogenetic mechanism in *C. pylori* infection is controversial, but MURAKAMI and his colleagues (1987a, b) have shown that ammonia can produce necrotic lesions in the rat stomach and that urease activity combined with high blood urea levels in patients with azotaemia leads to ammonia-induced damage of the gastric mucosa.

Other potential biochemical mechanisms by which the organism may cause mucosal damage are back-diffusion of hydrogen ions (HAZELL and LEE 1986), proteolytic degradation of mucus (SLOMIANY et al. 1987) and the production of toxins (LEUNK et al. 1988).

The relative importance of these mechanisms is not clear but they offer a more than adequate explanation for *C. pylori* as a cause of mucosal injury. Such injury might not only be manifest as a chronic gastritis but in combination with acid attack can lead to erosion and ulceration. There is evidence that *C. pylori*-associated gastritis may be involved in up to 70% of gastric ulcers (O'CONNOR et al. 1987).

2.5 Treatment Studies

If *C. pylori* is indeed the principal aetiological factor in type B chronic gastritis then eradication of the organism should result in symptomatic and histological improvement. While it has been shown that certain antimicrobials known to be effective against *C. pylori*, such as metronidazole and furazolidone, will bring about the healing of gastroduodenal ulcers (DIAZ and ESCOBAR 1986; ZHENG et al. 1985), their efficacy in chronic gastritis has not been investigated. Other potentially effective antibiotics, such as erythromycin (MCNULTY et al. 1986) and nitrofurantoin (GILMAN et al. 1987), have been tried but with variable results. Bismuth-containing compounds, alone amongst the ulcer-healing agents, are bactericidal for *C. pylori*, and several studies (MCKENNA et al. 1987; ROKKAS et al. 1987) have investigated the value of colloidal bismuth subcitrate in the treatment of gastritis. These studies using bismuth alone, and others using combinations of bismuth compounds with antibiotics (BORODY et al. 1988; RAUWS et al. 1988), have consistently shown that eradication of *C. pylori* is accompanied by symptomatic improvement and a significant reduction or resolution in histological gastritis. Thus treatment studies tend to endorse a pathogenetic role for *C. pylori*.

2.6 Conclusion

On the basis of this accumulated experience, I regard the evidence in favour of *C. pylori* having a pathogenetic role in chronic gastritis as very persuasive. Whether or not this role is primary or secondary is more debatable. The epidemiological data indicate a steadily increasing prevalence of *C. pylori* with advancing age; this is unusual for a primary infection spread by the oral route, and it still remains a possibility that *C. pylori* is an 'opportunistic' pathogen that follows in the wake of some (but not all) kinds of mucosal injury and initiates and perpetuates chronic inflammation. There are other workers in this area, however, who have no doubt that *C. pylori* is a primary pathogen, and yet others who consider the organism to be simply a 'passenger' carried by an abnormal gastric mucosa. The debate continues!

3 Type A Chronic Gastritis

Classically the appearances in type A gastritis are those of gastric atrophy affecting body mucosa. The mucosa is thinned, and there is virtually complete loss of specialised cells with apparent replacement of glands by downward extension of the proliferative compartment. This feature allied to widespread intestinal metaplasia gives an appearance of villi and elongated pits which can resemble small intestinal mucosa. Chronic inflammatory cells are generally scanty and polymorphs are absent, and the lamina propria may show infiltration by fat cells. These classical appearances, however, are found in less than half of patients with pernicious anaemia (PA) (JOSKE et al. 1955), while conversely end-stage gastric atrophy can be found in the absence of other features of PA (CHELI and GIACOSA 1983). The antral mucosa in PA is usually described as normal or shows less gastritis than the body. The fact that antral gastritis is common in the general population suggests that when antral involvement is found in patients with PA it represents coincidence of type A and type B gastritis. If this was the case one would expect to find *Campylobacter* organisms in the involved antrum.

3.1 Campylobacter Status

We examined the *Campylobacter* status in antral and body biopsies from 14 patients with PA and compared them with age- and sex-matched patients with peptic ulcer disease (O'CONNOR et al. 1984). As expected, all but one of the latter group had *C. pylori* whereas only three of the PA group had the organisms and in two of these they were scanty. The organisms were found on antral mucosa in two cases; thus the prevalence of antral *Campylobacter*-associated gastritis in this admittedly small series of PA patients was only 14%. A serological study of patients with low levels of vitamin B_{12} and positive intrinsic factor and parietal cell antibodies has independently confirmed the low prevalence of *C. pylori* antibodies amongst this group (RATHBONE et al. 1989). A more complete histological study has recently been reported by FLEJOU and colleagues (1989), who examined antral and body biopsies from 45 patients with PA. All had chronic atrophic gastritis in the body and gastritis was found in the antrum in 16 cases (36%). Only one patient with antral gastritis was colonised by *C. pylori*, giving a prevalence of 6%, far below that found in type B gastritis. These authors concluded that the antrum in PA is resistant to colonisation by *C. pylori* and their findings argue against coincidence of type A and type B gastritis. Thus, whatever the cause of the antral gastritis in PA, it does not involve *C. pylori*.

3.2 Pathogenesis

While an auto-immune pathogenesis for PA seems firmly established and the disease has been produced experimentally by serial injections of auto-antigens (ANDRADA et al. 1969) and auto-antibody (INADA and GLASS 1975), its distinction from 'environmental' gastritis is not clear-cut. In a prolonged follow-up study of chronic gastritis conducted by IHAMAKI et al. (1985), a considerable proportion of patients who showed diffuse (antral and body) gastritis 10 years before, exhibited a 'pure' body gastritis at follow-up, "obviously due to regression of the antral process", which gave rise to a phenotype characteristic of PA. Likewise the development of end-stage atrophic gastritis was significantly associated with the presence of parietal cell antibodies. Thus their findings indicate the existence of an alternative route for the development of type A gastritis from a pre-existing diffuse chronic atrophic gastritis (CAG). KAYE (1987) has gone even further in stating that "there is little reason to doubt that CAG and PA share a common aetiology and pathogenesis." Such a conclusion is difficult to reconcile with the striking differences in the prevalence of *C. pylori* found in these two conditions.

3.3 ECL Cells and Polyps

The parietal cell antibodies characteristic of PA are thought to have both direct cytotoxic effects and a blocking action on gastrin receptors on parietal cells. These effects and the consequent hypochlorhydria result in a 'negative feedback' stimulation of gastrin production (KAYE 1987). Thus, in a 'typical' case where the antrum is uninvolved there is G cell hyperplasia and hypergastrinaemia. The raised gastrin levels are in turn held to be responsible for proliferation of enterochromaffin-like cells in the body part of the stomach so that some patients with PA exhibit diffuse argyrophil cell hyperplasia (RODE et al. 1986) or develop carcinoid tumors (HARVEY et al. 1985) or both (BÖRCH et al. 1985).

Carcinoid polyps are increasingly recognised in PA, but they are by no means the commonest form of polyp encountered in these patients. Despite the claim by IKEDA and colleagues (1985) that gastric 'pseudopolyps' are "a new clinical manifestation of type A gastritis", multiple small sessile polyps have long been associated with pernicious anaemia and are observed in about one-third of patients (ELSBORG et al. 1977; VARIS et al. 1979: STOCKBRUGGER et al. 1983). Histologically they are described as hyperplastic but some might simply represent, as IKEDA suggests, residual islands of relatively normal mucosa thrown into relief by the surrounding mucosal atrophy.

4 Lymphocytic Gastritis

In our experience less than 10% of biopsies showing active chronic gastritis are *C. pylori* negative. While a few negative biopsies can be explained on the basis of sampling error, the majority cannot. We were intrigued by these 'active negative' cases and on review noted that some showed unusually marked lymphocytic infiltration of the surface and foveolar epithelium corresponding to an entity recently described as lymphocytic gastritis (HAOT et al. 1986 a, b).

4.1 Relationship to Varioliform Gastritis

Excessive lymphocytic infiltration of the gastric epithelium appears to have been first described in 1985 by HAOT et al., and by RUBIO et al. who observed it in a Japanese patient with peptic ulceration. HAOT and his collegues (1986 a, b) subsequently detailed the clinicopathological aspects in 46 patients and emphasised its relationship to 'varioliform gastritis'. The latter term was introduced in 1947 when it was applied by MOUTIER and MARTIN to the gross appearances in two cases of gastritis characterised by widespread nodular and eroded lesions running along the gastric rugae (Fig. 5). Two similar cases were described in the same year by ALBOT et al.

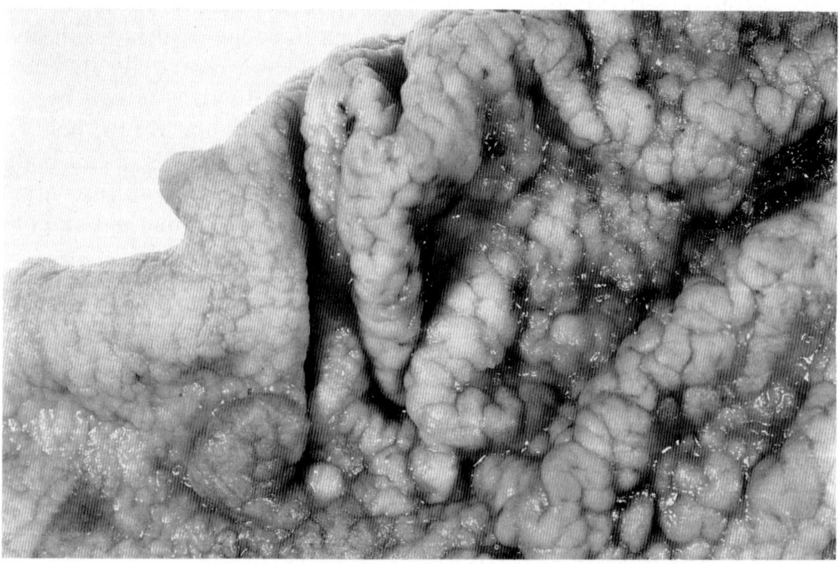

Fig. 5. Lymphocytic gastritis. Part of a gastrectomy specimen removed for early gastric cancer showing prominent mucosal folds in the body part of the stomach. The mucosa has a coarsely nodular or mamillated appearance. This proved to be lymphocytic gastritis on microscopy. We believe the two lesions to be unrelated

'Varioliform gastritis' as an endoscopic diagnosis seems to have been rather loosely applied to any condition in which there are multiple 'chronic' erosions, so that the reported histological findings are in disarray. Some authors describe foveolar hyperplasia and fibrosis (GREEN et al. 1977; FRANZIN et al. 1984) while others lay emphasis on dense mononuclear cell infiltration of the lamina propria (O'BRIEN et al. 1972; ELTA et al. 1983; GALLAGHER et al. 1987). A proportion of the latter patients will have lymphocytic gastritis. As I have argued elsewhere (WYATT and DIXON 1988), there appear to be three histological patterns associated with chronic erosive gastritis; strictly antral (prepyloric) chronic erosions usually show fibrosis and foveolar hyperplasia, whereas erosions maximal in the body are more likely to be lymphocytic gastritis. Other erosions, mainly antral, result from focally severe type B chronic gastritis.

4.2 Prevalence

Once one is aware of the entity of lymphocytic gastritis, the histological picture is readily recognised. On the basis of exceptional numbers of intra-epithelial lymphocytes in the surface and foveolar epithelium we identified 17 cases from amongst 382 (4.5%) otherwise straightforward cases of active chronic gastritis (DIXON et al. 1988). At low magnification the epithelium is crowded with nuclei (Fig. 6) which at higher power are seen to belong to mature-looking lymphocytes, many of which are surrounded by a clear halo typical of normal intra-epithelial lymphocytes (Fig. 7). On

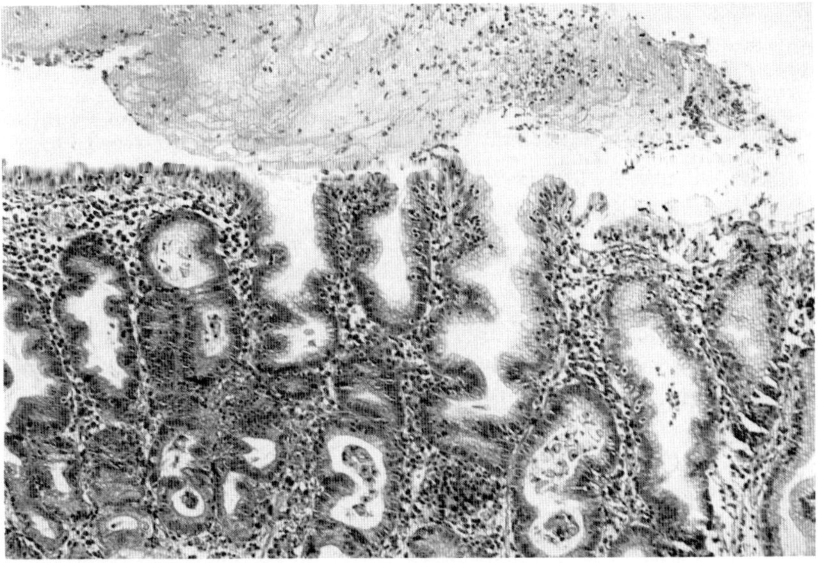

Fig. 6. Lymphocytic gastritis showing superficial erosion in a biopsy specimen

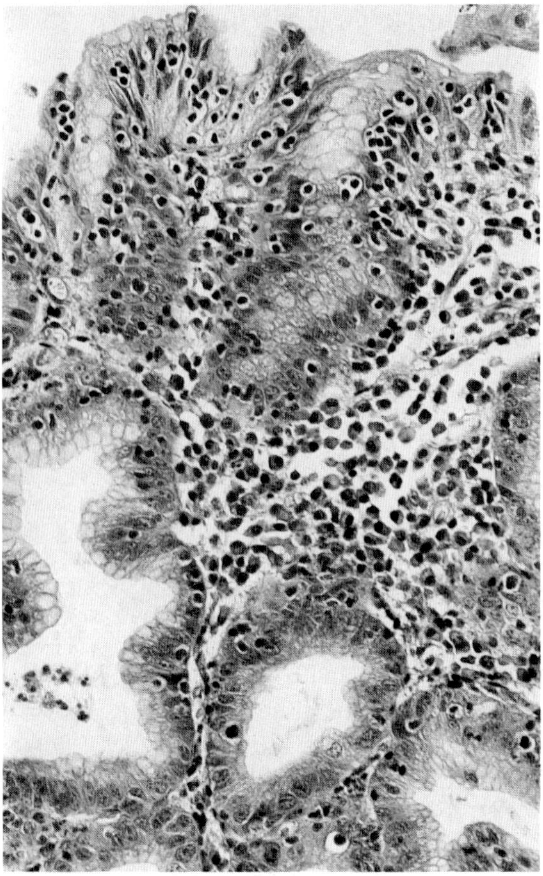

Fig. 7. Lymphocytic gastritis. Higher power view showing the prominent plasma cell content of the lamina propria and marked lymphocytic infiltration of the surface and foveolar epithelium. Many of the lymphocytes are of the 'halo' type characteristic of normal intra-epithelial T-cells

immunostaining these are exclusively of T cell type. The number of intra-epithelial lymphocytes in lymphocytic gastritis is increased by 10–15 times that found in active chronic gastritis; 55.3 ± 19.5 (mean $\pm$ SD) versus 3.7 ± 1.3 in our series.

While endoscopy in the classical case reveals multiple small nodules each surmounted by a shallow aphthoid or erupting erosion maximal in the body part of the stomach, only a minority of our cases showed this fully-developed picture. Therefore, in the same way that not all endoscopic varioliform gastritis is 'lymphocytic', not all histological lymphocytic gastritis is 'varioliform'.

4.3 Campylobacter Status

When we examined the *Campylobacter* status of our cases. Only seven of the patients (41%) were *C. pylori* positive compared with over 90% in the generality of active type B gastritis. However, the relationship was not clear-cut: four of the *C. pylori*-negative patients had antibody titres in the positive range, indicating previous infection; in two patients there were neither organisms nor serological evidence of infection; and in two cases an apparent change from *C. pylori* negative to positive on follow-up biopsy was not accompanied by any substantial change in the intra-epithelial lymphocyte counts.

4.4 Aetiology

The aetiology of lymphocytic gastritis remains obscure. Previous speculation on the pathogenesis of varioliform gastritis has centred on it being an allergic reaction. LAMBERT et al. (1978) reported finding increased numbers of IgE-positive cells in the lamina propria using immunofluorescence, but this has not been our experience in a small number of cases of lymphocytic gastritis investigated by immunohistology. In keeping with an allergic aetiology, ANDRE et al. (1982) have demonstrated the efficacy of sodium cromoglycate treatment, and a case of varioliform gastritis has been described in which the condition followed the drinking of a herb-tea mixture (PERARNAU et al. 1984). The histological picture of large numbers of T-lymphocytes infiltrating the surface epithelium is reminiscent of coeliac disease. Although the gastric epithelium does not show lymphocytic infiltration in gluten-sensitive enteropathy (HANSKY and SHINER 1983; GILLBERG et al. 1985), the similarity between the two conditions suggests that they may have a common immunopathological basis in sharing an abnormal response to some local antigen to which the patient has become sensitised. The nature of the antigen in lymphocytic gastritis is not clear; while *C. pylori* is a possible candidate, the tendency for the disease to affect the body rather than the antrum of the stomach is difficult to explain.

5 Reflux Gastritis

The General Infirmary at Leeds has a long tradition of expertise in gastric surgery culminating in recent years in the introduction of the highly selective vagotomy for duodenal ulcer (JOHNSTON and WILKINSON 1970). This in turn has led to considerable interest in the 'postoperative stomach' and in particular in enterogastric reflux of bile and its relationship to symptoms and gastritis. Among several studies on this topic, we have compared the severity of 'conventional' (type B) chronic gastritis with the levels of intragastric bile acids in patients who have undergone a variety of operations for duodenal (DEWAR et al. 1983) and gastric ulcer (DEWAR et al. 1984) and found there to be no correlation. However, during the course of these

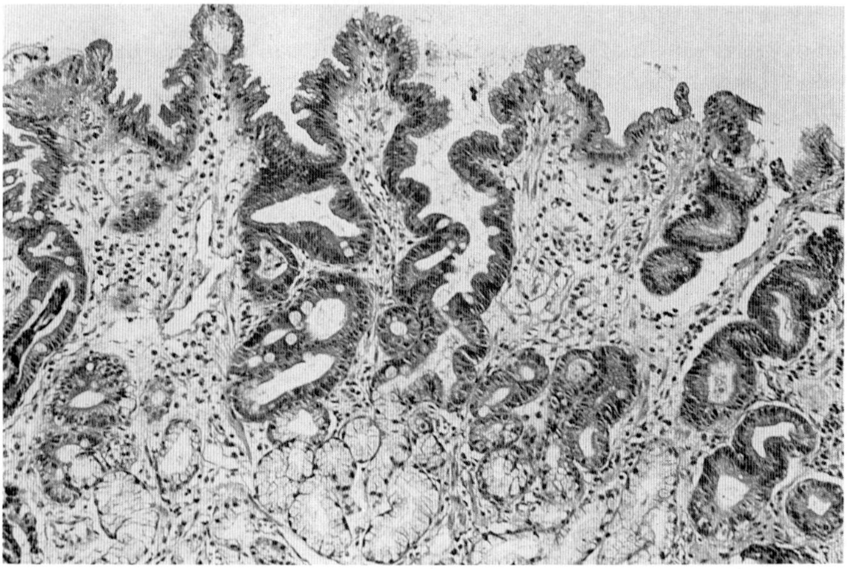

Fig. 8. Tpye C gastritis due to reflux. Antral biopsy from a patient who had undergone truncal vagotomy and pyloroplasty some years before. There is foveolar hyperplasia, increased vascularity and increased numbers of smooth muscle fibres but normal numbers of chronic inflammatory cells

studies I became increasingly convinced that some patients with reflux exhibited a distinctive form of 'gastritis' which did not fit into the usually accepted categories. These biopsies showed marked foveolar hyperplasia, oedema, vasodilatation and increased smooth muscle fibres in the lamina propria, and a *paucity* of acute and chronic inflammatory cells (Fig. 8). It should be emphasised that these appearances were found in widely separated areas in the gastric remnant and were not merely confined to the peristomal area where these changes, together with cystic dilatation, distortion and atrophy of glands, are well recognised. In a subsequent study we were able to demonstrate by allocating each patient a reflux score based on these histological criteria that there was a significant link between high reflux scores and abnormal bile acid levels and hypochlorhydria in samples of fasting gastric juice (DIXON et al. 1986). We therefore concluded that there is a distinct histological picture associated with alkaline enterogastric reflux which can be termed reflux gastritis.

5.1 Foveolar Hyperplasia

The concept of a reflux 'gastritis' without inflammatory cells is a difficult one for many histopathologists to accept. Indeed this reluctance to accept the term gastritis led DU PLESSIS, a pioneer in this field, to abandon the term 'proliferative gastritis' (DU PLESSIS and LAWSON 1974) in favour of 'chronic gastric mucosal reaction' (DU PLESSIS 1977), but even with this amended name the lesion remained largely ignored. It was LAWSON who first drew attention to foveolar hyperplasia as a feature of enterogastric reflux in describing a 'hypertrophic gastritis' which developed in dogs subjected to partial gastrectomy (LAWSON 1965), and further support for this being a major consequence of reflux has come from experimental (MENGUY and MAX 1970; DELANEY et al. 1975; ROBBINS et al. 1976) and clinical studies (DRAPANAS and BETHEA 1974; LOUP et al. 1978; RITCHIE 1980). These studies have been extended more recently by MOSIMANN and his colleagues, who in an investigation of duodenogastric reflux in vagotomised dogs found that foveolar hyperplasia was the only microscopic lesion induced by reflux (MOSIMANN et al. 1984) and that the hyperplasia regressed or disappeared after the correction of reflux (FONTOLLIET et al. 1984). In keeping with these findings, cell kinetic investigations reveal increased proliferation in the presence of duodenogastric reflux (LANGHANS et al. 1984a). Subsequent to publication of our study, BECHI et al. (1987) investigated partially gastrectomised patients for histological features of reflux and concluded that hyperplasia of the foveolar epithelium was reflux related whereas there was no relationship between chronic atrophic gastritis and reflux.

5.2 Paucity of Inflammatory Cells

Both DU PLESSIS and MOSIMANN have expressed misgivings over the significance of the inflammatory cell infiltrate in reflux; the former found the infiltrate to be frequently absent in symptomatic patients (DU PLESSIS 1977) while the latter stated that the infiltrate "does not regress significantly in humans after remedial surgery. This tends to deny reliability to this criterion for the diagnosis of reflux gastritis." (MOSIMANN et al. 1981). I would go further and claim that chronic inflammatory cell infiltration is not an integral part of the response to reflux and that previous attempts to correlate chronic superficial and atrophic gastritis with the degree of reflux have been misplaced. When chronic inflammatory cells are present in biopsies from a patient with reflux they are likely to represent coexistent type B chronic gastritis or the legacy of a pre-existing type B gastritis.

5.3 Hyperaemia

While the reluctance to accept inflammation *sine* inflammatory cells is understandable, it is surprising that histopathologists have been slow to acknowledge that lamina propria oedema and congestion represent the vascular component of an inflammatory response rather than biopsy artifact. It is surprising because mucosal hyperaemia has long been considered by endoscopists to be an important indicator of reflux gastritis, and a significant correlation has been found between hyperaemia and the concentration of bilirubin in gastric juice (KEIGHLEY et al. 1975). Furthermore, erythema and oedema almost invariably disappear following the creation of a Roux-en-Y limb (RITCHIE 1984). Histologically, both oedema (SCUDAMORE et al. 1973) and congestion (DRAPANUS and BETHEA 1974) have been mentioned but without special emphasis. More recently a careful study by EMMANOUILIDIS and colleagues (1984) gave rise to the observation that "marked oedema of the lamina propria with lack of inflammatory infiltration was a very characteristic finding in bile gastritis."

5.4 Pathogenesis

The injurious agent in enterogastric reflux remains a subject of debate. The refluxate contains alkaline pancreatico-duodenal secretions as well as bile acids, bile salts and lysolecithin, the latter being produced by the action of phospholipase in pancreatic juice on the lecithin in bile. The damaging action of lysolecithin (DAVENPORT 1970; ORCHARD et al. 1977) and bile salts (EASTWOOD 1975) has been long recognised, and more recently CARTER et al. (1984) have demonstrated exfoliation of surface cells following topical application of bile acids in an acid milieu. Just as we have proposed with aspirin-induced injury (BERRISFORD et al. 1985), it appears that increasing concentrations of taurocholic acid evoke a sequential response in the surface epithelium from an initial increased release of mucus through to massive cell exfoliation consequent upon disruption of the mucus barrier. Others have demonstrated that isolated pancreatic reflux gives rise to more antral erosions than isolated bile reflux, although the latter produced more fundal lesions (DISERENS et al. 1984). However, ARMSTRONG et al. (1988) have more recently demonstrated that bile acids, lysolecithin and gastric luminal pH, but not pancreatic enzymes, are major determinants of gastrotoxicity in the rat. Whatever the relative importance of these agents in man, it seems reasonable to argue that reflux leads to an essentially 'chemical' injury which results in disruption of the mucus barrier and directly affects the mucosa but also permits acid attack (REES and RHODES 1977). The combined injury leads to accelerated exfoliation of surface epithelial cells, and a histamine-mediated vascular response manifest as oedema and hyperaemia, without (presumably) the production of leucotaxins or the need for a local immune response which would entail the participation of acute and chronic inflammatory cells. Repetition of the injury might lead to the release of other soluble factors, such as platelet-derived growth factor, which stimulates smooth muscle and, later on, fibroblastic proliferation. I would argue that the finding of hyperaemia and interstitial fluid exudation, despite the absence of cellular exudation, justifies the term 'reflux gastritis' rather than the more cumbersome 'gastropathy'; furthermore reflux gastritis is now firmly established in clinical terminology.

5.5 Specificity

The individual histological features seen in association with alkaline reflux are in no way specific. Foveolar hyperplasia is simply a response to excessive cell exfoliation from the surface epithelium and as such is seen in all types of active gastritis. Likewise, hyperaemia and oedema are part of any inflammatory process. Indeed, the proposition that a combination of these features together with a paucity of inflammatory cells constitutes a distinct entity is only valid insofar as they indicate a distinctive response of the gastric mucosa to repeated 'chemical' injury. Thus identical appearances can be found following repeated drug injury to the mucosa, notably that caused by long-term treatment with NSAIDs (LAINE et al. 1988), and in some alcoholic patients (PARL et al. 1979). Thus, in the absence of precise clinical information, the histopathologist faced with these appearances might do better to employ a diagnostic term wich indicates that the picture is that of a 'chemically induced' chronic gastritis rather than to assume the cause to be 'reflux'. It seems logical therefore to employ the term 'type C' (Chemical) gastritis for this category.

5.6 Campylobacter Status

With regard to the relationship between enterogastric reflux and gastric *Campylobacter* organisms, we have investigated *C. pylori* status in patients with unoperated duodenal ulcer (DU) and several groups of postoperative DU patients, one group treated by highly selected vagotomy (HSV), and the others comprising patients who had undergone various operations which removed or bypassed the pylorus (O'CONNOR et al. 1986b). The preoperative DU group showed 97% *C. pylori* positivity and the HSV group 94% positivity, while the other postoperative groups had an overall positivity of 42%. In keeping with a previous study (O'CONNOR et al. 1986a) we found that *C. pylori* negativity was significantly linked to high histological reflux scores and high intragastric bile acid levels. Thus we concluded that many patients with DU must undergo a change from a *C. pylori*-positive chronic gastritis to a *C. pylori*-negative reflux gastritis following operations which permit enterogastric reflux. This means that for a variable time after surgery there must be a transitional phase during which biopsies will reveal a mixed picture of foveolar hyperplasia and chronic inflammatory cell infiltration. Only later will the more characteristic picture associated with reflux emerge. A more recent study (GUSTAVSSON et al. 1987) identified *C. pylori* in 6 of 24 partial gastrectomy patients. Interestingly, four of nine patients without symptoms were positive, whereas only 2 of 15 with symptoms attributed to 'alkaline reflux gastritis' had *C. pylori*. The disappearance of *C. pylori* in reflux is likely to be a consequence of disruption of the mucus-bicarbonate barrier (RITCHIE 1977) and the bile intolerance of the organism (TOMPKINS and WEST 1987). HSV appears to protect against reflux but the *C. pylori*-positive chronic gastritis persists in these patients.

5.7 Reflux in the Intact Stomach

Although our published work has been largely concerned with postoperative patients in whom the presence of reflux has been substantiated by intragastric bile acid measurements, I have frequently encountered similar,

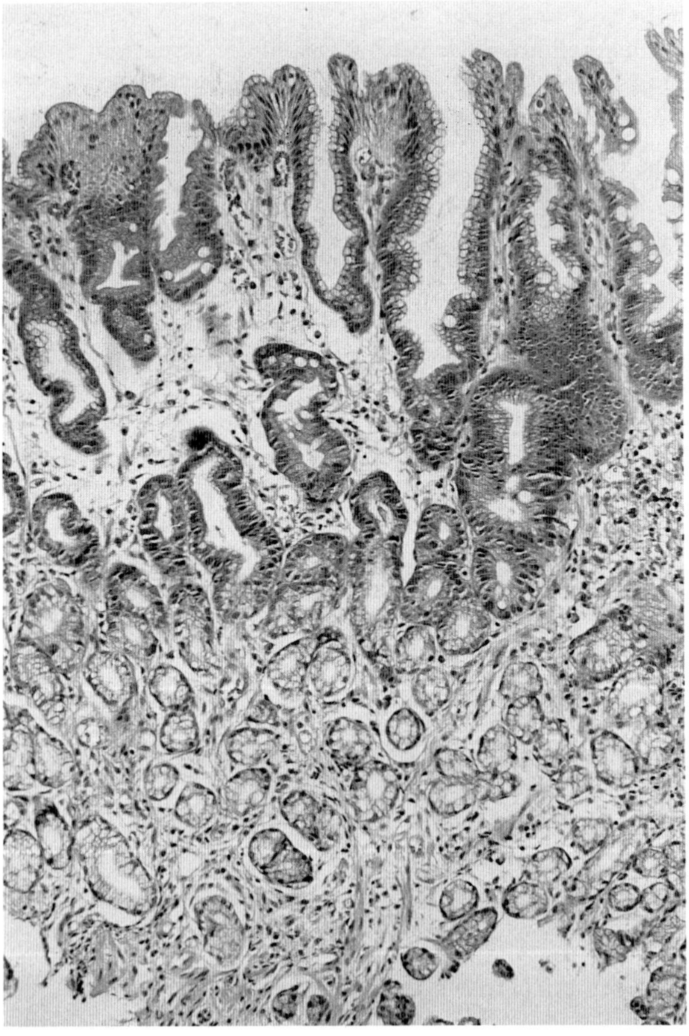

Fig. 9. Type C gastritis in the intact stomach. There is prominent foveolar hyperplasia, oedema and congestion of the lamina propria and a paucity of chronic inflammatory cells

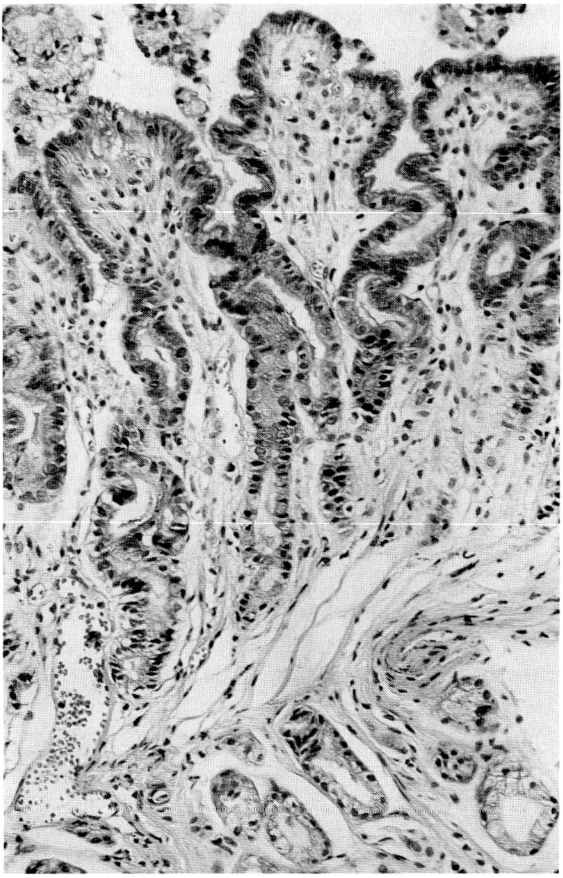

Fig. 10. Type C gastritis in the intact stomach. Biopsy from another case showing foveolar hyperplasia, capillary congestion and an increase in smooth muscle fibres in the lamina propria. There was no history of NSAID ingestion or alcohol abuse in either case

albeit milder, changes in intact stomachs (Figs. 9, 10). If ingestion of NSAIDs and alcohol abuse can be excluded, then I would claim that the finding of severe degrees of epithelial hyperplasia, congestion and lamina propria oedema, with no increase in chronic inflammatory cells, is indicative of reflux gastritis. 'Spontaneous' enterogastric reflux is less widely acknowledged than that following gastric surgery, and yet its occurrence in unoperated gastric ulcer patients (THOMAS 1984) and in 'gallstone dyspepsia' and post-cholecystectomy patients (SVENSSON et al. 1986) is well documented. After these associations have been eliminated there remains a substantial proportion of patients with demonstrable reflux who are assumed to have a motor disturbance of pyloro-antral function which can be termed 'primary or idiopathic enterogastric reflux' (FISHER 1985). This condition may or may not be part of a wider disturbance of gastrointestinal motility which overlaps with the irritable bowel syndrome, and recent experimental work indicates that the fault lies in decreased antral motility (DEFILIPPI et al. 1987).

The relationship between histology and reflux in the intact stomach has been explored recently by NIEMELA et al. (1987), and these authors found that reflux was associated with infiltration of mononuclear cells, neutrophils and eosinophils as well as foveolar hyperplasia. The possibility that many patients aged over 40 with demonstrable duodenogastric reflux will already have a type B chronic gastritis does not appear to have been taken into account in this study. Future studies on the intact stomach will have to ascertain the *C. pylori* status and examine correlations with reflux *within* positive and negative categories.

5.8 Reflux and Ulceration

Under most circumstances the increased rate of cell loss at the surface is compensated for by foveolar hyperplasia, but where the injury is particularly severe, erosions will develop, and the lesion may even progress to chronic gastric ulceration. Although enterogastric reflux has not been widely considered as a predisposing factor in antral (prepyloric) erosions and ulcers, from the foregoing and a consideration of their histological appearances it seems likely that reflux rather than type B gastritis reduces mucosal resistance and leads to erosion without a requirement for hyperacidity. Some support for this view comes from the finding that acid production in patients with antral erosive changes is within the normal range (NESLAND and BERSTAD 1985; GUSLANDI and BALLARIN 1986) and that the volume of duodenogastric reflux (FRIZIS et al. 1987) and gastric bile acid concentration (GOTTHARD et al. 1985) is high in patients with prepyloric ulcers. The role of bile reflux in gastric ulceration has been disputed (SCHINDLBECK et al. 1987) but histological studies suggest that duodenogastric reflux may be a factor in the production of about 30% of all gastric ulcers (O'CONNOR et al. 1987). Indeed, reflux might act together with type B gastritis to further reduce mucosal integrity and increase its susceptibility to acid attack so that a larger proportion of gastric ulcers may result from their combined effects (KARTTUNEN and NIEMELA 1988).

5.9 Hyperplasia Versus Dysplasia

Wider recognition of a 'chemical' (type C) gastritis may help in a fuller understanding of non-ulcer dyspepsia, and in postoperative patients will indicate those patients who are most likely to benefit from revisionary surgery to divert bile away from the stomach. Of more relevance to the histopathologist, however, is the distinction between foveolar hyperplasia and premalignant dysplasia. There is a tendency for histopathologists to interpret marked foveolar hyperplasia in the absence of inflammatory cells as dysplasia when the same cytological appearances in the presence of inflammatory cells would be termed 'reactive' or 'regenerative'. Thus a failure to appreciate the nature of the mucosal response to reflux probably underlies the high prevalence of low grade (mild and moderate) dysplasia reported in some studies on the postoperative stomach (LANGHANS et al. 1984 b; PICKFORD et al. 1984; THOMAS et al. 1984) and explains the rarity of progression to severe dysplasia and carcinoma found in follow-up studies on low grade dysplasia (OFFERHAUS et al. 1984). We believe that most diagnoses of low grade dysplasia in postoperative biopsies are examples of foveolar hyperplasia and not true (premalignant) dysplasia, a view endorsed by the findings of WEINSTEIN et al. (1985).

5.10 Gastric Antral Vascular Ectasia

An exaggerated form of the histological picture seen in reflux has been recently described in the uncommon condition of gastric antral vascular ectasia (GAVE). As the name implies, the most important feature is increased vascularity with capillary ectasia, but biopsies also show foveolar hyperplasia, fibromuscular hyperplasia in the lamina propria and a paucity of inflammatory cells, together with fibrin thrombi in mucosal capillaries (SUIT et al. 1987) (Figs. 11, 12). Endoscopically, one sees prominent longitudinally running mucosal folds each showing a band of intense hyperaemia running along the crest of the fold, which has given rise to the alternative description of 'watermelon stomach' (JABBARI et al. 1984). The

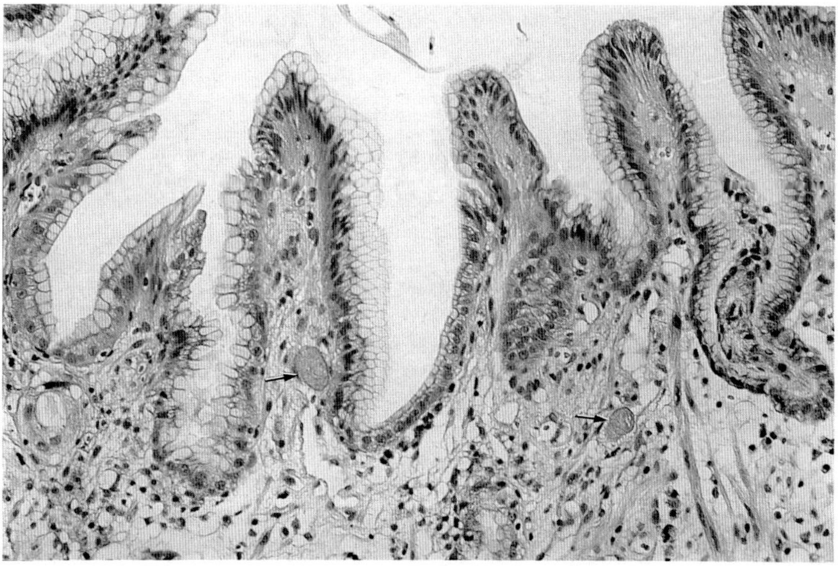

Fig. 11. GAVE. Antral biopsy showing oedema and smooth muscle fibres in the lamina propria together with fibrin thrombi in capillaries (*arrowed*)

presence of these superficial ectatic vessels predisposes to chronic blood loss from the mucosa and patients with this condition invariably have iron-deficiency anaemia.

The cause of GAVE is unknown. While I have drawn attention to the similarities with reflux gastritis, others have attributed the changes to mucosal prolapse (JABBARI et al. 1984) and drawn analogies with prolapse in the rectum (GARDINER et al. 1985). Yet another group (SUIT et al. 1987) state that "prolapse was not a prominent feature in our series" and suggest that vigorous antral contraction might be the cause. The similarity between the changes seen in reflux, GAVE and mucosal prolapse elsewhere in the gastrointestinal tract might simply reflect the limited repertoire of response to chemical and mechanical injury. Certainly, gastroduodenal prolapse is poorly documented in cases of GAVE. More recently, RODE et al. (1988) have incriminated excessive production of 5-hydroxytryptamine and vaso-acitve intestinal polypeptide in the pathogenesis of GAVE, arguing that these two hormones are potent mediators of vasodilatation. Obviously, further investigations are required to clarify the pathogenesis of this intriguing condition.

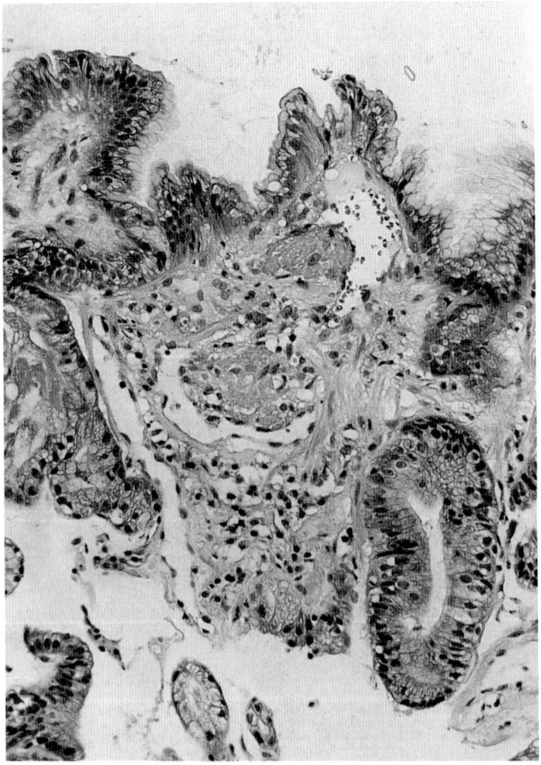

Fig. 12. GAVE. Ectatic capillaries in the superficial lamina propria containing fibrin/platelet thrombi undergoing early organisation

6 Pathogenetic and Diagnostic Classification of Gastritis

In a previous review (WYATT and DIXON 1988) we put forward a pathogenetic classification of chronic gastritis based on our recently acquired knowledge of *C. pylori* and gastritis related to enterogastric reflux. As stated above, I feel that the reflux type should be expanded to take account of identical appearances produced by other forms of chemical injury to the gastric mucosa, and advocate as an omnibus term ‘type C gastritis’ (Table 3).

The identification of type A gastritis is very much a clinicopathological diagnosis but it is suggested when the severity of body gastritis exceeds that found in the antrum. Its severity is best assessed in terms of the degree of glandular atrophy.

Type B gastritis is divided into *superficial* and *atrophic* forms on the basis of the absence or presence of glandular loss. The degree of atrophy can be used to designate mild, moderate and severe categories. It is also of interest to identify *active* and *inactive* cases according to the presence of polymorph infiltration.

The severity of type C gastritis is reflected in the degree of epithelial degeneration but this feature is best appreciated by an assessment of the degree of compensatory foveolar hyperplasia. The latter feature should be used to allocated biopsies into mild, moderate and severe categories.

Table 3. Major forms of chronic gastritis

Diagnosis	Pathogenesis	Aetiology
Type A	*A*uto-immunity	?
Type B	*B*acterial infection	*C. pylori*
(Lymphocytic gastritis –	? atypical response to	*C. pylori*)
Type C	*C*hemical injury	Enterogastric reflux NSAIDs Alcohol

7 Duodenitis

While inflammation in the duodenum resulting from specific infective causes and its involvement by coeliac disease and Crohn’s disease are well recognised, the vast majority of duodenitis is ‘non-specific’. The entity of non-specific chronic duodenitis is a controversial one; its histological definition has been ambiguous, and its clinical status and relationship to duodenal ulcer is disputed.

7.1 Duodenitis and Duodenal Ulcer

The most substantive recent work which explores the natural history of duodenitis is a study by SIRCUS (1985), who followed the progress and response to therapy of 219 subjects who had various combinations of non-erosive and erosive duodenitits and duodenal ulceration. His study revealed that the great majority of patients (82%) develop one or more duodenal ulcers sooner or later and concluded that most subjects display a spectrum of appearances at endoscopy reflecting stages of activity and severity of the inflammatory process. He found that erosive duodenitis with or without an ulcer was associated with significantly higher maximal acid secretion than was the non-erosive disease, and interestingly, found a highly significant difference between the good response to cimetidine of the ulcer craters and the poor response of erosive duodenitis both when this was alone or when accompanying an ulcer crater. Nevertheless, SIRCUS concluded that "both non-erosive and erosive duodenitis are components of the response of the mucosa of the duodenal bulb to the peptic process". However, others take a contrary view. GUSLANDI (1985) claims that many patients with chronic duodenitis, even when this is erosive, do not have hyperchlorhydria, and he underlines the discrepant response to H_2 blockers in arguing that there is an 'autonomous' erosive duodenitis in which gastric acidity plays only a minor pathogenetic role. Thus, he proposes that there are two subtypes of erosive duodenitis, one accompanying or following duodenal ulceration, and the other, autonomous erosive duodenitis, "a distinct disorder differing from peptic ulcer in regard to pathogenesis and therapy."

The fact that acid is by no means the sole factor in duodenal ulceration has been emphasised by COLIN-JONES (1986). He drew attention to the efficacy of anti-ulcer treatments, such as colloidal bismuth and sucralfate, that do not inhibit gastric acid secretion. Furthermore, ulcers which are resistant to cimetidine can be healed with colloidal bismuth (LAM et al. 1984), and patients with DU treated with bismuth exhibit a lower relapse rate than those treated with H_2 blockers (MARTIN et al. 1981; LEE et al. 1984).

It would appear from all this evidence that there are likely to be two major factors operating in duodenitis and duodenal ulcer which produce a spectrum of changes by virtue of their interplay. The first factor is a mucosal lesion, chronic duodenitis, which is not itself caused by hyperacidity, and the second is acid attack. Thus if the duodenitis is severe this could lead to erosions independent of acid, whereas if there is only mild duodenitis but high acid levels reaching the duodenum then erosion and crater formation can ensue; a combination of moderate duodenitis and a modest elevation in acid could also result in ulceration. A dual mechanism would appear to explain the clinical and endoscopic findings and the variable response to treatment with antacids, but poses the question as to the cause of the underlying duodenitis.

7.2 Histopathological Aspects

Early descriptions of duodenitis based on biopsies obtained by capsule first appeared in the 1950s (SHINER 1956; DONIACH and SHINER 1957) but its clinical significance was not adequately explored until the study of BECK et al. (1965). These authors clearly demonstrated a correlation between chronic duodenitis and symptomatology, but their histological categories were based predominantly on mononuclear cell density and paid scant attention to villous changes and polymorph infiltration. The latter feature, indicating 'active' duodenitis, was sought in the first endoscopically based study (COTTON et al. 1973), which found such activity in 44% of abnormal duodenal bulbs and in none of the control group, but it was WHITEHEAD and his colleagues (1975) who attempted to define grades of duodenitis using inflammatory cell infiltration together with villous and surface epithelial changes. They distinguished mild, moderate and severe categories, but advocated separate consideration of polymorph infiltration

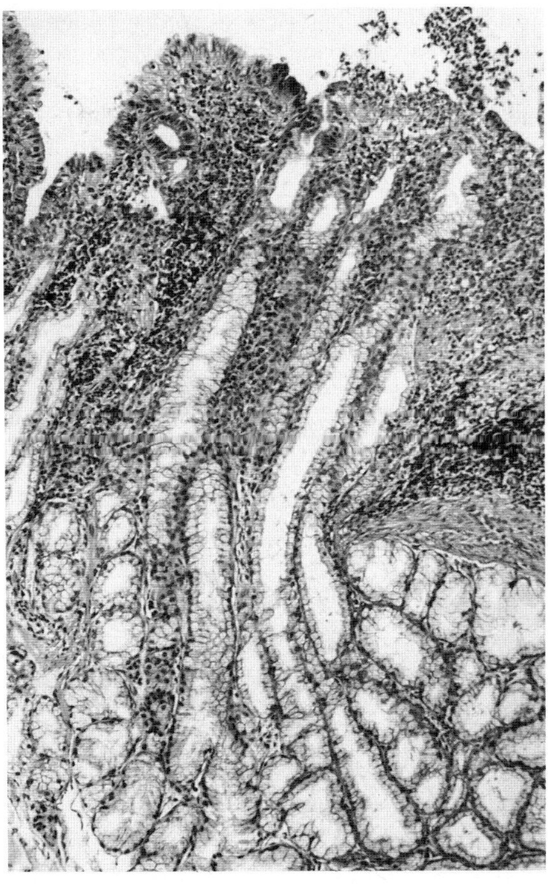

Fig. 13. Active chronic duodenitis showing dense chronic inflammatory cell infiltration of the lamina propria with focal erosion

as this could be found (albeit with diminishing intensity) in moderate and mild grades. However, a shortcoming of this study was the absence of any correlation between clinical features and histological grade. More recently using a quantitative approach, TOUKAN et al. (1985) have shown that the mean counts of neutrophil polymorphs and mononuclear cells are significantly higher in dyspeptic patients than controls.

The most important recent advance in the histopathological interpretation of duodenitis has been provided by JENKINS et al. (1985), who performed a detailed quantitative study in which the morphometric results were subjected to cluster and discriminant analysis which allowed allocation of the biopsies to one of three categories. Their *normal* category included many cases which would be classified as mild duodenitis according to Whitehead's criteria, and the authors suggest that this represents the extreme of the normal range. The second category, *mild* duodenitis, exhibits increased numbers of plasma cells and oedema, and usually, but not always, some polymorph response and increased gastric metaplasia. The third category, *severe* duodenitis, shows a large number of intraepithelial and lamina propria polymorphs but decreased plasma cells, together with severe villous atrophy (Fig. 13, 14). All except one patient in the latter group had either an ulcer or severe erosions at endoscopy, suggesting that this pattern of mucosal reaction represents a stage before ulceration. By analysing the interrelations between the histomorphometric features in a correlation matrix, JENKINS et al. suggest a dual pattern of response in duodenitis, one being an immune response reflected in

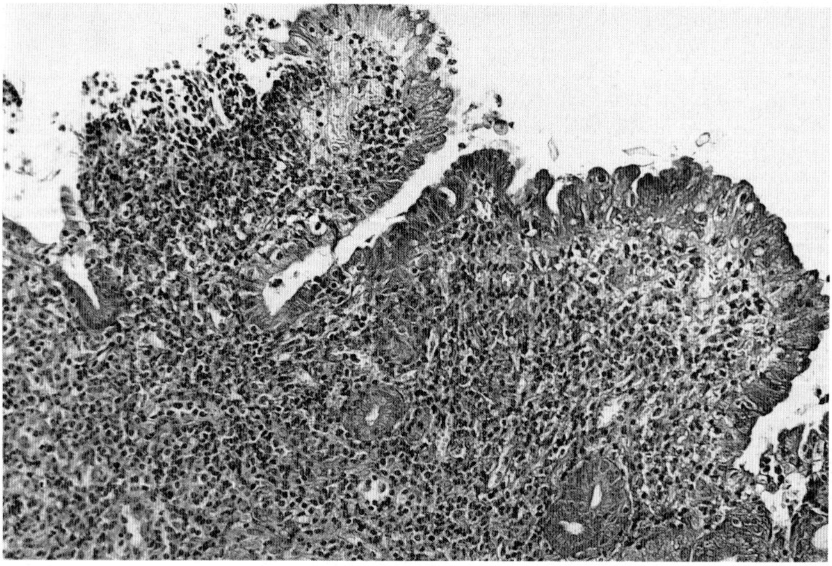

Fig. 14. Active chronic duodenitis. High power view of the same biopsy showing erosion and polymorph infiltration in an area of gastric metaplasia

changes in plasma cell population, and the other being an acute inflammatory response closely related to the indicators of epithelial damage, namely gastric metaplasia and villous atrophy.

7.3 Gastric Metaplasia and C. pylori

Campylobacter pylori do not colonise normal duodenal mucosa. It was MARSHALL et al. (1985 b) who first suggested that *C. pylori* was responsible for duodenitis by colonising 'antral type' mucosa in the duodenal cap. However, these authors considered the presence of gastric epithelium as a 'primary', presumably congenital, phenomenon rather than accepting its metaplastic development. While heterotopic gastric mucosa can be found in the duodenum (HOEDEMAEKER 1970), this term is better reserved for mucosa complete with gastric-type specialised glands and as such represents an uncommon finding. We regard the presence of surface gastric epithelium alone as a metaplastic process, and recent ultrastructural work has demonstrated transition from undifferentiated stem cells through to mature gastric-type cells in the vicinity of duodenal ulcers (GREGORY and SPITAELS 1987).

Gastric metaplasia occurring in the vicinity of peptic ulcers has been long recognised (BLOMQUIST 1956) and subsequent authors have suggested that the change is a defence response to high acid levels in the duodenum (JAMES 1964; PATRICK et al. 1974). However, its appearance is not necessarily a consequence of hyperacidity as it is frequently encountered in the small intestine in Crohn's disease; it must therefore represent a nonspecific response to continued injury and healing. Nevertheless, it seems reasonable to conclude that the most likely cause of such injury in the proximal duodenum is acid attack. We examined the relationship between fasting gastric juice pH and gastric metaplasia in 55 patients with non-ulcer dyspepsia (WYATT et al. 1987) and found metaplasia in 20/42 patients with a pH < 2.5 but none in 13 patients with a fasting pH greater than 2.5. Gastric metaplasia involving more than 5% of the surface epithelium was associated with a pH less than 2.0 in 10/11 cases.

Although gastric metaplasia can be found in otherwise normal duodenal mucosa (KREUNING et al. 1978), its relationship to duodenitis and in particular to active duodenitis is well established. SHOUSHA et al. (1983) noted the predilection of polymorphs for areas of gastric metaplasia but were at a loss to explain the phenomenon. It now seems likely that the polymorph response is directed towards *C. pylori* on the metaplastic epithelium. Even before MARSHALL's revelations, STEER (1975) had described the migration of polymorphs through gastric epithelium at the sites of bacterial attachment, and his later work established the presence of similar organisms and the associated polymorph response in gastric metaplasia (STEER 1984, 1985). More recently, JOHNSTON et al. (1986 a) reported that *C. pylori* were frequently found on metaplastic epithelium which was infiltrated by polymorphs. We have recently investigated the relationship between duodenitis, gastric metaplasia and *C. pylori*-associated antral gastritis in paired duodenal and gastric biopsies from 290 patients. There was concurrence of *C. pylori*-positive gastritis and > 5% gastric metaplasia in 30/34 (88%) patients with active duodenitis, 3/21 (14%) with chronic duodenitis, and only 1/235 (0.43%) with normal or minor changes (Wyatt et al. 1987). Our findings are therefore consistent with the hypothesis that gastric metaplasia in the presence of *C. pylori*-associated antral gastritis permits colonisation of the duodenum and these organisms elicit an acute inflammatory response.

7.4 Conclusions

We have proposed a sequence of events which point to a role for *C. pylori* in duodenal ulceration (Wyatt et al. 1988). The initial event is acid-induced gastric metaplasia in the duodenum. We have established in previous studies that there is almost invariably a *C. pylori*-positive antral gastritis in DU patients. The coexistence of *C. pylori* gastritis and gastric metaplasia permits colonisation of the duodenum. The organisms give rise to an active chronic duodenitis which is exactly analogous to type B gastritis in eliciting an immune response involving an increase in all plasma cell types. The correlation between the number of IgG plasma cells and the 'acute' features of intraepithelial polymorphs and mucosal oedema observed by Jenkins et al. can be explained by complement activation following coating of bacteria by IgG. The fact that this acute response was also related to epithelial degenerative features, gastric metaplasia and villous atrophy may also reflect aspects of the subsequent acid attack on the now susceptible mucosa.

Thus *C. pylori* infection is arguably the cause of the background (autonomous?) duodenitis. This infection is paradoxically facilitated by a defence response to hyperacidity, gastric metaplasia, but once established the infection weakens the mucosal defence to acid attack and leads to ulceration. That *C. pylori* infection is present in the ulcerated duodenum has been confirmed by Malfertheiner et al. (1987) and Daskalopoulos et al. (1987), the latter finding the organisms in biopsies from the ulcer rim in 24 of 28 patients. Gastric metaplasia was identified at the ulcer edge in 27 of these patients. Involvement of *C. pylori* in duodenal ulceration is also supported by the response to therapy. Colloidal bismuth is bactericidal for *C. pylori* and this could explain its efficacy in duodenitis (Johnston et al. 1986b) and in the healing of antacid-resistent ulcers, but the drug also stimulates alkaline secretion through a prostaglandin-dependent mechanism (Konturek et al. 1987) so this alternative explanation cannot be discounted. Even more persuasive is the finding that significantly more patients who remained *C. pylori* positive after healing of a DU relapsed in the first year after treatment than patients in whom the organism was eradicated (Coghlan et al. 1987).

Despite all these arguments and the plausibility of this line of reasoning, there are those who faced with the same evidence conclude that "this bacterium is irrelevant to ulcer disease" (WORMSLEY 1987). My thoughts on this dilemma are summed up by the expression *"Se non è vero, è molto ben trovato"* – if it is not true, it is a happy invention (ANON).

Acknowledgments. The writing of this review and my previous contributions to the literature on gastritis would not have been possible without the help and stimulus of a number of celleagues. I am very grateful to David Johnston, Tony Axon and Val Heatley for giving me access to clinical material and for initiating some of the projects with which I have collaborated. More especially, I would like to thank Paxton Dewar, Humphrey O'Connor, Barrie Rathbone and Judy Wyatt, compared to whose ideas and enthusiasm my own contribution has been a slender one. I am also very grateful to Peter Jackson, Declan Lunny and Sally Gray for technical assistance, to Samantha Hessey for the electron micrographs and to Stephen Toms for photographic assistance.

References

Ahmed A, Vaira D, Cairns SR, Holton J, Fulzon M, Polydorus A, Salmon PR (1987) Increased formation of leucotriene C_4 (LTC_4) in *Campylobacter pyloridis* associated gastritis. Gut 28:1405–1406A

Albot G, Leger L, Tricard A (1947) Formations polypoides a sommet ombliqué de la muqueuse gastrique. Presse Med 55:190–191

Andersen LP, Holck S, Povlsen CO, Elsborg L, Justesen T (1987) *Campylobacter pyloridis* in peptic ulcer disease. Scand J Gastroenterol 22:219–224

Andrada JA, Rose NR, Andrada EC (1969) Experimental autoimmune gastritis in the rhesus monkey. Clin Exp Immunol 4:293–310

Andre C, Gillon J, Moulinier B, Martin A, Fargier MC (1982) Randomised placebo-controlled double blind trial of two dosages of sodium cromoglycate in treatment of varioliform gastritis: comparison with cimetidine. Gut 23:348–352

Armstrong D, Murphy GM, Dowling RH (1988) The relative gastrotoxicity of duodenal juice components; acute studies in the rat. Gastroenterology 94:A13

Baskerville A, Newell DG (1988) Naturally occurring chronic gastritis and *C. pylori* infection in the rhesus monkey, a potential model for gastritis in man. Gut 29:465–472

Bechi P, Amorosi A, Mazzanti R, Romagnoli P, Tonelli L (1987) Gastric histology and fasting bile reflux after partial gastrectomy. Gastroenterology 93:335–343

Beck IT, Kahn DS, Lacerte M, Solymar J, Callegarini U, Geokas MC (1965) 'Chronic duodenitis': a clinical pathological entity? Gut 6:376–383

Berrisford RG, Wells M, Dixon MF (1985) Gastric epithelial mucus – a densitometric histochemical study of aspirin-induced damage in the rat. Br J Exp Pathol 66:27–33

Blaser MJ (1987) Gastric *Campylobacter*-like organisms, gastritis, and peptic ulcer disease. Gastroenterology 93:371–383

Blomquist HE (1956) Incidence of metaplasia around and at varying distance from chronic duodenal and gastric ulcers with special reference to differences between young and old persons. Acta Chir Scand 3:465–474

Borch K, Renvall H, Liedberg G (1985) Gastric endocrine cell hyperplasia and carcinoid tumors in pernicious anaemia. Gastroenterology 88:638–648

Borody T, Cole P, Noonan S, Morgan A, Ossip G, Maysey J, Brandl S (1988) Long-term *Campylobacter pylori* recurrence post-eradication. Gastroenterology 94:A43

Burnie J, Lee W, McNulty C, Dent J (1988) Virulence of *Campylobacter* strains and degree of gastritis. Lancet I:302

Carter KJ, Farley PC, Ritchie WP (1984) Effect of topical bile acids on gastric surface epithelial cells. Surgery 96:196–203

Cheli R, Giacosa A (1983) Chronic atrophic gastritis and gastric mucosal atrophy – one and the same. Gastrointest Endosc 29:23–25

Chen XG, Correa P, Offerhaus J et al. (1986) Ultrastructure of the gastric mucosa harboring *Campylobacter*-like organisms. Am J Clin Pathol 86:575–582

Coghlan JG, Gilligan D, Humphries H, McKenna D, Dooley C, Sweeney E, Keane C, O'Morain C (1987) *Campylobacter pylori* and recurrence of duodenal ulcers – a 12-months follow-up study. Lancet II:1109–1111

Colin-Jones DG (1986) There is more to healing ulcers than suppressing acid. Gut 27:475–480

Correa P (1980) The epidemiology and pathogenesis of chronic gastritis: three etiologic entities. Front Gastrointest Res 6:98–108

Cotton PB, Price AB, Tighe JR, Beales JSM (1973) Preliminary evaluation of 'duodenitis' by endoscopy and biopsy. Br Med J III:430–433

Czinn SJ, Dahms BB, Jacobs GH, Kaplan B, Rothstein FC (1986) *Campylobacter*-like organisms in association with symptomatic gastritis in children. J Pediatr 109:80–83

Daskalopoulos G, Carrick J, Borody T, Hazell S, Ralston M (1987) Do *Campylobacter pyloridis* and gastric metaplasia have a role in duodenal ulceration? Gastroenterology 92:1363A

Davenport HW (1970) Effect of lysolecithin, digitonin and phospholipase A upon the dog's gastric mucosal barrier. Gastroenterology 59:505–509

Defilippi C, Mamani N, Gomez E (1987) Relationship between antropyloric and intestinal motility and duodenogastric reflux in fasting dogs. Dig Dis Sci 32:171–176

Delaney JP, Broadie TA, Robbins PL (1975) Pyloric reflux gastritis; the offending agent. Surgery 77:764–772

Dewar EP, Dixon MF, Johnston D (1983) Bile reflux and degree of gastritis after highly selective vagotomy, truncal vagotomy, and partial gastrectomy for duodenal ulcer. World J Surg 7:743–750

Dewar EP, Dixon MF, Johnston D (1984) Bile reflux and degree of gastritis in patients with gastric ulcer: before and after operation. J Surg Res 37:277–284

Diaz MQ, Escobar AS (1986) Metronidazole versus cimetidine in treatment of gastroduodenal ulcer. Lancet I:907

Diserens H, Krstic R, Burri B, Mosimann F, Mosimann R (1984) The gastric mucosa in experimental duodenogastric reflux: a scanning electron microscope study. Scand J Gastroenterol 19 [Suppl 92]: 133–135

Dixon MF, O'Connor HJ, Axon ATR, King RFJG, Johnston D (1986) Reflux gastritis: distinct histopathological entity? J Clin Pathol 39:524–530

Dixon MF, Wyatt JI, Burke DA, Rathbone BJ (1988) Lymphocytic gastritis – relationship to *Campylobacter pylori* infection. J Pathol 154:125–132

Doniach I, Shiner M (1957) Duodenal and jejunal biopsies II. Histology. Gastroenterology 33:71–86

Drapanas T, Bethea M (1974) Reflux gastritis following gastric surgery. Ann Surg 179:618–627

Drumm B, Sherman P, Cutz E, Karmali M (1987) Association of *Campylobacter pylori* on the gastric mucosa with antral gastritis in children. N Engl J Med 316:1557–1561

du Plessis DJ, Lawson HH (1974) Gastric mucosal alterations: benign and malignant. Surg Ann 6:73–101

du Plessis DJ (1977) Consequences of bile reflux. In: Truelove SC, Lee EG (eds) Topics in gastroenterology, vol 5. Blackwell, Oxford, p 239

Eastwood GL (1975) Effect of pH on bile salt injury to mouse gastric mucosa: a light and electron microscope study. Gastroenterology 68:1456–1465

Elsborg L, Andersen D, Myhre-Jensen O, Bastrup-Madsen P (1977) Gastric mucosal polyps in pernicious anaemia. Scand J Gastroenterol 12:49–52

Elta GH, Fawaz KA, Dayal Y et al. (1983) Chronic erosive gastritis – a recently recognised disorder. Dig Dis Sci 28:7–12

Emmanouilidis A, Nicolopoulou-Stamati P, Manousos O (1984) The histologic pattern of bile gastritis. Gastrointest Endosc 30:179–182

Fisher RS (1985) Gastroduodenal motility distrubances in man. Scand J Gastroenterol 20 [Suppl 109]:59–68

Flejou PF, Bahame P, Smith A, Stockbrugger RW, Rode J, Price AB (1989) Pernicious anaemia and Campylobacter-like organisms: Is the gastric antrum resistant to colonisation? Gut 30:60–64
Fontolliet C, Mosimann F, Diserens H, Burri B, Loup PW, Mosimann R (1984) Modifications of the gastric mucosal barrier induced by experimental duodenogastric reflux: an electron microscopic study. Scand J Gastroenterol 19 [Suppl 92]:75–77
Fox JG, Edrise BM, Cabot EB, Beaucage C, Murphy JC, Prostak KS (1986) *Campylobacter* like organisms isolated from gastric mucosa of ferrets. Am J Vet Res 47:236–239.
Franzin G, Manfrini C, Musola R, Rodella S, Fratton A (1984) Chronic erosions of the stomach – a clinical, endoscopic and histological evaluation. Endoscopy 16:1–5
Frizis HI, Whitfield PF, Hobsley M (1987) Maximal gastric secretion and duodenogastric reflux in patients with gastric or duodenal ulcer and in control subjects. Br J Surg 74:106–109
Gallagher CG, Lennon JR, Crowe JP (1987) Chronic erosive gastritis: a clinical study. Am J Gastroenterol 82:302–306
Gardiner GW, Murray D, Prokipchuk EJ (1985) Watermelon stomach, or antral gastritis. J Clin Pathol 38:1317–1318
Gillberg R, Kastrup W, Mobacken H, Stockbrugger R, Ahren C (1985) Gastgric morphology and function in dermatitis herpetiformis and in coeliac disease. Scand J Gastroenterol 20:133–140
Gilman R, Leon-Barua R, Ramirez-Ramos A et al. (1987) Efficacy of nitrofurans in the treatment of antral gastritis associated with *Campylobacter pyloridis*. Gastroenterology 92:1405A
Glass GBJ, Pitchumoni CS (1975) Atrophic gastritis. Hum Pathol 6:219–250
Gledhill T, Leicester RJ, Addis B et al. (1985) Epidemic hypochlorhydria. Br Med J 290:1383–1386
Goodwin CS, Blincow ED, Warren JR, Waters TE, Sanderson CR, Easton L (1985) Evaluation of cultural techniques for isolating *Campylobacter pyloridis* fron endoscopic biopsies of gastric mucosa. J Clin Pathol 38:1127–1131
Goodwin CS, Armstrong JA, Marshall BJ (1986) *Campylobacter pyloridis*, gastritis and peptic ulceration. J Clin Pathol 39:353–365
Gotthard R, Bodemar G, Tjadermo M, Tobiasson P, Walan A (1985) High gastric bile acid concentrations in prepyloric ulcer patients. Scand J Gastroenterol 20:439–446
Graham DY, Klein PD, Evans DG, Opekun AR, Evans DG, Alpert LC, Boutton TW (1987) *Campylobacter pylori* detected noninvasively by the ^{13}C-urea breath test. Lancet I:1174–1177
Gray SF, Wyatt JI, Rathbone BJ (1986) Simplified techniques for identifying *Campylobacter pyloridis*. J Clin Pathol 39:1280
Green PHR, Fevre DI, Barrett PJ, Hunt JH, Gillespie PE, Nagy GS (1977) Chronic erosive (verrucous) gastritis. A study of 108 patients. Endoscopy 9:74–78
Gregory MA, Spitaels J M (1987) Variations in the morphology of villous epithelial cells within 8 mm of untreated duodenal ulcers. J Pathol 153:109–119
Guslandi M (1985) Duodenitis. Lancet II:1437
Guslandi M, Ballarin E (1986) Luminal leakage of HCO_3^- in chronic antral erosions. Hepatogastroenterology 33:221–222
Gustavsson S, Phillips SF, Malagelada J-R. Rosenblatt JE (1987) Assessment of *Campylobacter*-like organisms in the postoperative stomach, iatrogenic gastritis, and chronic gastroduodenal disease: preliminary observations. Mayo Clin Proc 62:265–268
Hansky J, Shiner M (1963) Gastric studies in idiopathic steatorrhoea. Gastroenterology 45:49–56
Haot J, Wallez A, Jouret-Mourin A, Hardy N (1985) La gastrite “à lymphocytes”. Une nouvelle entité? Acta Endosc 15:187–188
Haot J, Delos M, Wallez L, Hardy N, Lenzen B, Jouret-Mourin A (1986 a) Intraepithelial lymphocytes in inflammatory gastric pathology. Acta Endosc 16:61–67
Haot J, Jouret-Mourin A, Delos M et al. (1986 b) Anatomo-clinical study of a series of chronic gastritis characterized by intraepithelial lymphocytic infiltration. Acta Endosc 16:69–74
Harvey RF, Bradshaw MJ, Davidson CM, Wilkinson SP, Davies PS (1985) Multifocal gastric carcinoid tumours, achlorhydria, and hypergastrinaemia. Lancet I:951–954

Hazell SL, Lee A (1985) The adaption of motile strains of *Campylobacter pyloridis* to gastric mucus and their association with gastric epithelial spaces. *Campylobacter* III: Proceedings of the Third International Workshop on *Campylobacter* Infections. Public Health Laboratory Service, London, p 189

Hazell SL, Lee A (1986) *Campylobacter pyloridis*, urease, hydrogen ion back-diffusion and gastric ulcers. Lancet II:15–17

Hazell SL, Hennessy WB, Borody TJ, Carrick J, Ralston M, Brady L, Lee A (1987) *Campylobacter pyloridis* gastritis II: distribution of bacteria and associated inflammation in the gastroduodenal einvironment. Am J Gastroenterol 82:297–301

Hoedemaeker PJ (1970) Heterotopic gastric mucosa in the duodenum. Digestion 3:165–173

Hopwood D (1988) A histometric analysis of gastric biopsies from patients treated with Gastritex: a new drug active against acute or chronic gastritis. J Pathol 154:86A

Howden CW, Hunt RH (1987) Relationship between gastric secretion and infection. Gut 28:96–107

Ihamaki T, Kekki M, Sipponen P, Siurala M (1985) The sequelae and course of chronic gastritis during 30- to 34-year bioptic follow-up study. Scand J Gastroenterol 20:485–491

Ikeda T, Sennoue I, Hara M, Tsutsumi Y, Harasawa S, Miwa T (1985) Gastric pseudopolyposis: a new clinical manifestation of type A gastritis. Am J Gastroenterol 80:82–90

Inada M, Glass GBJ (1975) Effect of prolonged administration of homologous and heterologous intrinsic factor antibody on the parietal and peptic cell masses and the secretory function of the rat gastric mucosa. Gastroenterology 69:396–408

Isaacson P (1982) Immunoperoxidase study of the secretory immunoglobulin system and lysozyme in normal and diseased gastric mucosa. Gut 23:578–588

Jabbari M, Cherry R, Lough JO, Daly DS, Kinnear DG, Goresky CA (1984) Gastric antral vascular ectasia: the watermelon stomach. Gastroenterology 87:1165–1170

James AH (1964) Gastric epithelium in the duodenum. Gut 5:285–294

Jenkins D, Goodall A, Gillet FR, Scott BB (1985) Defining duodenitis: quantitative histological study of mucosal responses and their correlations. J Clin Pathol 38:1119–1126

Jiang SJ, Liu WZ, Zhang DZ, Shi Y, Xiao Sd, Zhang ZH, Lu DY (1987) *Campylobacter*-like organisms in chronic gastritis, peptic ulcer, and gastric carcinoma. Scand J Gastroenterol 22:553–558

Johnston BJ, Reed PI, Ali MH (1986 a) *Campylobacter* like organisms in duodenal and antral endoscopic biopsies: relationship to inflammation. Gut 27:1132–1137

Johnston BJ, Reed PI, Ali MH (1986 b) Relationship between the presence of duodenal *Campylobacter*-like organisms and duodenal ulcer healing. Gut 27:607–608A

Johnston D, Wilkinson AR (1970) Highly selective vagotomy without a drainage procedure in the treatment of duodenal ulcer. Br J Surg 57:289–296

Jones DM, Lessels AM, Elridge J (1984) *Campylobacter*-like organisms on the gastric mucosa: culture, histological, and serological studies. J Clin Pathol 37 1002–1006

Jones DM, Elridge J, Fox AJ, Sethi P, Whorwell PJ (1986) Antibody to the gastric *Campylobacter*-like organism ("*Campylobacter pyloridis*") – clinical correlations and distribution in the normal population. J Med Microbiol 22:57–62

Joske RA, Finckh ES, Wood IG (1955) Gastric biopsies. Q J Med 24:269–94

Kaldor J, Tee W, McCarthy P, Watson J, Dwyer B (1985) Immune response to *Campylobacter pyloridis* in patients with peptic ulceration. Lancet I:921

Karttunen T, Niemela S (1988) *Campylobacter pylori* and duodenogastric reflux in peptic ulcer disease and gastritis. Lancet I:118

Karttunen T, Niemela S, Lehtola J, Heikkala J, Maentausta O, Rasanen O (1987) *Campylobacter*-like organisms and gastritis: histopathology, bile reflux, and gastric fluid composition. Scand J Gastroenterol 22:478–486

Kaye MD (1987) Immunological aspects of gastritis and pernicious anaemia. Bailliere's Clinical Gastroenterology: International Practice and Research 1:487–506

Keighley MRB, Asquith P, Alexander-Williams J (1975) Duodeno-gastric reflux: a cause of gastric mucosal hyperaemia and symptoms after operations for peptic ulceration. Gut 16:28–32

Kekki M, Siurala M, Varis K, Sipponen P, Sistonen P, Nevanlinna HR (1987) Classification principles and genetics of chronic gastritis. Scand J Gastroenterol 22 [Suppl 141]:1–28

Konturek SJ, Bilski J, Kwiechien N, Obtulowicz, Kopp B, Olesky J (1987) De-Nol stimulates gastric and duodenal alkaline secretion through prostaglandin dependent mechanism. Gut 28:1557–1563

Kreuning J, Bosman FT, Kuiper G, v d Wal AM, Lindeman J (1978) Gastric and duodenal mucosa in 'healthy' individuals. J Clin Pathol 31:69–77

Laine L, Marin-Sorensen M, Weinstein WM (1988) The histology of gastric erosions in patients taking non-steroidal anti-inflammatory drugs (NSAIDs): a prospective study. Gastroenterology 94:A247

Lam SK, Lee NW, Koo J, Hui WM, Fok KH, Ng M (1984) Randomised cross-over trial of tripotasium dicitrato bismuthate versus high dose cimetidine for duodenal ulcers resistant to standard of cimetidine. Gut 25:703–706

Lambert JR, Borromeo M, Turner H, Korman MG, Hansky H (1987) Colonisation of gnotobiotic piglets with *Campylobacter pyloridis*. Gastroenterology 92:1489A

Lambert R, Andre C, Moulinier B, Bugnon B (1978) Diffuse varioliform gastritis. Digestion 17: 159–167

Langhans P, Bues M, Heger RA, Hohenstein J, Korfsmeier KH (1984 a) Cell-kinetic investigations in the operated rat stomach to show the influence of duodenogastric reflux. Scand J Gastroenterol 19 [Suppl 92]:87–90

Langhans P, Bues M, Bunte H (1984 b) Morphological changes in the operated stomach under the influence of duodenogastric reflux: clinical follow-up over 20 years. Scand J Gastroenterol 19 [Suppl 92]:145–148

Lawson HH (1965) The effect of duodenal contents on the gastric mucosa under experimental conditions. S Afr J Surg 3:79–92

Lee FI, Samloff IM, Hardman M (1984) Comparison of tripotassium dicitrato bismuthate tablets with ranitidine in healing and relapse of duodenal ulcers. Lancet I:1299–1302

Leunk RD, Johnson PT, David BC, Kraft WG, Morgan DR (1988) Cytotoxic activity in broth-culture filtrates of *Campylobacter pylori*. J Med Microbiol 26:93–99

Loup P, Fontolliet C, Gonvers JJ, Realini S, Birchler R, Pusztaszeri G, Fasel J (1978) Realité de la gastrite postoperatoire par reflux. Schweiz Med Wochenschr 108:1129–1135

Mahony MJ, Wyatt JI, Littlewood JM (1987) *Campylobacter* associated gastritis in children. Gut 28:A1357

Malfertheiner P, Bode G, Vanek E, Stanescu A, Lutz E, Blessing J, Ditschuneit H (1987) *Campylobacter pylori* – is there a connection with peptic ulcer? Dtsch Med Wochenschr 112:493–497

Marshall BJ, Armstrong JA, McGechie DB, Glancy RJ (1985 a) Attempt to fulfil Koch's postulates for pyloric *Campylobacter*. Med J Aust 142:436–439

Marshall BJ, McGechie DB, Rogers PA, Glancy RJ (1985 b) Pyloric *Campylobacter* infection and gastroduodenal disease. Med J Austr 142:439–444

Martin DF, Hollanders D, May SJ, Ravenscroft MM, Tweedle DEF, Miller JP (1981) Difference in relapse rates of duodenal ulcer after healing with cimetidine or tripotassium dicitrato bismuthate. Lancet I:7–10

McKenna D, Humphreys H, Dooley C, Bourke S, Keane C, Sweeney E, O'Morain C (1987) *Campylobacter pyloridis* and histological gastritis in duodenal ulcer: a controlled prospective randomised trial. Gastroenterology 92:1528 A

McNulty CAM (1986) *Campylobacter pyloridis*-associated gastritis. J Infection 13:107–113

McNulty CAM, Gearty JC, Crump B, Davis M, Donovan IA, Manhart MD, Wise R (1986) Successful therapy of *Campylobacter gastritis*. Gastroenterology 91:1547 A

Menguy R, Max MH (1970) Influence of bile on the canine gastric-antral mucosa. Am J Surg 119:177–182

Morgan DR, Kraft WG, Leunk RD, Krakowka GS (1988) A non-primate animal model for gastritis induced by *C. pyloridis*. In: *Campylobacter* IV: Proceedings of the IVth International Workshop on *Campylobacter* infections

Morris A, Nicholson G (1987) Ingestion of *Campylobacter pyloridis* causes gastritis and raised fasting gastric pH. Am J Gastroenterol 82:192–199

Morris A, Arthur J, Nicholson G (1986 a) *Campylobacter pyloridis* infection in Auckland patients with gastritis. NZ Med J 99:353–355

Morris A, McIntyre D, Rose T, Nicholson G (1986 b) Rapid diagnosis of *Campylobacter pyloridis* infection. Lancet I:149

Mosimann F, Burri B, Diserens H, Fontolliet C, Loup P, Mosimann R (1981) Enterogastric reflux; experimental and clinical study. A preliminary report. Scand J Gastroenterol 16 [Suppl 67]:149–152

Mosimann F, Burri B, Diserens H, Fontolliet C, Loup PW, Mirkovitch V, Mosimann R (1984) A long-term study of experimental duodenogastric reflux on the vagotomised stomach in dogs. Scand J Gastroenterol 19 [Suppl 92]:136–137

Moutier F, Martin J (1947) Deux cas de gastrite varioliforme. Arch Mal Appar Dig 36:155–161

Murakami M, Yoo JK, Mizuno M, Saita H, Inada M, Miyake T (1987 a) Effects of ammonia, urea, and urease on the rat gastric mucosa. Gastroenterology 92:1544 A

Murakami M, Yoo JK, Mizuno M, Saita H, Inada M, Miyake T (1987 b) Role of ammonia, urea and urease in gastric mucosal lesions in azotemia. Gastroenterology 92:1545 A

Nesland A, Berstad A (1985) Erosive prepyloric changes in persons with and without dyspepsia. Scand J Gastroenterol 20:222–228

Niedobitek F, Grosse G, Taube F, Volkheimer G, Fehrenbach FJ, Werner E (1987) Bacterial colonization of the gastric mucosa. Z Gastroenterol 25:98–106

Niemela S, Karttunen T, Heikkila J, Lehtola J (1987) Characteristics of reflux gastritis. Scand J Gastroenterol 22:349–354

O'Brien K, Saunders DR, Templeton FE (1972) Chronic gastric erosions and oral aphthae. Dig Dis 178:447–454

O'Connor HJ, Axon ATR, Dixon MF (1984) *Campylobacter*-like organisms unusual in type A (pernicious anaemia) gastritis. Lancet II:1091

O'Connor HJ, Wyatt JI, Dixon MF, Axon ATR (1986 a) *Campylobacter* like organisms and reflux gastritis. J Clin Pathol 39:531–534

O'Connor HJ, Dixon MF, Wyatt JI, Axon ATR, Ward DC, Dewar EP, Johnston D (1986 b) Effect of duodenal ulcer surgery and enterogastric reflux on *Campylobacter pyloridis*. Lancet II:1178–1181

O'Connor HJ, Dixon MF, Wyatt JI, Axon ATR, Dewar EP, Johnston D (1987) *Campylobacter pylori* and peptic ulcer disease. Lancet II:633

Offerhaus GJA, Stadt Jvd, Huibregtse K, Tytgat GNJ (1984) Endoscopic screening for malignancy in the gastric remnant: the clinical significance of dysplasia in gastric mucosa. J Clin Pathol 37:748–754

Orchard R, Reynolds K, Fox B, Andrews R, Parkins RA, Johnson AG (1977) Effect of lysolecithin on gastric mucosal structure and potential difference. Gut 18:457–461

Owen RJ, Martin SR, Borman P (1985) Rapid urea hydrolysis by gastric campylobacters. Lancet I:111

Parl FF, Lev R, Thomas E, Pitchumoni CS (1979) Histologic and morphometric study of chronic gastritis in alcoholic patients. Hum Pathol 10:45–56

Patrick WJA, Denham D, Forrest APM (1974) Mucous change in the human duodenum: a light and electron microscopic study and correlation with disease and gastric acid secretion. Gut 15:767–776

Perarnau J-M, Métais P, Schaeffer M, Raabe J-J, Courrier A, Arbogast J (1984) Gastrite varioliforme avec test de dégranulation des basophiles humains positif vis-à-vis d'une mélange de tisanes. Gastroenterol Clin Biol 8:676

Peterson W, Lee E, Skoglund M (1987) The role of *Campylobacter pyloridis* in epidemic gastritis with hypochlorhydria. Gastroenterology 92 1575

Pickford IR, Craven JL, Hall R, Thomas G, Stone WD (1984) Endoscopic examinaiton of the gastric remnant 31–39 years after subtotal gastrectomy for peptic ulcer. Gut 25:393–397

Price AB, Levi J, Dolby JM, Dunscombe PL, Smith A, Clark J, Stephenson ML (1985) *Campylobacter pyloridis* in peptic ulcer disease: microbiology, pathology and scanning electron microscopy. Gut 26:1183–1188

Ramsey EJ, Carey KV, Peterson WL (1979) Epidemic gastritis with hypochlorhydria. Gastroenterology 76:1449–1457

Rathbone BJ, Wyatt JI, Heatley RV (1986 a) *Campylobacter pyloridis* – a new factor in peptic ulcer disease? Gut 27:635–641

Rathbone BJ, Wyatt JI, Tompkins DS, Heatley RV, Losowsky MS (1986 b) Diagnostic IgG ELISA for gastric *Campylobacter pyloridis* infection using serum samples. Dig Dis Sci 31:1523

Rathbone BJ, Wyatt JI, Worsley BW, Shires SE, Trejosiewicz LK, Heatley RV, Losowsky MS (1986c) Systematic and local antibody responses to gastric *Campylobacter pyloridis* in non-ulcer dyspepsia. Gut 27:642–647

Rathbone BJ, Shires SE, Townsend C, Wyatt JI, Heatley RV, Losowsky MS (1988) Serum *Campylobacter pyloridis* specific IgG ELISA as a marker of colonisation in prevalence studies. IN: *Campylobacter* IV: Proceedings of the IVth International Workshop on *Campylobacter* Infections University of Gothenburg Press, p 182

Rathbone BJ, Trejosiewicz LK, Heatley RV, Losowsky MS (1989) Mucosal T-cell subjets in normal gastric antrum and C pylori associated chronic gastritis. Gut 29:A1438

Rauws EAJ, Langenberg W, Houthoff HJ, Zanen HC, Tytgat GNJ (1988) *Campylobacter pyloridis*-associated chronic active antral gastritis: a prospective study of its prevalence and the effects of antibacterial and antiulcer treatment. Gastroenterology 94:33–40

Rawles JW, Paull G, Yardley JH et al. (1986) Gastric *Campylobacter*-like organisms in a US hospital population. Gastroenterology 91:15599A

Rawles JW, Harris ML, Paull G et al. (1987) Antibody to *Campylobacter pyloridis* in endoscopy personnel, patients and controls. Gastroenterology 92:1589A

Rees W, Rhodes J (1977) Bile reflux in gastro-oesophageal disease. Clin Gastroenterol 6:179–200

Ritchie WP (1977) Bile acids, the "barrier", and reflux related clinical disorders of the gastric mucosa. Surgery 82:192–200

Ritchie WP (1980) Alkaline reflux gastritis: an objective assessment of its diagnosis and treatment. Ann Surg 192:288–298

Ritchie WP (1984) Alkaline reflux gastritis: a critical appraisal. Gut 25:975–987

Robbins PL, Broadie TA, Sosin H, Delaney JP (1976) Reflux gastritis. The consequences of intestinal juice in the stomach. Am J Surg 131:23–29

Rode J, Dhillon AP, Papadaki L, Stockbrugger R, Thompson RJ, Moss E, Cotton PB (1986) Pernicious anaemia and mucosal endocrine cell proliferation of the non-antral stomach. Gut 27:789–798

Rode J, Lowes JR, Moss E (1988) Neuroendocrine cell proliferations in gastric antral vascular ectasia. J Pathol 350A

Rokkas T, Pursey C, Simmons NA, Filipe MI, Sladen GE (1987) Non-ulcer dyspepsia and colloidal bismuth subcitrate therapy: the role of *Campylobacter pyloridis*. Gastroenterology 92:1599A

Rollason TP, Stone J, Rhodes JM (1984) Spiral organisms in endoscopic biopsies of the human stomach. J Clin Pathol 37:23–26

Rubio CA, Kato Y, Sugano H (1985) The lymphoepithelial phenomenon in the gastric mucosa. Pathol Res Pract 180:612–614

Savage D (1970) Associations of indigenous microorganisms with gastrointestinal mucosal epithelia. Am J Clin Nutr 23:1495–1501

Schindlbeck NE, Heinrich C, Stellaard F, Paumgartner G, Muller Lissner SA (1987) Healthy controls have as much bile reflux as gastric ulcer patients. Gut 28:1577–1583

Scudamore HH, Eckstam EE, Fencil WJ, Jaramillo CA (1973) Bile reflux gastritis: diagnosis, medical and surgical therapy. Am J Gastroenterol 60:9–22

Shiner M (1956) Duodenal biopsy. Lancet I:17–19

Shousha S, Spiller RC, Parkins RA (1983) The endoscopically abnormal duodenum in patients with dyspepsia: biopsy findings in 60 cases. Histopathology 7:23–34

Shousha S, Bull TR, Parkins RA (1984) Gastric spiral bacteria. Lancet II:101

Sircus W (1985) Duodenitis: a clinical, endoscopic and histopathological study. Q J Med 56:593–600

Slomiany BL, Bilski J, Sarosiek J et al. (1987) *Campylobacter pyloridis* degrades mucin and undermines gastric mucosal integrity. Biochem Biophys Res Commun 144:307–314

Steer HW (1975) Ultrastructure of cell migration through the gastric epithelium and its relationship to bacteria. J Clin Pathol 28:639–646

Steer HW (1984) Surface morphology of the gastroduodenal mucosa in duodenal ulceration. Gut 25:1203–1210

Steer HW (1985) The gastroduodenal epithelium in peptic ulceration. J Pathol 146:355–362

Stockbrugger RW, Menon GG, Bielby JOW, Mason RR, Cotton PB (1983) Gastroscopic screening in 80 patients with pernicious anaemia. Gut 24:1141–1147

Strickland RG, Mackay IR (1973) A reappraisal of the nature and significance of chronic atrophic gastritis. Dig Dis 18:426–440

Suit PF, Petras RE, Bauer TW, Petrini JL (1987) Gastric antral vascular ectasia: a histologic and morphometric study of 'the watermelon stomach'. Am J Surg Pathol 11:750–757

Svensson JO, Gelin J, Svanvik J (1986) Gallstones, cholecystectomy, and duodenogastric reflux of bile acid. Scand J Gastroenterol 21:181–187

Thomas JE, Elliot TSJ, Eastham EJ, Berkely D, Jones D (1988) The incidence of *Campylobacter pylori* associated gastritis in a paediatric population and its relationship to symptoms. J Med Microbiol 25:pt 4, iv

Thomas WEG (1984) The possible role of duodenogastric reflux in the pathogenesis of both gastric and duodenal ulcers. Scand J Gastroenterol 19 [Suppl 92]:155–155

Thomas WEG, Cooper MJ, Mortensen NJM, Burton PA, Davies ER (1984) The clinical assessment of duodenogastric reflux by scintigraphy and its relation to histological changes in gastric mucosa. Scand J Gastroenterol 19 [Suppl 92]:195–199

Tompkins DS, West AP (1987) *Campylobacter pylori*, acid, and bile. J Clin Pathol 40:1387

Toukan AU, Kamal MF, Amr SS, Arnaout MA, Abu-Romiyeh AS (1985) Gastroduodenal inflammation in patients with nonulcer dyspepsia: a controlled endoscopic and morphometric study. Dig Dis Sci 30:313–320

Tricottet V, Bruneval P, Vire O, Camilleri JP (1986) *Campylobacter*-like organisms and surface epithelium abnormalities in active, chronic gastritis in humans: an ultrastructural study. Ultrastruct Pathol 10:113–122

Valnes K, Brandzaeg P, Elgjo K, Stave R (1984) Specific and non-specific humoral defence factors in the epithelium of normal and inflamed gastric mucosa. Gastroenterology 86:402–412

Varis K, Ihamaki T, Harkonen M, Samlof IM, Siurala M (1979) Gastric morphology, function and immunology in first degree-relatives of probands with pernicious anaemia and controls. Scand J Gastroenterol 14:129–139

Villako K, Tamm A, Savisaar E, Ruttas M (1976) Prevalence of antral and fundic gastritis in a randomly selected group of an Estonian rural population. Scand J Gastroenterol 11:817–22

Villako K, Kekki M, Tamm A, Savisaar E (1986) Development and progression of chronic gastritis in the antrum and body mucosa: results of long term follow-up examinations. Ann Clin Res 18:121–123

Warren JR, Marshall B (1983) Unidentified curved bacilli on gastric epithelium in active chronic gastritis. Lancet I:1273–1275

Weinstein WM, Buch KL, Elashoff J, Reedy T, Tedesco FJ, Samloff IM, Ippoliti AF (1985) The histology of the stomach in symptomatic patients after gastric surgery: a model to assess selective patterns of mucosal injury. Scand J Gastroenterol 20 [Suppl 109):77–89

Whitehead R, Truelove SC, Gear MWL (1972) The histological diagnosis of chronic gastritis in fibreoptic gastroscope biopsy specimens. J Clin Pathol 25:1–11

Whitehead R, Roca M, Meikle DD, Skinner J, Truelove SC (1975) The histological classification of duodenitis in fibreoptic biopsy specimens. Digestion 13:129–136

Wormsley KG (1987) Ulcer disease: epidemiology. Curr Opin Gastroenterol 3:944–951

Wyatt JI, Dixon MF (1988) Chronic gastritis – a pathogenetic approach. J Pathol 154:113–124

Waytt JI, Rathbone BJ (1988) Immune response of the gastric mucosa to *Campylobacter pylori*. Scand J Gastroenterol 23 [Suppl 142]:44–49

Wyatt JI, Rathbone BJ, Heatley RV (1986) Local immune response to gastric *Campylobacter* in non-ulcer dyspepsia. J Clin Pathol 39:863–870

Wyatt JI, Rathbone BJ, Dixon MF, Heatley RV (1987) *Campylobacter pyloridis* and acid-induced metaplasia in the pathogenesis of duodenitis. J Clin Pathol 40:841–848

Wyatt JI, Rathbone BJ, Dixon MF, Heatley RV, Axon ATR (1988 a) *Campylobacter pylori* and development of duodenal ulcer. Lancet I:118–119

Waytt JI, Primrose J, Dixon MF (1988 b) Distribution of *Campylobacter pylori* in gastric biopsies. J Pathol 350A

Zheng ZT, Wang ZY, Chu YX (1985) Double blind short term trial of furazolidone in peptic ulcer. Lancet I:1048–1049

Precancerous Lesions of the Gastrointestinal Tract

A Barrett's Oesophagus

F. POTET and V. DUCHATELLE

1 Introduction

Barrett's oesophagus or columnar epithelial lined lower oesophagus (CELLO) is usually considered to be an acquired disorder complicating prolonged reflux oesophagitis. In 1953, ALLISON and JOHNSTONE described hiatal hernia with oesophageal stricture, below which the oesophagus was lined with gastric epithelium. In 1957, BARRET described the columnar-lined oesophagus and its complications such as ulcer, stricture and carcinoma. At the same time, LORTAT-JACOB et al. (1957) described this entity under the term "endobrachyoesophage". CELLO consists of several types of columnar epithelium, one of which is the very distinctive "specialised columnar type". The latter resembles intestinal metaplasia (IM) of the stomach. Barrett's oesophagus is a condition of considerable interest because several authors have reported a high incidence of adenocarcinoma arising in CELLO.

2 Definition

Barrett's oesophagus is defined as a columnar epithelium lining a variable length of the lower oesophagus. The major diagnostic difficulty is to determine precisely the anatomical border between the stomach and the oesophagus. Although theoretically this is the cardia, marked anatomically by the lower oesophageal sphincter and endoscopically by the Z line, in reality the squamocolumnar junction does not always coincide with the lower oesophageal sphincter. Moreover, the junction of the two epithelial

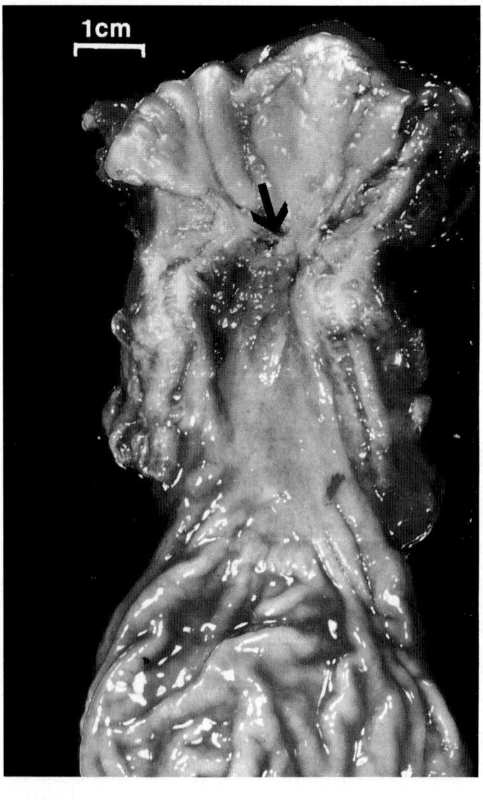

Fig. 1. Photograph of a specimen of Barrett's oesophagus: CELLO is extended over 4 cm with peptic ulcer and stricture at the squamous and columnar epithelium junction (*arrow*)

types is often irregular, showing little "tongues" of columnar epithelium spreading 1–2 cm up the oesophagus. HERLIHY et al. (1984) use the term CELLO or Barrett's oesophagus when the columnar epithelium extends to at least 3 cm. According to these authors, there are two types of CELLO of equal frequency: the *circumferential type*, involving a continuous circumferential area (Fig. 1), and *the island type* where the columnar epithelium is seen as one or more islands of red mucosa which are located just above the gastro-oesophageal junction. This latter type is often associated with "tongues" of gastric epithelium arising from the Z line. CELLO is easily identified endoscopically by its prominent red colour, which contrasts with the adjacent light-pink colour of the squamous epithelium.

3 Pathogenesis

Controversy has existed about the pathogenesis of CELLO. ALLISON and JOHNSTONE (1953) suggested that gastro-oesophageal reflux may be responsible for this abnormality. On the other hand, BARRETT (1957) postulated a congenital origin: the developing oesophagus in the embryo is lined by columnar epithelium (BOZYMSKI et al. 1982; SJØGREN and JOHNSON 1983) which is completely replaced at birth by squamous epithelium. Moreover, BARRETT (1957) postulated that this replacement may be altered, resulting in the persistence of columnar epithelium in the lower oesophagus.

There is now strong evidence supporting the acquired origin of CELLO by the replacement in peptic oesophagitis of the ulcerated squamous epithelium by a metaplastic columnar epithelium. NAEF et al. (1975) and WINTERS et al. (1987) found a high prevalence of CELLO in gastro-oesophageal reflux disease (11% and 12.4% respectively). HAMILTON and YARDLEY (1977) studied the lower oesophagus of 17 patients who had undergone oesophagogastrostomy: CELLO was demonstrated in the region of the anastomosis in ten of these patients. It is still unknown why columnar epithelium develops only in a small number of patients with reflux oesophagitis. Another unresolved question is the cellular origin of CELLO; proposed candidates include oesophageal gastric glands, gastric mucosa, congenital rests of columnar cells or an undefined primordial stem cell (SJØGREN and JOHNSON 1983).

4 Microscopic Features

4.1 Histological Features

PAULL et al. (1976) were the first to describe, in patients with CELLO, one or a combination of three types of columnar epithelium: a distinctive "specialised epithelium", a junctional type and a gastric fundic type. Many authors (SJØGREN and JOHNSON 1983; SPECHLER et al. 1984; ZWAS et al. 1986) have confirmed these histological patterns:

- The *specialised type epithelium* appears to be a particular variant of incomplete IM (Fig. 2). The surface is almost villous and lined by columnar and goblet cells. The columnar cells usually resemble gastric mucus-secreting pit cells rather than intestinal absorptive cells, interspersed with sparse goblet cells. Deep in the mucosa there are some clear mucus-secreting glands with EC cells and rare gastrin and somatostatin-containing endocrine cells (BUCHAN et al. 1985).
- The *junctional type epithelium* resembles normal cardiac epithelium, with the surface and pits lined by typical mucus-secreting cells.
- The *gastric fundic type epithelium* resembles the epithelium found in the gastric body, and is characterised by mucus cells on the surface with chief and parietal cells in the deep part. If compared with normal fundic mucosa, the fundic type of CELLO appears slightly atrophic.

When two or more types of mucosa coexist, they generally have a specific relationship with the specialised type adjacent to the squamous area, the junctional type below this and the fundic type in the most distal zone. In our experience of 34 CELLO, we found 23 with specialised type, 25 with junctional type and 9 with gastric fundic type. Ten CELLO were lined with only one type of epithelium (six junctional and four specialised); in three cases all three epithelial types were present. There is no evidence of regression of CELLO with medical or surgical treatment (POPE 1985).

4.2 Ultrastructural Studies

Ultrastructural studies (BERENSON et al. 1974; TRIER 1985) show that the specialised epithelium has a uniform aspect: although the cells resemble gastric foveolar cells, their microvilli are longer and more numerous and they contain fewer mucus secretory vesicles than normal gastric foveolar cells. On the other hand, the goblet cells of the specialised type closely resemble the goblet cells of normal intestinal epithelium. Study of the mucosal surface by scanning electron microscopy reveals a morphological heterogeneity which is not seen by light microscopy (ZWAS et al. 1986).

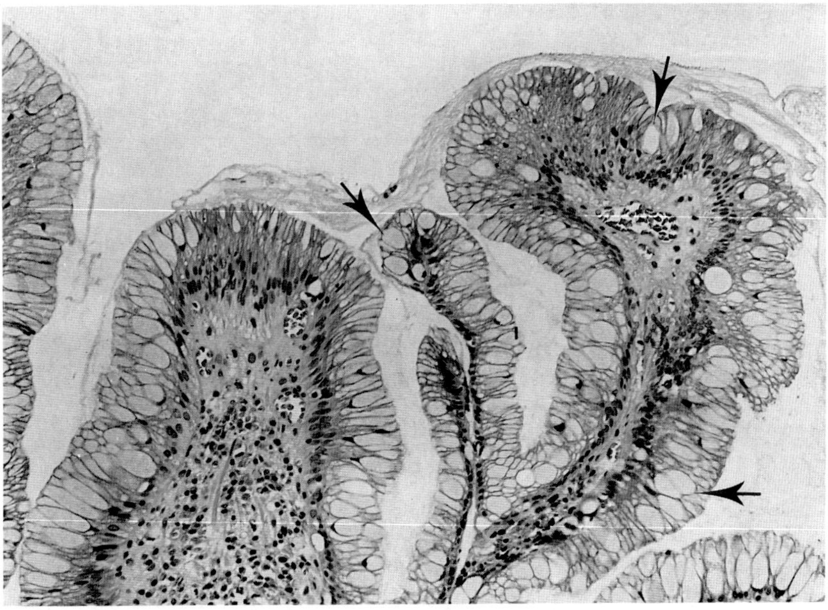

Fig. 2. Specialised columnar epithelium with villous appearance. Some cells resemble gastric mucus-secreting pit cells. Intestinal type goblet cells are also present (*arrows*). HE, × 120

5 Adenocarcinoma in Patients with CELLO

5.1 Frequency

In several series, the premalignant character of CELLO, has been established with a 10%–15% prevalence of adenocarcinoma (range 0%–46.5%). In our experience (at Beaujon hospital), we have found a 10% prevalence in a biopsy series of 44 cases.

However, *prevalence* is defined as the total number of patients with adenocarcinoma in a series of CELLO without distinction of the time of their occurrence. We believe that the risk of carcinoma in CELLO is better estimated by considering the *incidence*, which expresses the number of new cases per year. In the literature three sets of data are available (SPECHLER et al. 1984; SPRUNG et al. 1984; CAMERON et al. 1985) concerning the incidence of oesophageal adenocarcinomas in CELLO. These are summarised in Table 1. Although the results appear different from those of studies reporting prevalence, the risk of malignancy in CELLO is about 30–40 times higher than in the general population.

Table 1. Incidence of oesophageal adenocarcinoma in patients with CELLO (modified from SPECHLER and GYAL 1986)

	SPECHLER et al. (1984)	CAMERON et al. (1985)	SPRUNG et al. (1984)
Total no. of patients	115	122	108
Prevalence of CELLO adenocarcinoma (%)	7	15	22
Number of cancer-free patients followed	105	104	41
Mean (range) length of follow-up (years)	3.3 (0.1–20)	8.5 (3–15)	4 (1–11)
Number of patients in whom cancer developed during follow-up	2	2	2
Incidence of oesophageal adenocarcinoma (cases/person-years)	1/175	1/441	1/81
Estimated increased risk above that in general population	40 times	30 times	

5.2 Definition

One of the difficulties is how to determine whether or not an adenocarcinoma is complicating CELLO. HAGGITT et al. (1978) define primary oesophageal carcinomas as tumours developing 75% or more within the oesophagus and reserve adenocarcinoma in CELLO for cases where the mucosa proximal to the tumour is columnar. In ten of our own cases, we have found the following combinations extending distally:

- Squamous epithelium, carcinoma, CELLO in three cases
- Squamous epithelium, CELLO, carcinoma, CELLO in five cases
- Squamous epithelium, CELLO and carcinoma in two cases

We believe that the difference between cardiac adenocarcinoma and adenocarcinoma in CELLO is the evident presence of columnar epithelium between the carcinoma and either the squamous epithelium or the cardiac line.

5.3 General Features

A review of 121 cases of adenocarcinoma developing in CELLO reported in the literature (SJØGREN and JOHNSON 1983) shows that the average age at diagnosis is 57 years and the male to female ratio is approximately 6:1. The main clinical symptoms are dysphagia and weight loss.

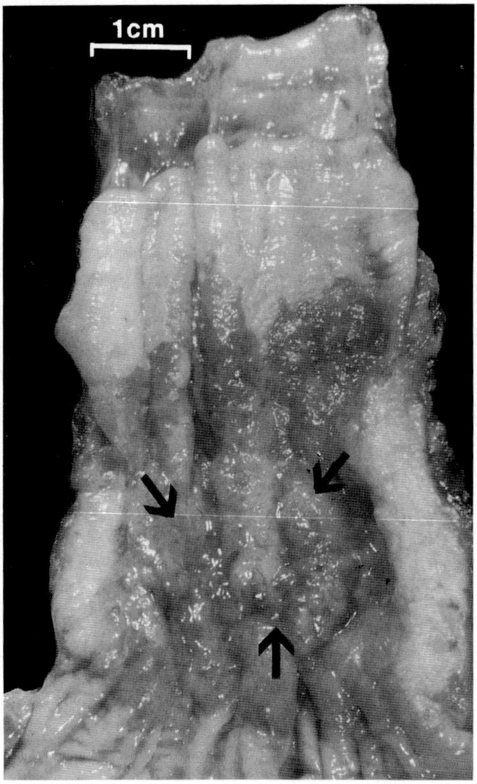

Fig. 3. Photograph of a specimen with an adenocarcinoma (*arrows*) arising in an extensive columnar metaplasia of the distal oesophagus

The localisation of the carcinoma is most often the lower third of the oesophagus (24 of 26 cases in SMITH et al. 1984). The tumour is frequently flat with surface ulceration (Fig. 3) and is polypoid in less than 35% of cases. The tumours measure from 0.6 to 9 cm.

5.4 Histology

Histologically, adenocarcinoma is the most common type of carcinoma in CELLO. All the patterns observed in gastric carcinoma can be seen but the most frequent is a well or moderately differentiated glandular pattern (Fig. 4) (HAGGITT and DEAN 1985). Other less frequent types are mucinous carcinoma, poorly differentiated carcinoma, adenosquamous (SMITH et al. 1984; PASCAL and CLEARFIELD 1987), adenocarcinoid or adenocarcinoma associated with squamous carcinoma (SMITH et al. 1984). The epithelium around the tumour is often dysplastic. In the series of 26 cases of SMITH et al. (1984), the carcinoma had extended through the oesophageal wall into the peri-oesophageal soft tissues in 23 cases, to the lymph nodes in 17 cases and to the surgical resection margins in 9 cases.

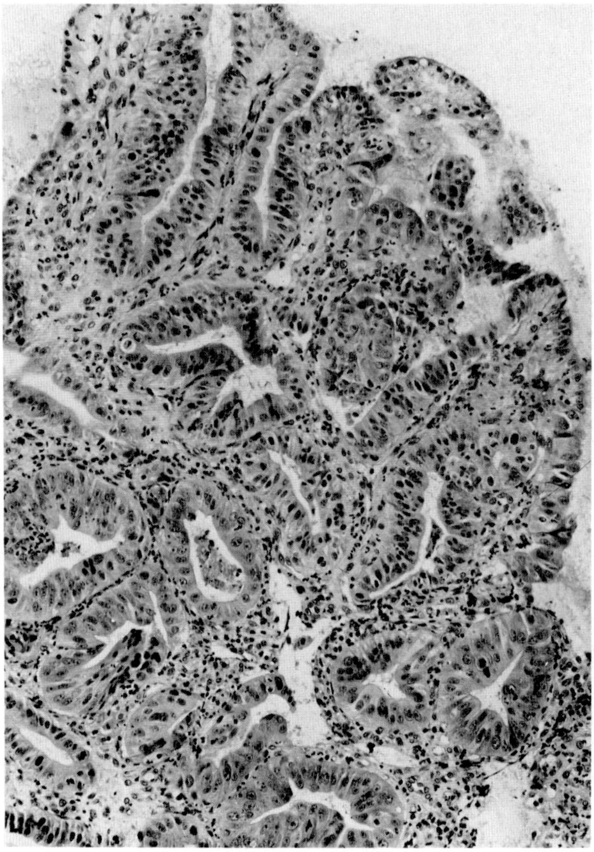

Fig. 4. Well differentiated adenocarcinoma: the well defined glands resemble those of an intestinal type gastric adenocarcinoma. HE, × 130

Infiltrating pattern, poor differentiation, positive lymph nodes and resection margin involvement explain the poor prognosis of these tumours: SMITH et al. (1984) reported a median survival of 23 ± 5 months for their 26 patients with adenocarcinoma in CELLO. The series of 32 cases of SANFEY et al. (1985) showed a 34% survival rate at 2 years and a 14.8% survival rate at 5 years.

5.5 Dysplasia and Adenocarcinoma in CELLO

Dysplastic Barrett's mucosa is generally considered as a precursor of adenocarcinoma in CELLO. This concept, based on the frequent presence of multifocal dysplasia in association with oesophageal adenocarcinoma, has been widely studied. Coexisting dysplasia has been diagnosed in 83% (HAGGITT et al. 1978) to 100% (THOMPSON et al. 1983) of the resected adenocarcinomas: these authors conclude that high grade dypslasia (HGD) indicates a high risk of developing carcinoma. This dysplastic pattern is mainly observed in the specialised type of Barrett's epithelium. It seems that the surveillance of dysplasia and carcinoma in patients with Barrett's oesophagus has much in common with that in chronic inflammatory bowel disease (HAMILTON and SMITH 1987). According to several studies (BERENSON et al. 1978; HAMILTON and SMITH 1987; REID et al. 1988), as well as our own experience, HGD proves to be a good marker indicating a high probability of coexisting invasive carcinoma. HAMILTON and SMITH (1987) suggest that prophylactic oesophagectomy is indicated in a patient with persistent HGD in oesophageal biopsy specimens of CELLO. We disagree with this recommendation and usually ask for repeat biopsies from the abnormal area until we are certain of malignancy. The important paper of REID et al. (1988) supports our policy. They describe four patients with HGD diagnosed in biopsy specimens who underwent subsequent oesophagectomy. All four resected specimens showed only HGD and two of the patients died post operatively. These authors found that HGD could exist for as long as 42 months without progressing to invasive carcinoma.

5.6 Superficial Adenocarcinoma in CELLO

BELLADONNA et al. (1974) found one mucosal carcinoma in CELLO using endoscopic cytology. The surveillance of patients with HGD allowed HAMILTON and SMITH (1987) to discover two superficial carcinomas amongst five patients with HGD. Of 130 patients in another endoscopic biopsy surveillance programme, REID et al. (1988) found eight patients with HGD (four) or early oesophageal adenocarcinoma, (four) diagnosed in biopsy specimens taken from mucosa without grossly recognisable tumoral lesions.

We have studied seven cases of superficial adenocarcinoma in CELLO diagnosed during surveillance of HGD. Macroscopically, the carcinomas had the same location as other carcinomas in CELLO. The mucosa appeared normal in two cases, opaque in one, verrucous in one and in the remaining three cases an erosive pattern was the main feature. The tumors ranged in size from 0·2 to 3 cm. Histologically, all the carcinomas were of glandular pattern; one was confined to the mucosa with partial extension into the muscularis mucosa while in the other six cases, the proliferation spread to the submucosa. Only one case, the largest identified carcinoma, showed a lymph node metastasis. The prognosis of these superficial carcinomas seems to be better than the infiltrative ones. In our group of patients, one patient died during the postsurgical period. The remaining six patients are still alive with follow-up periods ranging from 19 months to 4 years and 2 months. According to our experience the prevalence of superficial carcinoma is high (7 out of 32) in populations undergoing surveillance. This agrees with the results of ROSENBERG et al. (1985), who, using a staging system, found three intramucosal carcinomas out of nine CELLO carcinomas. However, the number of cases is small and additional prospective studies are needed to establish the value of routine surveillance in the diagnosis of early CELLO carcinomas.

5.7 Precancerous Conditions and Aetiological Factors

Hiatal hernia and reflux oesophagitis are often but not always present in patients who develop adenocarcinoma in CELLO. There is no evidence in the literature (ROSENBERG et al. 1985) to claim that duration and severity of oesophagitis are directly related to the malignant transformation. SKINNER et al. (1983) compared benign and malignant cases of CELLO and found no difference in the duration of symptoms of oesophagitis. There is also no correlation between the severity of oesophagitis and the stage of malignancy (ROSENBERG et al. 1985). In one series of 110 patients (WITT et al. 1983; ROSENBERG et al. 1985) who had a successful antireflux surgical procedure, none developed carcinoma, suggesting that oesophagitis could be involved not only in the aetiology of CELLO, but also in the development of adenocarcinoma in CELLO. However, HAMILTON and YARDLEY (1977) and SANFEY et al. (1985) report patients with CELLO who developed adenocarcinomas 5–8 years after surgical elimination of gastro-oesophageal reflux. Other factors may be involved, in association with oesophagitis: cigarette smoking and alcohol ingestion are found with higher frequency in patients with adenocarcinoma (ROSENBERG et al. 1985; KALISH et al. 1984; WANG et al. 1986; SANFEY et al. 1985) than in patients with CELLO alone (SKINNER et al. 1983).

The occurence of benign adenomatous polyps in CELLO is very unusual and available observations are rare. LEE (1986) described three cases of tubulovillous adenoma arising in specialised mucosa associated with dysplasia. He also found three similar reports in the literature (MCDONALD et al. 1977; THOMPSON et al. 1983). We have observed one case associated with HGD and invasive carcinoma. It is probable that an adenoma is not a frequent precursor of adenocarcinoma in CELLO.

5.8 Association with Extra-oesophageal Neoplasms

SPECHLER et al. (1984) found extra-oesophageal cancers in 25 patients out of 115 with CELLO (22%). SONTAG et al. (1985) described 29 out of 65 CELLO patients with benign (19) or malignant (10) colonic tumours. The frequency of colonic tumours was especially high (38%) in patients with CELLO aged 64 years or older. SYMONDS and RAMSEY (1980) described one case of pancreatic gastrinoma (Zollinger Ellison), associated with CELLO adenocarcinoma. This peculiar association warrants further investigation.

5.9 CELLO and Cardiac Adenocarcinomas

KALISH et al. (1984) and WANG et al. (1986) found that both CELLO and cardiac adenocarcinomas of the stomach have almost identical patterns of growth and differentiation. Reflux oesophagitis is noticed with equal frequency in both. PEUCHMAUR et al. (1984) found the same histochemical characteristics, with predominance of sulphomucins, in both CELLO and cardiac carcinomas. Furthermore, these carcinomas share certain common epidemiological features. WANG et al. (1986) suggest that proximal adenocarcinomas (of the distal oesophagus, gastro-oesophageal junction and cardia) may form a group with similar epidemiological and pathological features, such as increasing frequency, lower mean age, possible increased risk with smoking and alcohol use and greater frequency of concomitant hiatal hernia. These common features suggest that this group may be aetiologically distinct from the group of more distal gastric carcinomas (gastric body and antrum).

6 Precancerous Lesions and Precancerous Markers

Attempts have been made to identify structural and functional changes preceding the development of adenocarcinoma in CELLO, most of them investigating epithelial differentiation. Among the aspects studied are different types of dysplasia, patterns of epithelial mucins identified by histochemistry or immunohistochemisty, the detection of tumour markers, embryonal antigens or differentiation antigens, the measurement of the cell kinetics in the columnar epithelium with ^{3}H-thymidine, and flow cytometry.

6.1 Dysplasia

6.1.1 Definition and Classifications

According to RIDDELL (1985), dysplasia is defined as an unequivocal neoplastic alteration in CELLO. SCHMIDT et al. (1985) propose a classification of dysplasia in CELLO similar to that of dysplasia in inflammatory bowel disease. This classification consists of three groups: negative, indefinite and positive for dysplasia. The indefinite group is subdivided into probably negative, unknown and probably positive subgroups. The positive group comprises low grade dysplasia (LGD) and high grade dysplasia (HGD).

CELLO is considered as *negative for dysplasia* when it corresponds to a normal mucosa. Mucosal changes due to inflammatory or regenerative processes are also considered as negative for dypslasia. *Indefinite for*

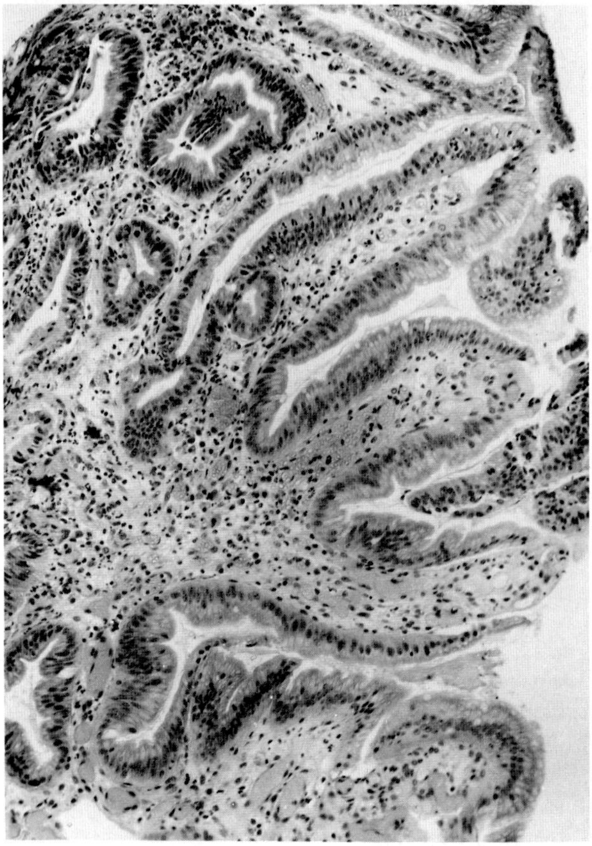

Fig. 5. Low grade dysplasia: enlarged nuclei with crowding and stratification. Compared with Fig. 2, there is a loss of mucin in the cytoplasm of the cells. HE, × 120

dysplasia is the term used to describe the mucosal changes in which it is not possible to decide whether the change is due to inflammation, regeneration or neoplasia. An epithelium which is unequivocally neoplastic is considered as *dysplastic*.

HAMILTON et al. (1987) classified dysplasia in CELLO into three grades: low, intermediate and high, similar to an international classification of gastric dysplasia, although they conceded that the intermediate grade could be included in the HGD category. For most authors, HGD includes also carcinoma in situ or grade 0. SCHMIDT et al. (1985) used two major types of dysplasia, LGD and HGD. In LGD, the nuclei are markedly enlarged, elongated and hyperchromatic with crowding and stratification. However, they are confined to the basal part of the cells. A loss of mucin in the cytoplasm is evident (Fig. 5) and there is mucosal thickening. In HGD, the changes are more severe and the nuclei extend up into the apical parts of the cells with a greater increase in the nuclear-cytoplasmic

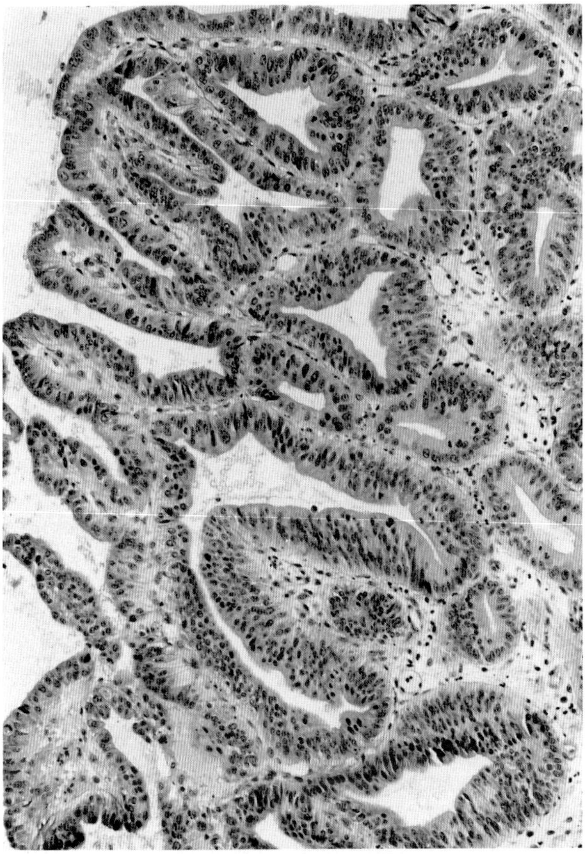

Fig. 6. Adenomatous dysplasia (type 1) high grade: the nuclei extend up into the apical part of the cells. The changes are more severe. The architecture of the glands is disorganised. HE, × 120

ratio (Fig. 6). For each grade of dysplasia, these authors describe two types. Type 1 is indistinguishable from adenomas found elsewhere in the gastrointestinal tract. Type 2 resembles the incomplete maturation described in colonic crypts in inflammatory bowel disease. It is characterised mainly by a lack of cytoplasmic maturation and large basal hyperchromatic nuclei. This latter type may be associated more often with adenocarcinoma in CELLO.

HGD arises from specialised (IM) mucosa in 75%, 93% and 100% of cases according to SCHMIDT et al. (1985), HAMILTON and SMITH (1987) and LEE (1985) respectively.

6.1.2 *Frequency of Dysplasia*

Approximately 10% of CELLO patients without adenocarcinoma develop LGD: 2 out of 38 (SCHMIDT et al. 1985), 3 out of 20 (HERLIHY et al. 1984), and 5 out of 44 in our series. HGD alone without carcinoma is extremely rare, as mentioned above (only one case was found in the preoperative biopsy series of HAMILTON and SMITH 1987). When HGD is present, there is a very high probability of coexistent invasive carcinoma.

6.1.3 *Surveillance of High Grade Dysplasia*

REID et al. (1988) recommend for all patients with CELLO an initial endoscopy with systematic sampling. The biopsy specimens should be obtained at least at 2 cm intervals. If HGD is diagnosed they recommend early re-endoscopy with multiple biopsies to rule out a coexisting adenocarcinoma. If no carcinoma is found at this second endoscopy, they suggest repeat endoscopy and biopsy twice at 3 month intervals and 6 monthly thereafter. They conclude that surveillance of CELLO is necessary and useful to detect adenocarcinoma before the invasive stage.

6.2 Histochemical Studies in CELLO

JASS (1981) showed that mucin histochemistry is helpful in further classifying the specialised columnar epithelium. He found in surgical specimens an incompletely differentiated variant of IM secreting sulphomucins, (type III) associated with well differentiated adenocarcinoma in CELLO. This had been previously recognised in the stomach by other authors. In a prospective study on biopsy material, we studied 38 patients with symptoms of reflux oesophagitis and CELLO. The results showed one case with IM type I, 12 with IM type II and 22 with IM type III (57.9%). Our results as well as those of other studies (LEE 1984; ROTHERY et al. 1986; ZWAS et al. 1986) show a high incidence of type III IM in CELLO. In dysplastic mucosa, histochemical stains for mucins show a decreased cytoplasmic secretion and a predominance of sulphomucins (LEE 1985; SCHMIDT et al. 1985; HAMILTON and SMITH 1987). These findings are consistent with the hypothesis that the patients with CELLO represent a very high risk group for adenocarcinoma of the lower oesophagus.

6.3 Other Lines of Research

6.3.1 Immunohistochemical Study of Mucins in CELLO

In an attempt to study the immunohistochemical profile of CELLO, we have used two antimucus antibodies: anti-LIMA (large intestine mucus antigen) and anti-SIMA (small intestine mucus antigen) generously provided by Dr. Ma (MA et al. 1982). In a preliminary (unpublished) study, we found that anti-LIMA labels the goblet and the intermediate cells in IM II and III while anti-SIMA labels only the goblet cells. Type II and III IM have a similar antigenic profile. The immunohistochemical profile of mucins in CELLO resembles the mucin profile in adenocarcinoma arising in CELLO.

6.3.2 Ornithine Decarboxylase

GAREWALL et al. (1988), found markedly elevated ornithine decarboxylase levels in biopsy specimens from 15 (71%) of 21 patients with CELLO, compared with control tissues.

6.3.3 Fluorescent Lectins

SCHIMAMOTO et al. (1985), using fluorescent lectins, have observed a modification of glycoconjugate expression in CELLO: minor changes were seen in the specialised epithelium, but much more pronounced alterations were observed in high grade dysplastic epithelium and in carcinoma arising on CELLO.

6.3.4 Measurement of Cell Proliferation in CELLO

Only two studies of cell proliferation in CELLO have been published with a method using ^{3}H-thymidine. In the first, HERBST et al. (1978) studied 11 patients, two of them with adenocarcinoma: they did not find important differences between the patients with or without adenocarcinoma. In the second study, PELLISH et al. (1980) found that the number of cells in the proliferative zone was significantly greater in both specialised and junctional type biospies compared with control fundic specimens.

6.3.5 Flow Cytometry in CELLO

Flow cytometry has been used to assess DNA content in CELLO. REID et al. (1987) studied biopsy specimens from 49 patients. Of 34 patients with specialised metaplastic epithelium, "negative for dysplasia", one had a single aneuploid peak of DNA. Of four with mucosa "indefinite for dysplasia", one had an increased G_2/tetraploid fraction. The remaining 11 patients with dysplasia or adenocarcinoma produced aneuploid peaks. These authors interpreted the results as showing that patients with CELLO develop genomic instability within their specialised epithelium, and that flow cytometry could contribute to the precise histological diagnosis of dysplasia or an equivalent of dysplasia. Patients with an aneuploid peak may benefit from more frequent endoscopic surveillance for early detection of adenocarcinomatous change.

Acknowledgment. The authors wish to thank G. Kharsa and W. Bogomoletz for reviewing the manuscript and Mr. Wolfelsperger for preparation of photomicrographs.

References

Allsion, Johnstone AS (1953) The esophagus lined with gastric mucous membrane. Thorax 8:87–101

Barrett NR (1957) The lower esophagus lined by columnar epithelium. Surgery 41:881–895

Belladonna JA, Hajdu SI, Bains MS (1974) Adenocarcinoma in situ of Barrett's esophagus diagnosed by endoscopic cytology. N Engl J Med 291:895–896

Berenson MM, Herbst JJ, Freston JW (1974) Enzyme and ultrastructural characteristics of esophageal columnar epithelium. Am J Dig Dis 19:895–907

Berenson MM, Riddell RH, Skinner DB, Freston JW (1978) Malignant transformation of esophageal columnar epithelium. Cancer 41:554–561

Bozymski EM, Herlihy KJ, Orlando RC (1982) Barrett's esophagus. Ann Intern Med 97:103–107

Buchan AMJ, Grant S, Freeman HJ (1985) Regulatory peptides in Barrett's oesophagus. J Pathol 146:227–234

Cameron AJ, Ott BJ, Payne WS (1985) The incidence of adenocarcinoma in columnar lined (Barrett's) esophagus. N Engl J Med 313:857–859

Garewal HS, Sampliner R, Gerner E, Steinbronn K, Alberts D, Kendall D (1988) Ornithine decarboxylase activity in Barrett's esophagus: a potential marker for dysplasia. Gastroenterolgy 94, 819–821

Haggitt RC, Dean PJ (1985) Adenocarcinoma in Barrett's epithelium. In: Spechler SJ, Goyal RK (eds) Barrett's esophagus, Elsevier, New York, pp 153–166

Haggitt RC, Tryzelaar J, Ellis FM, Colcher H (1978) Adenocarcinoma complicating columnar epithelium lined (Barrett's) esophagus. Am J Clin Pathol 70:1–5

Haggitt RH, Reid BJ, Rabinovitch PS, Rubin CE (1988) Barrett's Esophagus. Correlation between mucin histochemistry, flow cytometry and histologic diagnosis for predicting increased cancer risk. Am J Pathol 131,53–61

Hameeteman W, Tytgat GNJ, Houthoff HJ, Van Den Tweel JG (1989) Barrett's esophagus: development of dysplasia and adenocarcinoma. Gastroenterology 96,1249–1256

Hamilton SR, Smith RRL (1987) The relationship between columnar epithelial dysplasia and invasive adenocarcinoma arising in Barrett's esophagus. Am J Clin Pathol 87:301–312

Hamilton SR, Yardley JA (1977) Regeneration of cardia type mucosa and acquisition of Barrett mucosa after esophagogastrostomy. Gastroenterology 72:669–675

Hamilton SR, Hutcheon DF, Ravich WJ, Paulson M (1984) Adenocarcinoma of Barrett's esophagus after elimination of gastroesophageal reflux. Gastroenterology 86:356–360

Herbst JJ, Berenson MM, MCGloskey DW, Wise WC (1978) Cell proliferation in esophageal columnar epithelium (Barrett's esophagus). Gastroenterology 75:683–687

Herlihy KJ, Orlando RC, Bryson JC, Bozymski EM, Carney CN, Powell DW (1984) Barrett's esophagus: clinical, endoscopic, histologic, manometric and electrical potential difference characteristics. Gastroenterology 86:436–443

Jass JR (1981) Mucin histochemistry of the columnar epithelium of oesophagus: a retrospective study. J Clin Pathol 34:866–870

Kalish RJ, Clancy PE, Orringer MB, Appelman HD (1984) Clinical, epidemiologic, and morphologic comparison between adenocarcinomas arising in Barrett's esophagus and in the gastric cardia. Gastroenterology 86:461–467

Lee RG (1984): Mucins in Barrett's esophagus: a histochemical study. Am J Clin Pathol 81:500–503

Lee RG (1985): Dysplasia in Barrett's esophagus: a clinical pathologic study of six patients. Am J Surg Pathol 9,845–852

Lee RG (1986) Adenomas arising in Barrett's esophagus. Am J Clin Pathol, 85:629–632

Lortat-Jacob JL (1957) L'endobrachyoesophage. Ann Chir 11:1247–1254

Ma J, Deboer W, Nayman J (1982) Intestinal mucinous substances in gastric intestinal metaplasia and carcinoma studied by immunofluorescence. Cancer 49, 1664–1667

McDonald GB, Brand DL, Thorning DR (1977) Multiple adenomatous neoplasms arising in columnar lined (Barrett's) esophagus. Gastroenterology 72:1317–1321

Naef AP, Savary M, Ozello L (1975) Columnar lined lower esophagus: an acquired lesion with malignant predispositon: report on 140 cases of Barrett's esophagus with 12 adenocarcinomas. J Thorac Cardiovasc Surg 70:826–835

Pascal RR, Clearfield HR (1987): Mucoepidermoid (adenosquamous) carcinoma arising in Barrett's esophagus. Dig Dis Sci 32:428–432

Paull A, Trier JS, Dalton MO, Camp RC, Loeb P, Goyal RK (1976): The histological spectrum of Barrett's esophagus. N Engl J Med 295:476–480

Pellish LJ, Hermos JA, Eastwood GL (1980) Cell proliferation in three types of Barrett's epithelium. Gut 21, 26–31

Peuchmaur M, Potet F, Goldfain D (1984) Mucin histochemistry of the columnar epithelium of the oesophagus (Barrett's oesophagus): a prospective study. J Clin Pathol 37:607–610

Pope CE (1985) Regression of Barrett's epithelium. In Spechler SJ, Goyal RK (eds), Barrett's esophagus, Elsevier, New York, pp 224–229

Reid BJ, Haggitt RC, Rubin CE, Rabinovitch PS (1987) Barrett's esophagus. Correlation between flow cytometry and histology in detection of patients at risk for adenocarcinoma. Gastroenterology 93, 1–11

Reid BJ, Weinstein WM, Lewin KJ, Haggitt RC, VanDeventer G, DenBesten L, Rubin CE (1988) Endoscopic biopsy can detect high-grade dysplasia or early adenocarcinoma in Barrett's esophagus without grossly recognizable neoplastic lesions. Gastroenterology 94, 81–90

Riddell RH (1985) Dysplasia and regression in Barrett's epithelium. In Barrett's esophagus, Spechler SJ, Goyal RK (eds) Barrett's esophagus, Elsevier, New York, pp 143–152

Rosenberg JC, Budev H, Edwards RC, Singal S, Steiger Z, Sunderson AS (1985) Analysis of adenocarcinoma in Barrett's esophagus utilizing a staging system. Cancer 55:1353–1360

Rothery GA, Patterson JE, Stoddard CJ, Day DW (1986) Histological and histochemical changes in the columnar lined (Barrett's) oesophagus. Gut 27:1062–1068

Sanfey H, Hamilton SR, Smith RRL, Cameron JL (1985) Carcinoma arising in Barrett's esophagus. Surg Gynecol Obstet 161:570–574

Saubier EC, Gouillat C, Samaniego C, Guillaud M, Moulinier B (1985) Adenocarcinoma in columnar lined Barrett's esophagus. Analysis of 13 esophagectomies. Am J Surg 150:365–369

Schmidt HG, Riddell RH, Walther B, Skinner DB, Riemann JF (1985) Dysplasia in Barrett's esophagus. J Cancer Res Clin Oncol 110, 145–152

Shimamoto C, Weinstein WW, Boland CR (1985) Glyconjugate (GC) expression in metaplastic and dysplastic epithelium in Barrett's esophagus (BE). Gastroenterology 88, 1632 (abstr)

Sjøgren RW Jr, Johnson LF (1983) Barrett's esophagus: a review. Am J Med 74:313–321

Skinner DB, Walther BC, Riddell RH, Schmidt H, Iascone C, De Meester TR (1983) Barrett's esophagus: comparison of benign and malignant cases. Ann Surg 198:554–566

Smith RRL, Hamilton SR, Boitnott JK, Rogers El (1984) The spectrum of carcinoma arising in Barrett's esophagus: a clinicopathologic study of 26 patients. Am J Surg Pathol 8:563–573

Sontag SJ, Schnell TG, Chejfec G, O'Connell S, Stanley MM, Best W, Chintam R, Nemchausky B, Wanner J, Moroni B (1985) Barrett's oesophagus and colonic tumours Lancet I:946–949

Spechler SJ, Goyal RK (1986) Barrett's esophagus. N Engl J Med 315:362–371

Spechler SJ, Robbins AH, Rubins HB, Vincent ME, Heeren T, Doos WG, Colton T, Schimmel EM (1984) Adenocarcinoma and Barrett's esophagus: an overrated risk? Gastroenterology 87:927–933

Sprung DJ, Ellis FH, Gibb SP (1984) Incidence of adenocarcinoma in Barrett's esophagus. Am J Gastroenterol 79, 817 (abstr)

Steinbronn K, Alberts D, Gerner E (1987) Ornithine decarboxylase levels in Barrett's esophagus: correlation with dysplasia. Gastroenterology 92, 1400 (abstr)

Symonds DA, Ramsey ME (1980) Adenocarcinoma arising in Barrett's esophagus with Zollinger syndrome. Am J Clin Pathol 73:823–826

Thompson JJ, Zinsser KR, Enterline HT (1983) Barrett's metaplasia and adenocarcinoma of the esophagus and the gastroesophageal junction. Hum Pathol 14:42–61

Trier JS (1985) Morphology of the columnar cell-lined. (Barrett's) esophagus. In: Spechler SJ Goyal RK (eds) Barrett's esophagus, Elsevier, New York

Van der Veen AH, Dees J, Blankensteijn JD, Van Blankenstein M (1989) Adenocarcinoma in Barrett's oesophagus: an overrated risk. Gut 30, 14–18

Wang HH, Antonioli DA, Goldman H (1986) Comparative features of esophageal and gastric adenocarcinomas: recent changes in type and frequency. Hum Pathol 17:482–487

Winters C, Spurling TJ, Chobanian SJ, Curtis DJ, Esposito RL, Hacker JF, Johnson DA, Cruess DF, Cotelingam JD, Gurney MS, Cattau EL (1987) Barrett's esophagus. A prevalent, occult complication of gastroesophageal reflux disease. Gastroenterology 92:118–124

Witt TR, Bains MS, Zaman MB, Martini N (1983) Adenocarcinoma in Barrett's esophagus. J Thorac Cardiovasc Surg 85, 337–345

Zwas F, Shields HM, Doos WG, Antonioli DA, Goldman H, Ransil BJ, Spechler SJ (1986) Scanning electron microscopy of Barrett's epithelium and its correlation with light microscopy and mucin stains. Gastroenterology 90:1932–1941

B Gastric Dysplasia

P. SIPPONEN

1 Introduction

The correct diagnosis of dysplasia provides an opportunity for the identification and treatment of cancer in an early phase. It also provides the potential to recognise subjects who have a particularly high risk of cancer. Proper identification and management of dysplastic lesions have led to success in population-wide prevention of some common cancers, especially cancer of cervix and, to a lesser extent, cancer of colon and rectum. Less success has been achieved in the diagnosis and treatment of gastric dysplasia.

The histogenesis of gastric cancer is complex and it does not follow well recognised morphological stages as do the major proportion of colonic carcinomas or squamous carcinomas of cervix. The spectrum of the benign lesions in gastric mucosa is wide and manifold. Although some of the lesions, such as intestinal metaplasia and atrophic gastritis are probably related to the pathogenesis of gastric cancer, they are too common to advocate meaningful follow-up or treatment. On the other hand, severe, morphologically clear-cut, dysplastic lesions in the stomach, without a coexisting malignant tumour, are quite rare in everyday practice compared with the frequency of diagnoses of overt gastric cancer. This may suggest that clearly recognisable precancerous dysplastic lesions, as we understand them today, are short-lived, focal and very late phenomena in the morphogenesis of gastric carcinomas, or that the dysplastic lesions in the stomach are poorly recognised and understood. It is also possible that dysplastic alterations are patchy and only occasionally found by current biopsy and endoscopy procedures.

Although the diagnosis of dysplasia must be based on sound morphological criteria and techniques, it is the author's opinion that new ideas and methods in interpretation and identification of dysplastic, precancerous lesions are warranted. A target of these efforts could be the finding of techniques and criteria to identify cases in which the gastric mucosa shows an ongoing process of neoplastic transformation and replication, phenomena of which morphological tumours or advanced dysplastic lesions may be only late focal and patchy reflections. The modern immunochemical and the future molecular biological techniques may offer such opportunities. They may make it possible to identify objectively gene-based aberrations in differentiation and maturation of the epithelium. The pathogenesis of gastric cancer is affected by and dependent upon environmental, exogenous carcinogens and factors that may alter the genome of the cells. These changes must be important in the initiation, promotion and/or modulation of growth of the cancer. It would be logical to assume that the changes in the genome, and subsequently in the cell phenotype, reflect the early, incipient and dysplastic phases of gastric carcinogenesis.

In the present review, the author concentrates on the most recent reports on investigations of cellular alterations in dysplastic epithelium in the stomach. In addition, reference is made to the relatively few available studies in which the clinical value of gastric dysplasia has been investigated in reliable patient series by appropriate follow-up. The reader is advised to consult several earlier papers, reviews and books in which many other viewpoints on the histology and clinical significance of gastric dysplasia are presented and illustrated (NAGAYO 1971; SCHADE 1974; OEHLERT et al. 1975; GRUNDMANN 1975; KAWAI 1974; HEILMANN 1978; MEISTER et al. 1979; CUELLO et al. 1979; MING 1979; JASS 1983).

2 Definitions

Dysplasia is a premalignant lesion (precancerous lesion) which is characterised by abnormal, frequently tumorous growth of dedifferentiated, often immature epithelium and glands. The present understanding of dysplasia implies that it is a lesion in which transformation to neoplasia has occurred or is in progress. It may be considered to be an intraepithelial neoplasia with a particularly high tendency to malignant progression, the risk of which increases with increasing grade of the dysplasia.

Dysplastic lesions show a tendency to progress, although some dysplastic lesions, at least mild ones, may regress or remain stable for long periods. By analogy with the cervical and colorectal neoplasia, it seems reasonable to assume that a dysplasia-carcinoma sequence exists in the morphogenesis of gastric carcinoma, although this hypothesis can be and has been challenged. It is possible that dysplasia and carcinoma arise coincidently from the same cells in the proliferative zone of the neck area of glands, without any precursor lesions for either of them (HATTORI 1986). This view may be held to be supported by observations in experimental models in which benign atrophic, hyperplastic and/or dysplastic lesions arise synchronously with malignant tumours. In spite of this, dysplasia can be considered a marker of an increased risk for cancer.

3 Types and Grading

Wide agreement exists between pathologists in the classification of gastric dysplasia into two main morphogenetic types: intestinal and gastric (foveolar) (MORSON et al. 1980). This division follows the belief that a proportion of gastric carcinomas develop through dedifferentiation in intestinal metaplasia, or at least in close association with this change. In fact, intestinalised epithelium commonly coexists or precedes the intestinal type of cancer. A relationship also seems to exist between non-metaplastic gastric mucosa and the diffuse type of cancer, although cases with an opposite association may also occur.

Grading of dysplasia into three categories (mild, moderate or severe) is suggested by several authors. The grading is arbitrary and subjective. The principle, however, is that the severe grade indicates cases with the most advanced non-invasive dysplastic lesions, including those considered to be borderline lesions and those thought to be lesions of carcinoma in situ. The mild grade might be characterised in practice by cases in which the pathologist is convinced of the dysplastic nature of the lesion but in which difficulties nevertheless exist in its differentiation from simple regeneration, hyperplasia or mature metaplasia.

Histological interpretation and grading of dysplasia of metaplastic type may, in general, follow the principles of dysplasia in colonic adenomas or of dysplasia in ulcerative colitis. A proportion of gastric dysplasias of metaplastic type may indeed exhibit patterns, either elevated or flat, which strikingly resemble colonic adenomas. HERMANEK (1979) has estimated that a small proportion of intestinal-type gastric carcinomas may develop through this adenoma-carcinoma sequence. True adenomatous tumours (polyps) of gastric type also exist, but they are rare.

General guidelines for the interpretation of the dysplasia of gastric type are not widely available. This type of dysplasia appears as an abnormality of epithelial cells in the surface epithelium or in the regenerative zone (OEHLERT 1984). Dysplasia of the gastric type may predispose to gastric carcinoma of the diffuse type which may develop by invasion of the neoplastic mucus-secreting epithelial cells into the lamina propria. However, this phenomenon is also accompanied by changes in the morphological and staining properties of the intracellular mucus granules (see OEHLERT 1984).

4 Criteria

A diagnosis of dysplasia is justified by the presence of changes in architecture, cytology and differentiation of the epithelium and glands. Dysplasia is hardly to be considered if only one or two of the above-mentioned three criteria are present. For example, simple hyperplasia of the surface epithelium or hyperplastic polyps, although they show a distinct abnormality of architecture of the foveolae, exhibit normal differentiation and cytology of the epithelial cells and can hardly be considered dysplastic lesions. Striking atypia of nuclei and a high mitotic rate are features of a regenerative epithelium, as seen in gastritis, ulcer edges, erosions, and in the surface epithelium of the gastric remnant following partial gastrectomy. These lesions, however, show a straight and normal, although sometimes a corkscrew-like, structure of the foveoli, and are non-neoplastic.

A sample of illustration representing both the intestinal and the gastric types of dysplasia is presented in Figs. 1–3.

4.1 Architecture

Irregularity of the crypts, branching, budding and back-to-back formations of the glands, villous, adenomatous or cystic growth patterns of the epithelium, and a net-like anastomosing epithelium are architectural features suggestive of dysplasia. Dysplastic epithelium is characterised by increased cell proliferation (OEHLERT 1984) and by an abnormal upward shift of the proliferative compartment from the neck area of glands (OFFERHAUS et al. 1985). This may result in the formation of large irregular cystic epithelial remnants in the lower parts of the mucosa, a picture that is seen in the early phases of dysplastic growth in particular (FUJITA and HATTORI 1977; RUBIO et al. 1984).

4.2 Cytology

Cytological atypia includes features such as hyperchromasia and nuclear pleomorphism, abnormal staining and structure of the cell cytoplasm, and an increase and variation in the nuclear-cytoplasmic ratio. This cytological anaplasia may be particularly marked in dysplasia of the metaplastic type, less so in dysplasia of the gastric type, and this corresponds to differences in cell morphology between overt intestinal and diffuse types of gastric cancer cells (JOHANSEN 1981). According to a computer-aided morphomet-

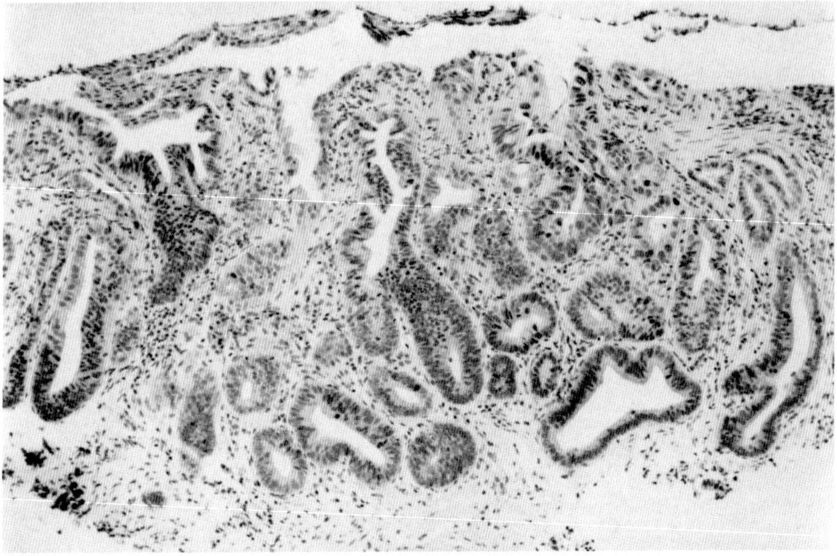

a

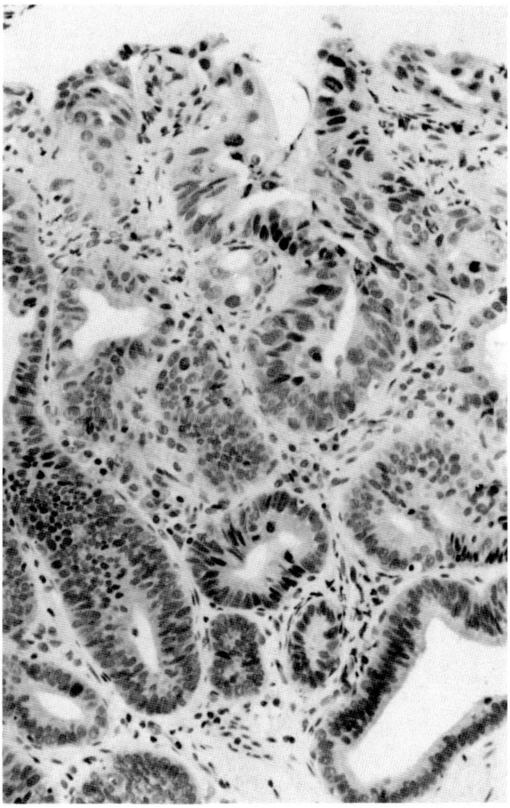

b

Fig. 1 a, b. Severe dysplasia of the intestinal type. **a** A low power view that demonstrates a clear-cut disarranged architecture of the glands (HE, × 150). **b** A high power view showing atypia in the epithelial cells, stratification of nuclei, and high number and abnormal distribution of the mitotic figures within the glands (HE, × 400)

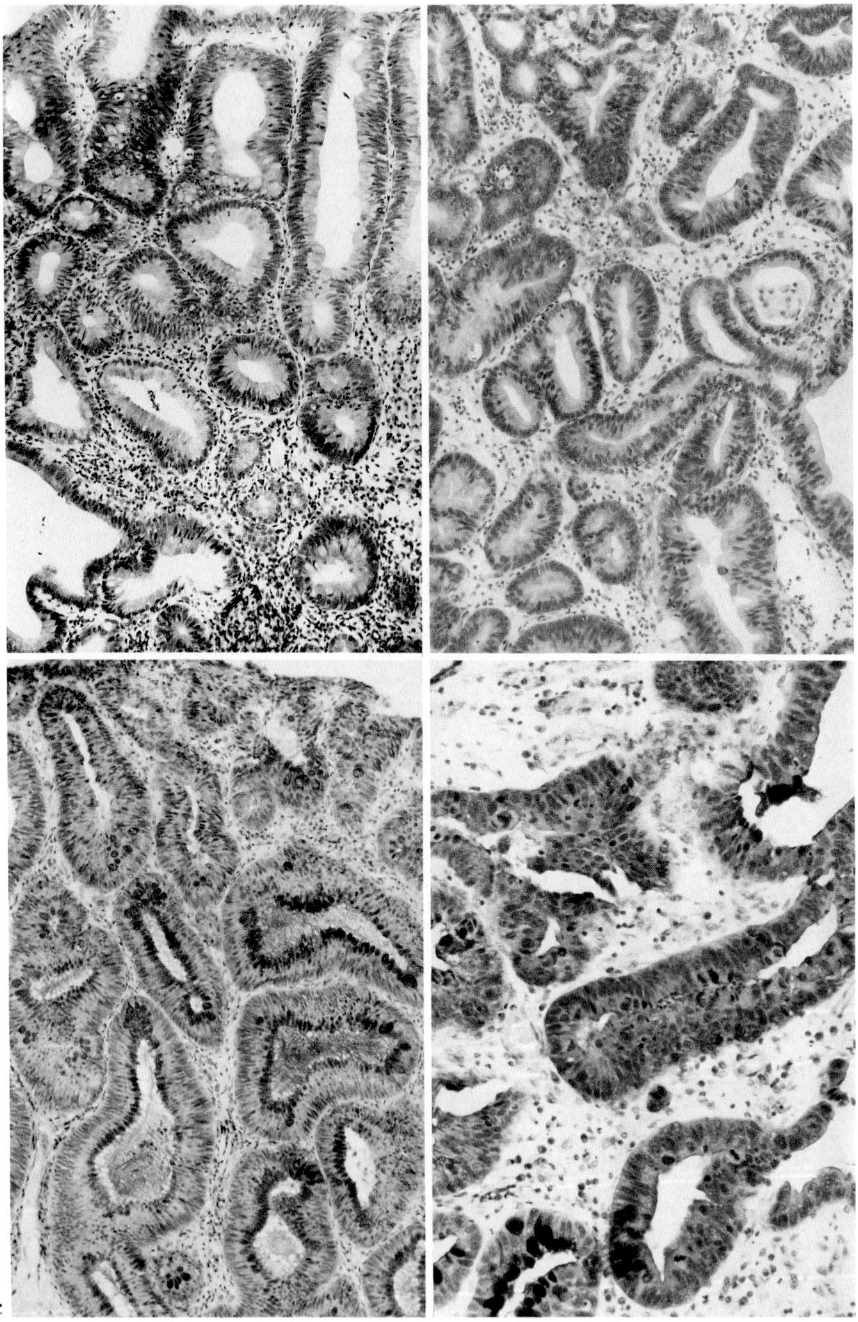

a b c d

Fig. 2a–d. A panel of lesions of dysplasia of the intestinal type. **a** Mild dysplasia with adenoma-like growth patterns (HE, × 250). **b** A dysplastic lesion interpreted as moderate (HE, × 250). **c, d** Dysplasia of severe degree [AB (pH 2.5)-PAS, × 250, × 350]

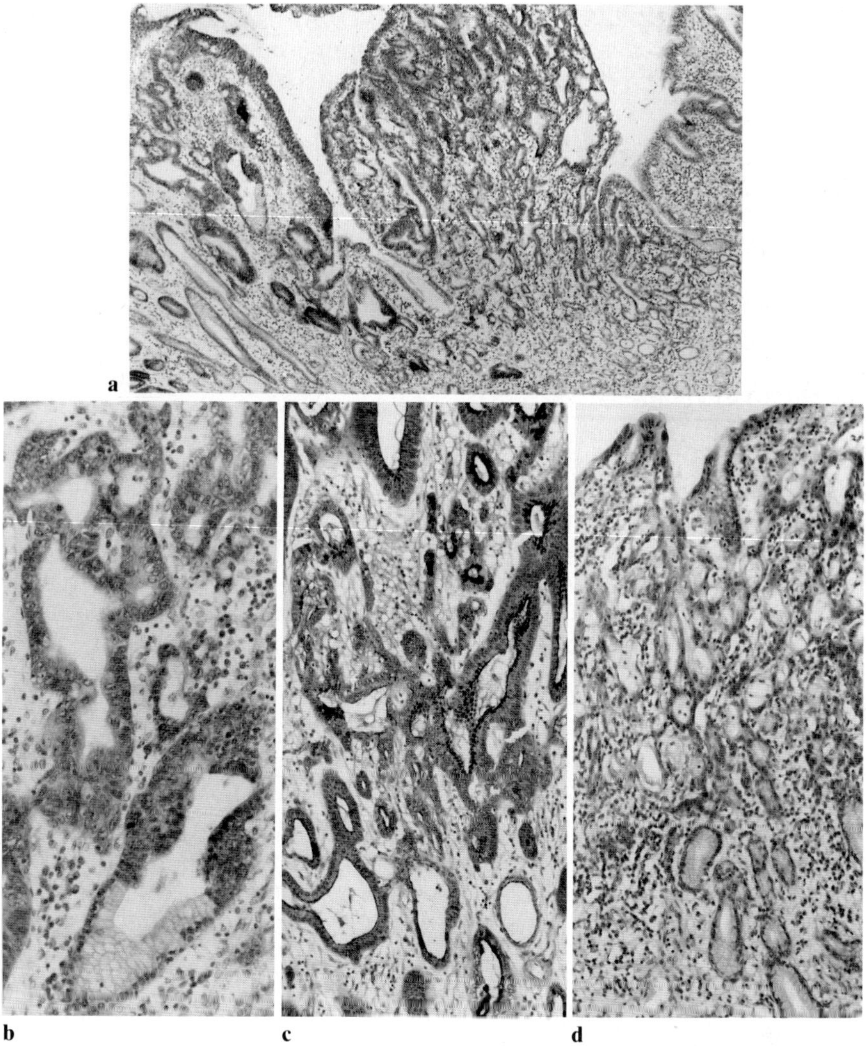

Fig. 3a–d. Severe dysplasia of the gastric type. A high power view of a polypoid lesion (**a**) and three details (**b–d**) of the tumour showing examples of disturbed architecture of the foveolae and of abnormal differentiation of the epithelium (**b**, **c**). A possible early invasion (**d**) of mucus-secreting cells into the lamina propria from the neck area of the glands. [**a**: HE, x 150; **b** and **d**: HE, × 250; **c**: AB (pH 2.5)-PAS, × 250]

ric study by JARVIS and WHITEHEAD (1985), nuclear size was found to be the parameter that best differentiated between dysplastic and benign lesions.

Quantitative analyses of nuclear DNA by cytophotometry have been used with some success in differentiating between benign and malignant or dysplastic cells in the stomach (SPRENGER and WITTE 1980; SZENTIR-

MAY et al. 1986; KORENAGA et al. 1986; MACARTNEY and CAMPLEJOHN 1986). DNA ploidy clearly correlates with chromosomal abnormalities, and an aneuploid pattern of cell nuclear DNA content is considered to reflect increased cancer risk. Unfortunately. however, only a limited proportion (20%–50%) of gastric carcinomas, as with malignant tumours in general, show an aneuploid DNA pattern (BARLOGIE 1984). Some overlap in DNA aneuploidy exists between neoplastic and obviously benign proliferative regeneration (SPRENGER and WITTE 1980), suggesting that analyses on cell DNA patterns are only of limited value as criteria in the diagnosis of gastric dysplasia.

4.3 Differentiation

Depletion and uneven distribution of goblet cells, disappearance of Paneth cells, stratification of the epithelial cells and poor development of the brush border are morphological alterations that indicate the presence of abnormal differentiation in dysplasia of the metaplastic type. Morphological interpretation of abnormal differentiation is more problematic in non-metaplastic epithelium. The diagnosis in these cases can be helped by observations on the synthesis and content of mucin granules in the cells. Loss of mucin granules combined with ultrastructural depletion and abnormality of rough endoplasmic reticulum and disturbance in the polarity or morphology of cell organelles occur both in dysplastic gastric surface epithelium and in overt cancer (RIEMANN et al. 1983).

An abnormal differentiation is regularly accompanied by an expression of unexpected, immature, foetal and/or abnormal antigens in dedifferentiated cells and their secretions (SAKAI et al. 1985, 1986; DENK 1979; FEIZI 1982; COON and WEINSTEIN 1986; KAPADIA et al. 1981; LIPKIN et al. 1985; FISCHER et al. 1984; HIGGINS et al. 1984; WESTERVELD et al. 1986; BLASZCZYK-THURIN et al. 1987; BORCH et al. 1987). This is a consequence of failure in expression or in the structure of the genes. There is, furthermore, a growing list of studies in the literature which show expression and amplification of oncogenes and abnormal gene fragments both in overt cancers (SEKI et al. 1985; FUKUSHIGE et al. 1986; NAKATANI et al. 1986; O'HARA et al. 1986; FERTI-PASSANTONOPOULOU et al. 1987) and in benign metaplastic and dysplastic gastric tissues (NOGUCHI et al. 1986; CICLITIRA et al. 1987; OCHUCHI et al. 1987), suggesting that the expression and amplification of abnormal genes or gene fragments are early fundamental phenomena in the pathogenesis of gastric cancer. Indeed, expression of the *ras* oncogene product p21 has been shown to be a universal phenomenon in gastric cancer tissue in a recent study by CZERNIAK et al. (1987).

Studies of the structure of the oligosaccharide moieties in glycocompounds of secretory mucus in surface epithelial cells could identify abnormal differentiation by using simple histochemical and immunohistochemical methods (see FEIZI 1982). Dedifferentiation of gastric epithelium commonly and typically shows the appearance of immature and unexpected blood group moieties in secretory mucus glycoproteins which may undergo further and inappropriate sialylation or sulphation. The resulting phenotype of the dedifferentiated epithelium may finally exhibit a mixture of expressions that range from mature elements to abnormal embryonal antigens even in the same cell or cell line. It is possible that these alterations are the very early signs of the dysplastic process, i.e., alterations in which the morphological changes of cells and epithelium may yet be slight or even absent. In a recent experiment with four adult dogs, HÄKKINEN et al. (1984) observed that foetal antigens may appear, without changes in microscopic morphology of the cells, in mature gastric surface epithelium within 36 months after a single dose (600 mg) of the carcinogen N-methyl-N'-nitro-N-nitrosoguanidine.

Simple histochemical and immunohistochemical techniques have been used with some practical success in the demonstration of abnormal differentiation in metaplastic gastric epithelium. These efforts follow the simple observation that intestinal metaplasia (IM) in the stomach is not a single entity but may occasionally occur as dedifferentiated forms and exhibit characteristics that are typical of foetal gut or normal colon. By

a 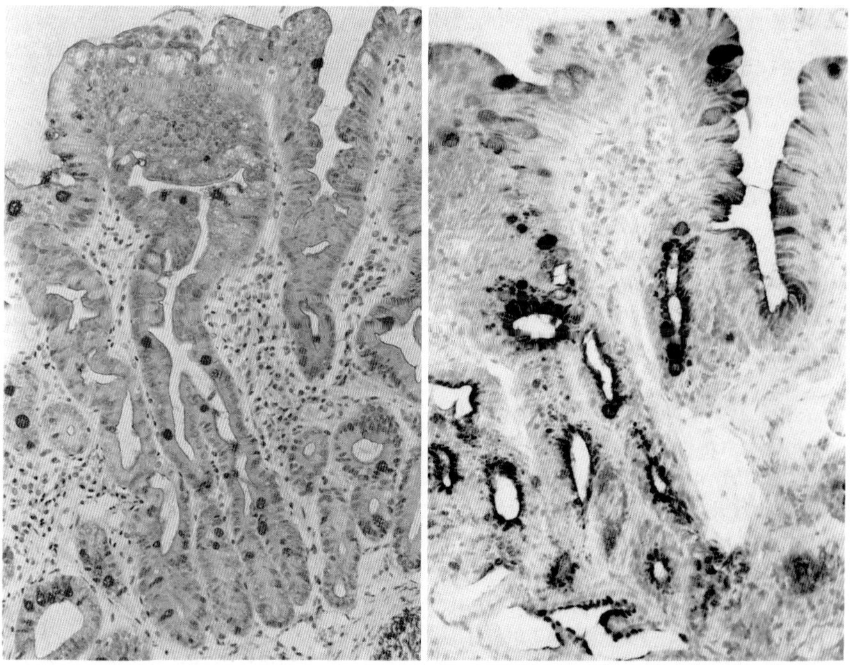 b

Fig. 4 a, b. Intestinal metaplasia of the colonic type. **a** An abnormal metaplastic gland showing sulphomucins in goblet cells, and **b** a metaplastic gland of typical "colonic type" (type III) showing an expression of sulphomucins in both goblet and columnar epithelial cells. (**a** and **b**: × 250; HID)

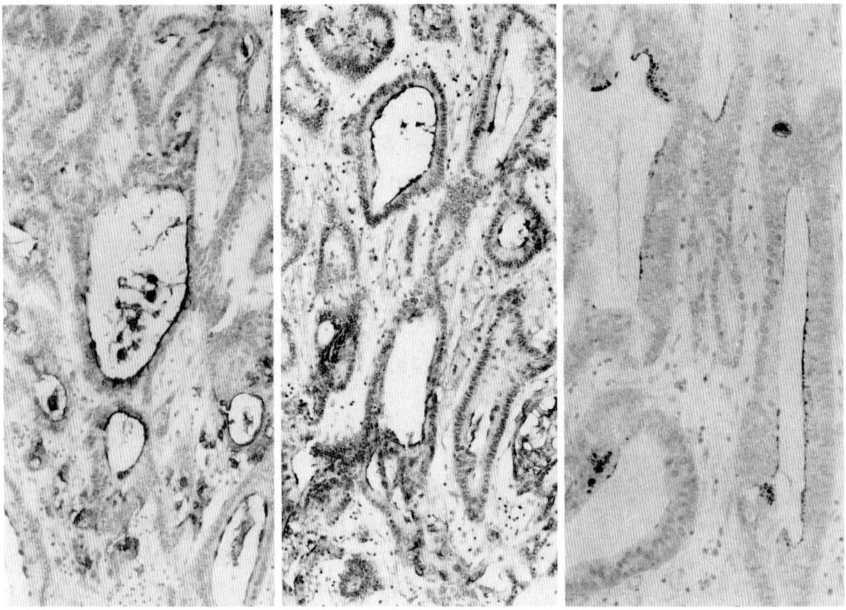

a b c

Fig. 5 a–c. Expression of inappropriate antigenic determinants in dysplasia of gastric type. An expression of the Lewis[a] antigen (**a**), CA 19–9 (sialylated Lewis[a] antigen) (**b**) and sulphomucins (**c**) in dysplastic epithelium of a subject of Lewis[b] genotype (Lewis[b] blood group who expresses Lewis[b] antigen in the non-dysplastic gastric epithelium). Same patient and lesion as in Fig. 3

analogy with the common presence of colon-like characteristics in overt gastric cancer tissue, the presence of such alterations in a non-cancerous stomach may be considered to be an indicator of an increased risk of cancer and a sign of disordered differentiation. A proportion of IMs express structures, mucins and antigens that resemble those of normal colon or foetal intestinal mucosa when examined by morphological, histochemical or immunohistochemical techniques (TEGLBJAERG and NIELSEN 1987; NARDELLI et al. 1983; LEI and YU 1984; KRALOVANSZKY et al. 1984; HIGGINS et al. 1984; TURANI et al. 1986). Histological criteria have been presented for such metaplasias of the immature or colonic type (incomplete sulphomucin-secreting IM; type III; see FILIPE et al. 1985; FILIPE and JASS 1986); they are characterised by a mixed growth of metaplastic goblet and columnar cells, both of which synthesise and secrete sulphomucins and other colon-like or embryonic glycoproteins. These lesions may be considered dysplastic (JASS et al. 1984), although their value in predicting gastric cancer risk in the short term might be low (ECTORS and DIXON 1986; RAMESAR et al. 1987). However, IM of colonic type occurs in 9,8% of all biopsies with IM, and it is more common (35%) in gastric cancer cases than in benign conditions (7%) (FILIPE et al. 1985; ROTHERY and DAY 1985). Moreover, it is more common than expected in precancerous conditions and in lesions that are considered dysplastic on pure morphological criteria (SIPPONEN et al. 1980; PAGNINI et al. 1983). An example of IM of the colonic type is presented in Fig. 4.

Although the intestinal and gastric types of gastric dysplasia have morphological characteristics of their own, similar patterns of abnormal antigen and mucin expressions may occur in both. None of the known tumour or embryonic markers or histochemical mucin patterns has been found to be limited solely to one of the dysplasia types. Colon-like histochemical properties, which are particularly common in dysplasia of the intestinal type, may also occur in dysplasia of the gastric type. Correspondingly, cancer cells in diffuse type tumours frequently exhibit sulphated, colon-like mucosubstances. An example of the coexisting presence of several in appropriate antigens in the same dysplastic lesion of gastric type is presented in Fig. 5.

5 Clinical Significance

The available published studies on the prevalence of dysplasia are few and report divergent results. All are based on series of symptomatic subjects, and our knowledge of the occurrence of dysplasia in the general population is scanty. Furthermore, very few of the available investigations are prospective and include follow-up data. A short synopsis of studies made in the last few years is presented in Table 1. At least some important general conclusions can be drawn:

1. Severe dysplasia is of high predictive value for gastric cancer, and it represents a short-lived, late phase in the process of gastric carcinogenesis. In fact, a high proportion of severe dysplasia cases either have a coexisting carcinoma or develop one within the next few months.
2. Dysplastic lesions seem to progress in severity. There is evidence that mild dysplasia may progress to more severe grades, suggesting that gastric dysplasia is a stepwise and time-related process.
3. Dysplastic lesions have a strong anatomical relationship to cancer, suggesting that dysplasia can be a precursor lesion of gastric cancer, and that at least a proportion of cancers develop by way of a dysplasia-cancer sequence.
4. Dysplasia does not seem to exist in the normal, non-gastritic stomach but arises in patient groups with a diseased gastric mucosa. In the study of 31 dysplasia patients without a coexisting cancer (SERCK-HANSSEN et al. 1984), an underlying gastritis was present in 16 patients, adenomatous polyps in ten patients and a benign ulcer in five patients. Correspondingly, the accumulation of dysplastic lesions in patient groups with chronic atrophic gastritis, ulcers or post-gastrectomy rem-

Table 1. Studies on the prevalence of dysplasia

Author(s)	Design of the study	Main results
ASTE et al. 1986	Endoscopic biopsy study of 694 patients with ulcer, polyp, fold or tumour	29 (4%) had moderate or severe dysplasia, of whom 8 (28%) had a coexisting gastric cancer. No further cancers were found in the short-term follow-up
STOCKBRUGGER et al. 1983	Endoscopic cross-section study of 80 patients with pernicious anaemia	Mild, moderate or severe dysplasia in 24, 6 and 3 patients, respectively. Carcinoma in one patient
NAGAYO 1986	Prospective study of over 16000 resection specimens	55 patients had severe dysplasia without coexisting ulcer or gastric cancer. Severe dysplasia outside the tumour area in 109 out of 5642 patients with carcinoma
GRAEM et al. 1984	Prospective endoscopic follow-up of patients with post-gastrectomy remnant	30% prevalence of dysplasia 22–30 years after the resection
ZHANG 1984	Prospective biopsy series of endoscoped and biopsied out-patients and patients with gastric cancer	Severe dysplasia in 42 out of 3272 endoscoped out-patients. Severe dysplasia in 41 out of 572 patients with gastric cancer
SERCK-HANSSEN et al. 1984	Prospective endoscopic biopsy material of 3921 specimens	Dysplasia (all grades) in 1.8% of the specimens. Severe dysplasia in 40 patients, of whom 22 had a coexisting gastric cancer or developed cancer within the next 3–60 months
CAMILLERI et al. 1984	Prospective endoscopic biopsy material from 12394 patients. Follow-up data for some patients	Moderate dysplasia in 430 patients, severe dysplasia in 34 patients. Among patients with severe dysplasia, gastric cancer was found within 2 years of the diagnosis in 6 patients. Dysplasia regressed in some patients
OFFERHAUS et al. 1984	Endoscopic biopsy screening of 504 patients with post-gastrectomy remnant	Dysplasia in 70 (14%) patients. Severe dysplasia in 5 patients. Three patients with severe dysplasia developed gastric cancer within the next 4 years. No progression in 22 mild or moderate dysplasias followed-up

nant is emphasised by the studies of ZHANG (1984) and CAMILLERI et al. (1984). Indeed, these observations suggest that precancerous conditions, such as atrophic gastritis or the post-gastrectomy remnant, are precursor states of gastric dysplasia. A practical consequence is that dysplastic lesions should be sought particularly in patients who have such gastric diseases or precancerous conditions. Correspondingly, dysplasia is highly improbable and rare in subjects with an endoscopically and histologically normal stomach.

The above conclusions suggest that the recognition of severe dysplasia demands consideration of surgical intervention or at least a careful endoscopic follow-up at intervals of a few months. Data on the prognostic value of mild or moderate dysplasia are, however, more controversial or uncertain (ANDERSSON et al. 1987). These lesions may regress and, in addition, their progression to higher grades and overt cancer is apparently very slow and may take several years or decades (FUJITA 1978; MORTENSEN et al. 1984). However, the cumulative risk of gastric cancer in such patients may also be increased, particularly if the subject is young and has a long life expectancy.

6 Summary

The morphological diagnosis of gastric dysplasia is based on the presence of changes in the architecture, cytology and differentiation of the epithelium and mucosal glands. Two morphological types exist: gastric (foveolar) and metaplastic. Definite morphological criteria for gastric dysplasias can be presented. The present morphological grading of dysplasia into mild, moderate or severe is, however, arbitrary and subjective. The available investigations show that dysplasia and overt carcinoma have several biological and epidemiological links that indicate that a dysplasia-cancer sequence operates in the pathogenesis of at least a proportion of gastric carcinomas. The data available in the literature strongly indicate that severe dysplasia is highly predictive for coexisting or shortly appearing carcinoma. The literature on the clinical significance of dysplasia of mild or moderate grade, however, is as yet scanty and inconsistent.

References

Andersson AP, Lauritsen KB, West F, Johansen A (1987) Dysplasia in gastric mucosa: prognostic significance. Acta Chir Scand 153:29–31

Aste H, Sciallero S, Pugliese V, Gennaro M (1986) The clinical significance of gastric epithelial dysplasia. Endoscopy 18:174–176

Barlogie B (1984) Abnormal cellular DNA content as a marker of neoplasia. Eur J Cancer Clin Oncol 20:1123–1125

Blaszczyk-Thurin M, Thurin J, Hindsgaul O, Karlsson KA, Steplewski Z, Koprowski H (1987) Y and blood group B type 2 glycolipid antigens accumulate in a human gastric carcinoma

cell line as detected by monoclonal antibody. Isolation and characterization by mass spectrometry and NMR spectroscopy. J Biol Chem 262:372–279
Borch K, Renvall H, Lundin C, Wahren B (1987) Evaluation of gastric carcinoembryonic antigen analysis as an aid during screening for gastric neoplasia in atrophic gastritis. Gut 28:26–32
Camilleri JP, Potet F, Amat C, Molas G (1984) Gastric mucosal dysplasia: preliminary results of a prospective study of patients followed for periods of up to six years. In: Ming S-C (ed) Precursors of gastric cancer. Praeger, New York, pp 83–92
Ciclitira PJ, Macartney JC, Evan G (1987) Expression of c-myc in non-malignant and premalignant gastrointestinal disorders. J Pathol 151:293–296
Coon JS, Weinstein RS (1986) Blood group-related antigens as markers of malignant potential and heterogeneity in human carcinomas. Hum Pathol 17:1089–1106
Correa P (1985) Mechanisms of gastric carcinogenesis. Int Congr Ser 685:109–115
Cuello C, Correa P, Zarama G, Lopez J, Murray J, Gordillo G (1979) Histopathology of gastric dysplasia: correlations with gastric juice histochemistry. Am J Surg Pathol 3:491–500
Czerniak B, Herz F, Koss LG, Schlom J (1987) *Ras* oncogene p21 as a tumor marker in the cytodiagnosis of gastric and colonic carcinomas. Cancer 60:2432–2436
Denk H, (1979) Blood group antigens and carcinoembryonic antigen in gastric cancer. In: Pfeiffer CJ (ed) Gastric cancer. Gerhard Witzstrock, New York, pp 191–208
Ectors N, Dixon MF (1986) The prognostic value of sulphomucin positive intestinal metaplasia in the development of gastric cancer. Histopathology 10:1271–1277
Feizi T (1982) Blood group antigens and gastric cancer. Med Biol 60:7–11
Ferti-Passantonopoulou AD, Panani AD, Vlachos JD, Paptis SA (1987) Common cytogenetic findings in gastric cancer. Cancer Genet Cytogenet 24:63–73
Filipe MI, Jass JR (1986) Intestinal metaplasia subtypes and cancer risk. In: Filipe MI, Jass JR (eds) Gastric cancer. Churchill Livingstone, Edinburgh, pp 87–115
Filipe MI, Potet F, Bogomoletz WV et al. (1985) Incomplete sulphomucin-secreting intestinal metaplasia for gastric cancer. Preliminary data from a prospective study from three centres. Gut 26:1319–1326
Fischer J, Klein PJ, Vierbuchen M, Skutta B, Uhlenbruck G, Fischer R (1984) Characterization of glycoconjugates of human gastrointestinal mucosa by lectins. I. Histochemical distribution of lectin binding sites in normal alimentary tract as well as in benign and malignant gastric neoplasms. J Histochem Cytochem 32:681–689
Fujita S (1978) Biology of early gastric carcinoma. Path Res Pract 163:297–309
Fujita S, Hattori T (1977) Cell proliferation, and migration in the gastric mucosa: a study on the background of carcinogenesis. In: Farber E (ed) Pathophysiology of carcinogenesis in digestive organs. University of Tokyo Press, Tokyo/University Park Press, Baltimore, pp 21–36
Fukushige S, Matsubara K, Yoshida M et al. (1986) Localization of a novel v-erb-related gene, c-erb-2, on human chromosome 17 and its amplification in a gastric cancer cell line. Mol Cell Biol 6:955–958
Graem N, Fischer AB, Beck H (1984) Dysplasia and carcinoma in Billroth II resected stomach 27–35 years postoperatively. Acta Pathol Microbiol Immunol Scand [A] 92:185–188
Grundmann E (1975) Histologic types and possible initial stages in early gastric carcinoma. Beitr Pathol 154:256–280
Häkkinen IP, Heinonen R, Isberg U, Järvi OH (1984) Canine gastric glycoprotein antigens in early carcinogenesis. Cancer 53:928–934
Hattori T (1986) Development of adenocarcinomas in the stomach. Cancer 57:1528–1534
Heilmann KL (1978) Gastritis-Intestinale Metaplasie-Karzinom. Thieme, Stuttgart
Hermanek P (1979) Gastric polyps and gastric carcinoma. In: Herfarth C, Schlag P (eds) Gastrin cancer. Springer, Berlin Heidelberg New York, pp 147–148
Higgins PJ, Correa P, Cuello C, Lipkin M (1984) Fetal antigens in the precursor stages of gastric cancer. Oncology 41:73–76
Jarvis LR, Whitehead R (1985) Morphometric analysis of gastric dysplasia. Pathol 147:133–138
Jass JR (1983) A classification of gastric dysplasia. Histopathology 7:181–193

Jass JR, Strudley I, Falady J (1984) Histochemistry of epithelial metaplasia and dysplasia in human stomach and colorectum. Scand J Gastroenterol 104:109–130

Johansen AB (1981) Early gastric cancer. A contribution to the pathology and to gastric cancer histogenesis. Bispebjerg Hospital, Copenhagen

Kapadia A, Feizi T, Jewell D, Keeling J, Slavin G (1981) Immunocytochemical studies of blood group A, H, I and i antigens in gastric mucosa of infants with normal gastric histology and of patients with gastric carcinoma and chronic peptic ulceration. J Clin Pathol 34:320–337

Kawai K (1974) Doubtful cases and precancerous lesions. In: Grundmann E, Gruntze H, Witte S (eds) Early gastric cancer. Springer, Berlin Heidelberg New York, pp 177–179

Korenaga D, Mori M, Okamura T, Sugimachi K, Enjoji M (1986) DNA ploidy in clinical malignant gastric lesions less than 5 mm in diameter. Cancer 58:2542–2545

Kralovanszky J, Szentirmay Z, Besznyak I, Eckhardt S (1984) Placental type alkaline phosphatase in possibly premalignant alterations of human gastric mucosa. Oncology 41:189–194

Lei DN, Yu JY (1984) Types of intestinal metaplasia in relation to the histogenesis of gastric carcinoma. Arch Pathol Lab Med 108:220–224

Lipkin M, Correa P, Mikol VB et al. (1985) Proliferative and antigenic modifications in human epithelial cells in chronic atrophic gastritis J Natl Cancer Inst 75:613–619

Macartney JC, Camplejohn RS (1986) DNA flow cytometry of histological material from dysplastic lesions of human gastric mucosa. J Pathol 150:113–118

Meister H, Holubarsch CH, Haferkamp O, Schlag P, Herfarth C (1979) Gastritis, intestinal metaplasia and dysplasia versus benign ulcer in stomach and duodenum and gastric carcinoma. A histotopographic study. Path Res Pract 164:259–269

Ming S-C (1979) Dysplasia of gastric epithelium. Front Gastrointest Res 4:164–172

Morson BC, Sobin LH, Grundmann E, Johansen A, Nagayo T, Serck-Hanssen A (1980) Precancerous conditions and epithelial dysplasia in stomach. J Clin Pathol 33:711–721

Mortensen NJ, Thomas WE, Jones SM, Savage A (1984) Endoscopic screening for premalignant changes 25 years after gastrectomy: results of a five-year prospective study. Br J Surg 71:363–367

Nagayo T, (1971) Histological diagnosis of biopsied gastric mucosae with special reference to that of borderline lesions. Gann Monogr 11:245–256

Nagayo T (1986) Histopathology of gastric dysplasia. In: Filipe MI, Jass JR (eds) Gastric cancer. Churchill Livingstone, Edinburgh, pp 116–131

Nakatani H, Tahara E, Yoshida T et al. (1986) Detection of amplified DNA sequences in gastric cancers by a DNA renaturation method in gel. Jpn J Cancer Res 77:849–853

Nardelli J, Bara J, Rosa B, Burtin P (1983) Intestinal metaplasia and carcinomas of the human stomach. An immunohistological study. J Histochem Cytochem 31:366–375

Noguchi M, Hirohashi S, Shimosato Y et al. (1986) Histologic demonstration of antigens reactive with anti P21 Ras monoclonal antibody (Rap-5) in human stomach cancers. J Natl Cancer Inst 77:379–385

Ochuchi N, Thor A, Nose M, Fukita J, Kyogoku M, Schlom J (1986) Tumor-associated glycoprotein (TAG-72) detected in adenocarcinomas and benign of the stomach. Int J Cancer 38:643–650

Ochuchi N, Hand PH, Merlo G et al. (1987) Enhanced expression of c-Ha-ras p21 in human stomach adenocarcinomas defined by immunoassays using monoclonal antibodies and in situ hybridization. Cancer Res 47:1413–1420

Oehlert W (1984) Preneoplastic lesions of the stomach. In: Ming S-C (ed) Precursors of gastric cancer. Praeger, New York, pp 73–82

Oehlert W, Keller P, Henke M, Strauch M (1975) Dysplasien der Magenschleimhaut. Dtsch Med Wochenschr 100:1950–1956

Offerhaus GJ, Huibregtse K, de Baer J, Verhoeven T, van Olffen GH, van de Stadt J, Tytgat GN (1984) The operated stomach: a premalignant condition? A prospective follow-up study. Scand J Gastronenterol 19:521–524

Offerhaus GJ, van de Stadt J, Samson G, Tytgat GN (1985) Cell proliferation kinetics in the gastric remnant. Eur J Cancer Clin Oncol 21:73–79

O'Hara BM, Oskarsson M, Tainsky MA, Blair DG (1986) Mechanisms of activation of human Ras genes cloned from a gastric adenocarcinoma and a pancreatic carcinoma cell line. Cancer Res 46:4695–4700

Pagnini CA, Farini R, Cardin F, Di Mario F, Rugge M, Naccarato R (1983) Gastric epithelial dysplasia and sulphomucin-type intestinal metaplasia. Tumori 69:355–357

Ramesar KCRB, Sanders DSA, Hopwood D (1987) Limited value of type III intestinal metaplasia in predicting risk of gastric carcinoma. J Clin Pathol 40:1287–1290

Riemann JF, Schmidt H, Hermanek P (1983) On the ultrastructure of the gastric "borderline lesion". J Cancer Res Clin Oncol 105:285–291

Rothery GA, Day DW (1985) Intestinal metaplasia in endoscopic biopsy specimens of gastric mucosa. J Clin Pathol 38:613–621

Rubio CA, Kato Y, Sugano H (1984) The intramucosal cysts of the stomach. VI. Their quantitative and qualitative characteristics in focal (elevated) neoplastic lesions. Path Res Pract 179:105–109

Sakai K, Mori S, Mori T, Kobori O, Morioka Y, Kano K (1985) Anomalous expression of HLA antigens in gastric cancer. Jpn J Cancer Res 30:162

Sakai K, Mori S, Kawamoto T et al. (1986) Expression of epidermal growth factor receptors on normal human gastric epithelia and gastric carcinomas. J Natl Cancer Inst 77:1047–1052

Schade ROK (1974) The borderline between benign and malignant lesions in the stomach. In: Grundmann E, Gruntze H, Witte S (eds) Early gastric cancer. Springer, Berlin, Heidelberg, New York, pp 45–53

Seki T, Fujii G, Mori S, Tamaoki N, Shibuya M (1985) Amplification of c-yes-1 proto-oncogene in a primary human gastric cancer. Jpn J Cancer Res 76:907–910

Serck-Hanssen A, Osnes M, Myren J (1984) Epithelial dysplasia in the stomach: the size of the problem and some preliminary results of a follow-up study. In: Ming S-C (ed) Precursors of gastric cancer. Praeger, New York, pp 53–71

Sipponen P, Seppälä K, Varis K, Hjelt L, Siurala M (1980) Intestinal metaplasia with colonic type sulphomucins in the gastric mucosa. Its association with gastric carcinoma. Acta Pathol Microbiol Scand [A]88:217–221

Sprenger E, Witte S (1980) The diagnostic significance of flow cytometric nuclear DNA measurement in gastroscopic diagnosis of the stomach. Path Res Pract 169:269–275

Stockbrugger RW, Menon GG, Beilby JO, Mason RR, Cotton PB (1983) Gastroscopic screening in 80 patients with pernicious anaemia. Gut 24:1141–1147

Szentirmay Z, Csuka O, Sugar J (1986) DNA and enzyme histochemistry of dysplasia and gastric cancer. In: Filipe MI; Jass JR (eds) Gastric cancer. Churchill Livingstone, Edinburgh, pp 68–86

Teglbjaerg PS, Nielsen HO (1978) "Small intestinal type" and "colonic type" intestinal metaplasia of the human stomach, and their relationship to the histogenetic types of gastric adenocarcinoma. Acta Pathol Microbiol Scand [A]86:351–355

Turani H, Lurie B, Chaimoff C, Kessler E (1986) The diagnostic significance of sulfated acid mucin content in gastric intestinal metaplasia with early gastric cancer. Am J Gastroenterol 81:343–345

Westerveld BD, Pals G, Defize J et al. (1986) Pepsinogen A polymorphism in gastric mucosa and urine, with special reference to patients with gastric cancer. Clin Genet 30:202–212

Zhang Y (1984) Epithelial dysplasia of the stomach and its relationship with gastric cancer. In: Ming S–C (ed) Precursors of gastric cancer. Praeger, New York, pp 41–52

C Duodenal and Peri-ampullary Adenomas

A. H. QIZILBASH

1 Introduction

Neoplasms of the small intestine are uncommon, representing approximately 1.5% of all gastrointestinal tumours (HANCOCK 1970). Most reports (WILSON et al. 1974; PERZIN and BRIDGE 1981) list adenocarcinoma as the commonest tumour. In one study (WILSON et al. 1974) 46% of the malignant small intestinal tumours were adenocarcinomas, 33% carcinoid tumours and 20% sarcomas. Although some authors (HANCOCK 1970) regard leiomyoma as the most frequent benign tumour, others (PERZIN and BRIDGE 1981) have found adenomas to be more common. In the latter report, 51 of the 196 benign small intestinal tumours were adenomas. There were 43 leiomyomas, 35 lipomas, 22 Brunner's gland adenoma, 21 lymphangiomas, 14 vascular tumours and 10 fibromas.

Adenomas are more frequent in the duodenum, especially at the papilla, and decrease in frequency in the jejunum and ileum. GOLDEN published the first case of villous adenoma of the duodenum (GOLDEN 1928), although PERRY in 1893 is credited with previously describing a broad-based cauliflower-like tumour in the duodenum as a papilloma (SCHULTEN et al. 1976). Approximately 85 well documented cases have been reported (COOPERMAN et al. 1978; EVERETT et al. 1981; HAUBRICH et al. 1973; KOMOROWSKI and COHEN 1981; PERZIN and BRIDGE 1981;

REDDY et al. 1981; RYAN et al. 1986; SCHULTEN et al. 1976; SPIRA and WOLFF 1977; UPPAPUTHANGKULE et al. 1976; WEISS and SEMERDJIAN 1986). Although most of the published reports refer to villous adenomas, tubular or non-villous lesions also occur and probably are more frequent. In one review (PERZIN and BRIDGE 1981) of 51 adenomas of the small intestine, 31 were reported as adenomas (adenomatous polyps or tubular adenomas) and 20 as papillary (villous) adenomas.

Peri-ampullary neoplasms include lesions arising in the ampulla of Vater, terminal panceratic duct and distal common bile duct and tumours arising from the duodenal mucosa adjacent to the ampulla. Separation of duodenal from peri-ampullary tumours is at times very difficult, especially in large lesions. The terminology used in the literature in describing lesions involving the ampulla is confusing. Terms used to describe benign tumours include polyps, adenomatoid hyperplasia, hamartomatous polyps, adenomyosis, adenomyoma, papilloma, adenoma and villous adenoma. Adenomatoid hyperplasia, hamartomatous polyps, adenomyosis and adenomyoma are terms used for specific non-neoplastic lesions. These have been reviewed elsewhere (QIZILBASH 1984) and will not be discussed here. The term polyp refers to any polypoid lesion which projects into the lumen of the duodenum. The lesion may be inflammatory, hyperplastic, hamartomatous or neoplastic and its use without further description is meaningless. Papilloma probably refers to polypoid adenoma and its use should be discouraged. Neoplastic polyps are best referred to as adenomas. CALZAVARA, in 1895, is credited with describing the first case of ampullary papilloma (SOBOL and COOPERMAN 1978). In 1965, OH and JEMERIN, reviewed the literature and collected 48 well documented examples under the term of adenomatous polyps of the papilla of Vater. Some of the illustrations and references included in this report represent villous adenomas. In 1981, PERZIN and BRIDGE reported 28 examples of adenomas involving the ampulla. Fourteen were examples of tubular and 14 villous adenomas. Thirty additional examples of villous adenoma of the ampulla of Vater have recently been reported (HASLETON et al. 1980; LEESE et al. 1986); DUPAS et al. 1977; OHMORI et al. 1976; ROSENBERG et al. 1986; RYAN et al. 1986; SOBOL and COOPERMAN 1978; STARLING and TURNER 1982; TAXIER et al. 1979).

A recent report (WARSHAW et al. 1987) documents an unusual case of villous adenoma of the duct of Wirsung in a 65-year-old man. The common bile duct and ampulla of Vater were not involved. The tumour could not be visualised at endoscopy and was revealed by a pancreatogram as a small rounded defect in the proximal pancreatic duct. At surgery a 1.0-cm villous adenoma attached to the pancreatic duct by a short stalk was excised via the transduodenal approach.

Duodenal adenomas are common in familial polyposis syndromes, and will not be discussed here. The polyposis syndromes are discussed on pp 323.

2 Classification

Adenomas of the small intestine have the same gross and histological features as their counterparts in the colorectum and are categorized into one of the following two subtypes: (a) tubular and (b) villous adenomas. Lesions with a mixture of glands and villous processes are classified according to the predominant pattern.

Since the normal small bowel mucosa has a villous pattern, adenomas arising in this site tend to be villous in comparison with adenomas which arise in the colorectum, where the predominant pattern is tubular. PERZIN and BRIDGE (1981) suggest that this is the result of lateral growth of the adenomatous epithelium along pre-existing small bowel villi with replacement of normal lining cells by the neoplastic epithelium.

3 Clinical Features

The patients range in age from 30 to 90 years, with the peak in the seventh decade. The sexes are equally affected. The signs and symptoms depend upon the location and type of the lesion.

3.1 Tubular Adenomas

In the duodenum, tubular adenomas generally present as asymptomatic lesions although larger lesions may be associated with abdominal pain and occult bleeding. There are no specific radiological or endoscopic appearances although small filling defects with or without a pedicle may give a clue to the diagnosis. At endoscopy the lesions appear as sessile or pedunculated tumours with a smooth or lobulated surface. The tumours are usually solitary, although multiple adenomas have been reported (PERZIN and BRIDGE 1981). Tubular adenomas tend to be small, varying from 0.5 to 3 cm in diameter. Larger tumours may be associated with ulceration and obstruction. Carcinoma is liable to develop in larger lesions.

In the ampulla of Vater and peri-ampullary region, tubular adenomas produce symptoms early, despite their small size. Jaundice, biliary colic, cholangitis, epigastric pain and bleeding are common. At endoscopy the tumour appears as a fleshy soft pink lesion filling the orifice of the papilla or projecting into the lumen of the duodenum. Endoscopic retrograde cholangiopancreatography (ERCP) and percutaneous transhepatic cholangiography are valuable in demonstrating the site of obstruction. Ultrasound and computed tomograms also play an important role in the diagnosis.

3.2 Villous Adenomas

Unlike tubular adenomas, villous tumours tend to be symptomatic and larger at the time of diagnosis. Symptoms include abdominal pain, gastrointestinal bleeding, intestinal obstruction, intussusception, jaundice and pancreatitis. In some patients the symptoms are vague and non-specific. Mucorrhoea and electrolyte loss are uncommon in villous adenomas of the duodenum. A recent report (WEISS and SEMERDJIAN 1986) documents mucoid diarrhoea in an 82-year-old woman with villous adenoma of the duodenum. After surgical excision of the tumour the diarrhoea stopped but recurred 6.5 years later. Endoscopic and radiographic examinations confirmed a large recurrent villous tumour in the duodenum. Following polypectomy, the diarrhoea promptly ceased, suggesting a cause and effect.

Barium X-ray studies of villous adenomas usually reveal a characteristic "soap bubble" appearance, although a correct preoperative diagnosis is made only in one-third of the cases (SCHULTEN et al. 1976). Endoscopy is diagnostic in most cases and very valuable in diagnosing smaller lesions that escape detection by barium studies. At endoscopy most of the lesions present as sessile multilobulated, soft tumours. Villous adenomas are usually solitary, although multiple tumours have been reported (COOPERMAN et al. 1978; HASLETON et al. 1980). Villous adenomas are usually larger than tubular adenomas and may attain a size of 8 cm or more, the average being 5 cm. (SCHULTEN et al. 1976). Carcinomas appear to develop more frequently in villous than in tubular adenomas.

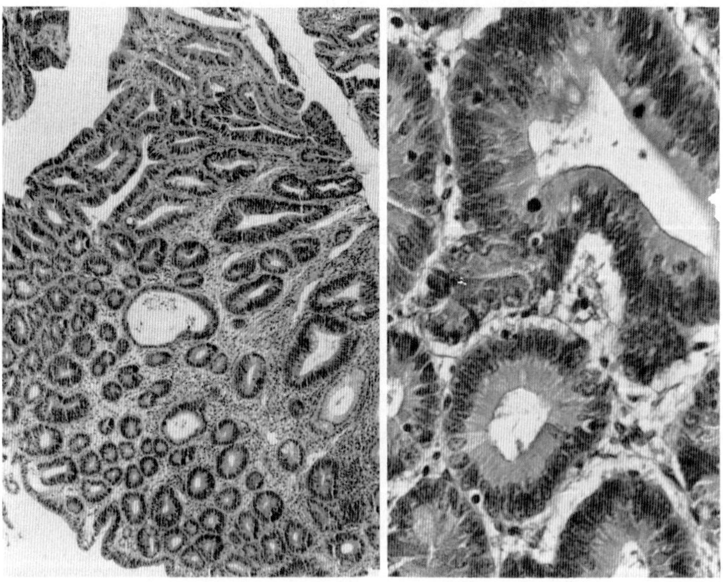

Fig. 1. Endoscopic biopsy of a small tubular adenoma. HE, × 50 *(left)*, × 300 *(right)*

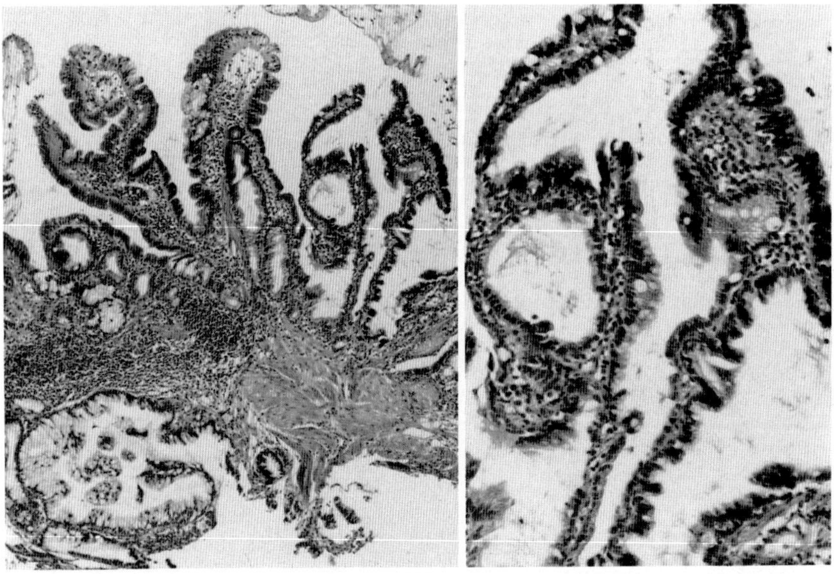

Fig. 2. Endoscopic biopsy of a small villous adenoma. HE, × 50 *(left)*, × 125 *(right)*

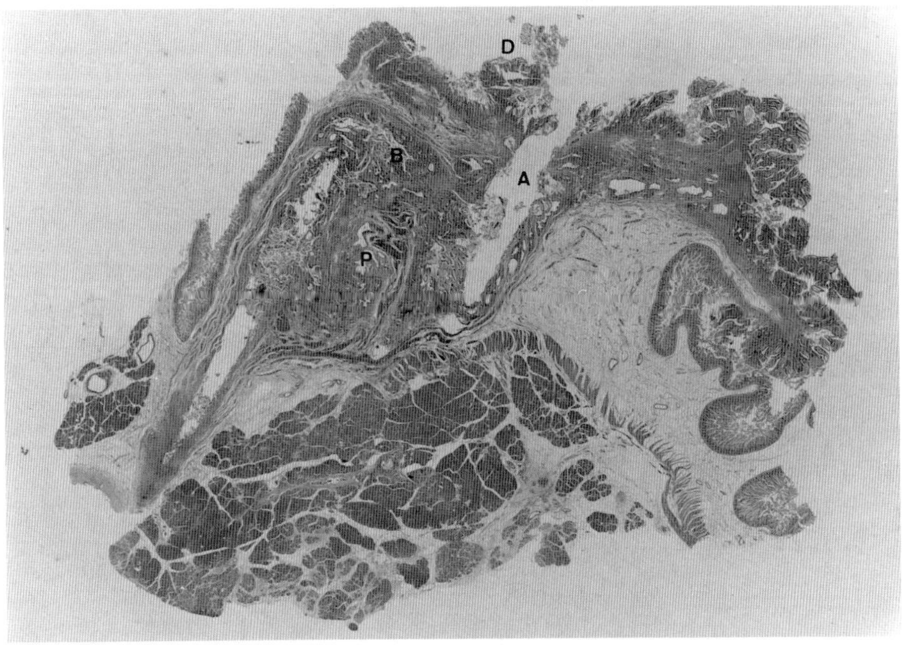

Fig. 3. Whole mount section of a tubular adenoma of the ampulla of Vater. Tumour is present in the distal common bile duct *(B)*, pancreatic duct *(P)*, ampulla of Vater *(A)* and duodenal mucosa *(D)*. HE, × 5

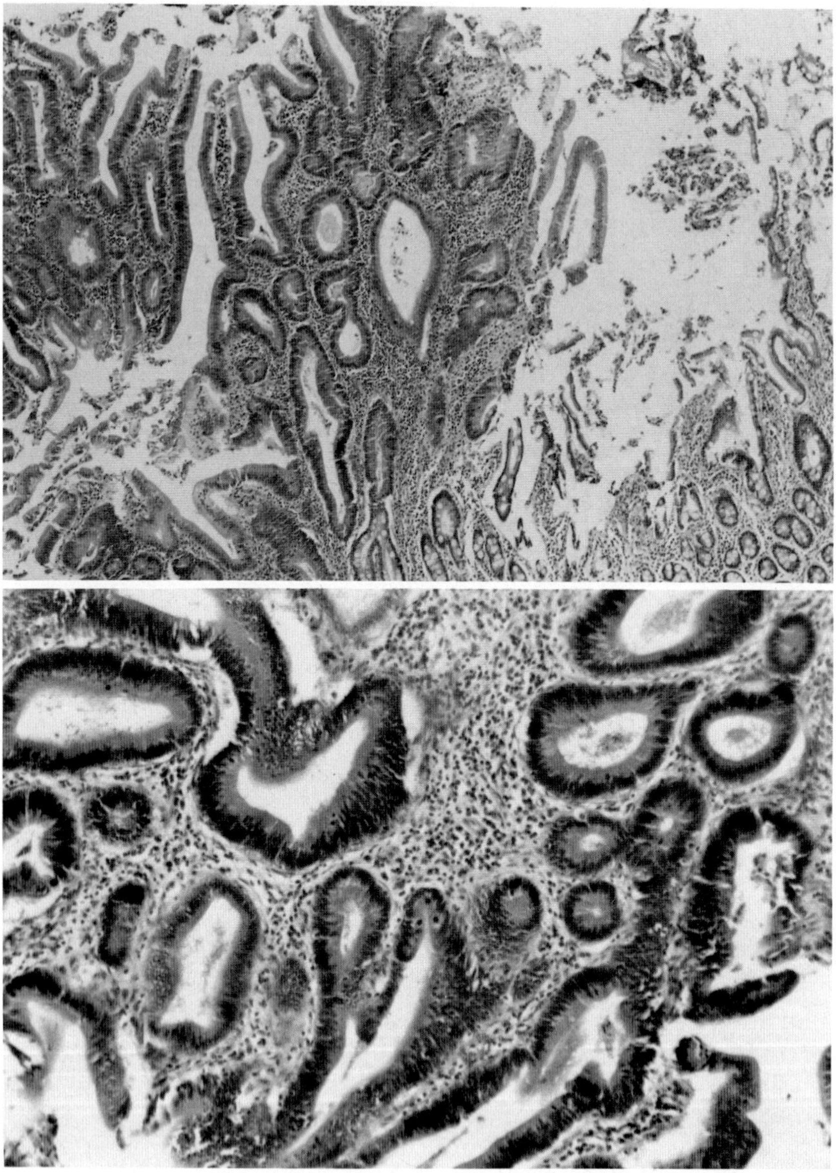

a

b

Fig. 4a, b. Higher magnifications of the lesions shown in Fig. 3. **a** From the peri-ampullary duodenal mucosa labelled as *(D)*. **b** From the distal end of the common bile duct labelled as (*B*). HE: **a** × 50, **b** × 125

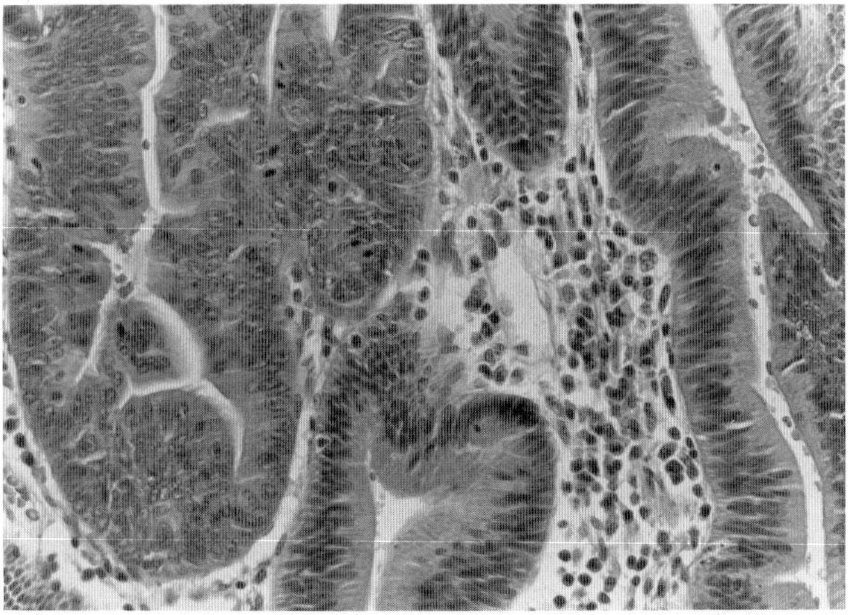

Fig. 5. Severe dysplasia/in situ carcinoma involving adenomatous epithelium of a villous adenoma of the duodenum. Early invasive carcinoma was present in this lesion. HE × 125

3.3 Location

Adenomas have been reported in all parts of the duodenum. In one review (SCHULTEN et al. 1976) approximately 74% were located in areas other than the second part of the duodenum, making them easily accessible to local excision. In another report (PERZIN and BRIDGE 1981) 28 of the 51 adenomas involved the ampullary region and 14 arose in extra-ampullary portions of the duodenum. Six of the remaining nine adenomas were located in the jejunum and three in the ileum.

4 Pathological Features

Gross examination shows duodenal adenomas to be pedunculated or sessile. The external surface of tubular adenomas is smooth or lobulated and pink to red in colour, while villous adenomas are soft, sessile tumours with an irregular external surface.

Microscopic examination of tubular adenomas reveals an appearance similar to tubular adenomas found elsewhere in the gastrointestinal tract. They are composed of neoplastic tubules lined by tall columnar stratified epithelium (Figs. 1, 3, 4) with scattered goblet cells. Mitoses are seen at

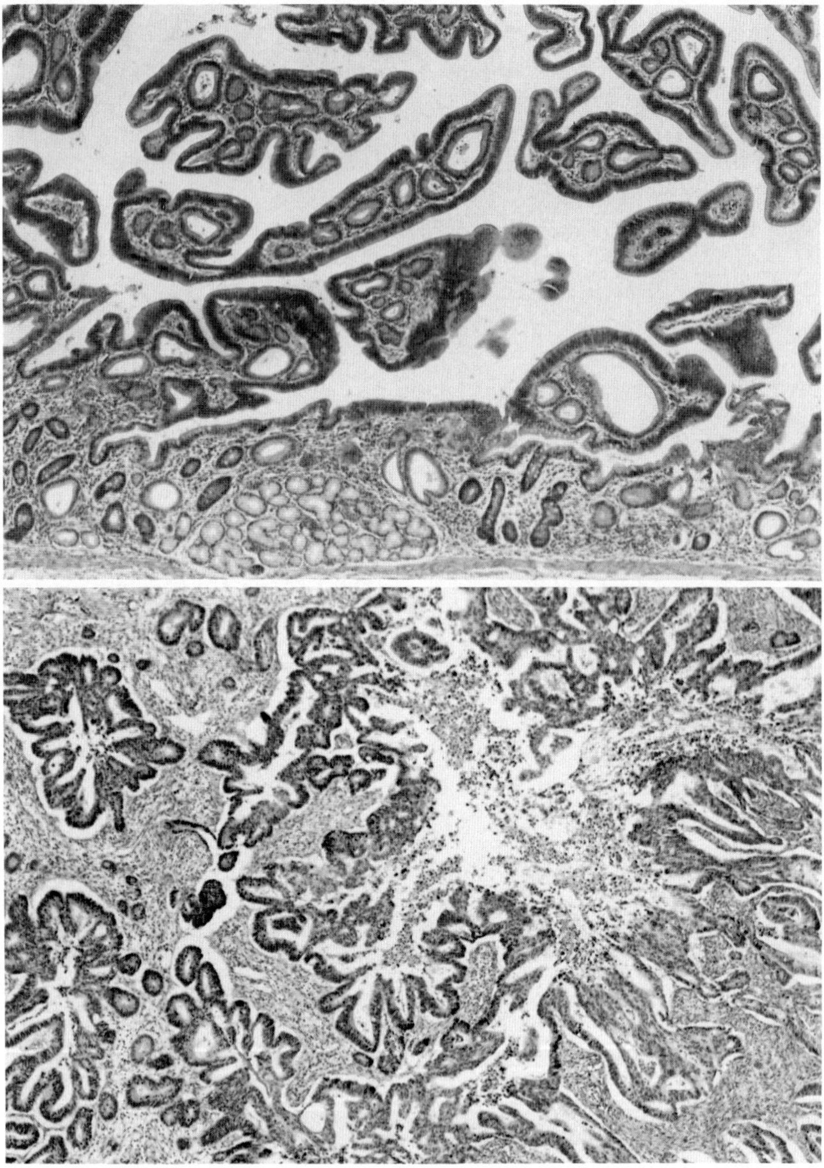

a

b

Fig. 6a, b. Carcinoma of the ampulla arising in villous adenoma. **a** Villous adenoma involving the peri-ampullary duodenal mucosa. **b** Invasive adenocarcinoma of the ampulla. HE: **a** × 50, **b** × 80

all levels of the lesion. Although a villous pattern may be present on the surface, the majority of the tumour should be composed of neoplastic tubules in order to classify a tumour as tubular adenoma. Villous adenomas are formed of finger-like villous or papillary processes of thin cords of fib-

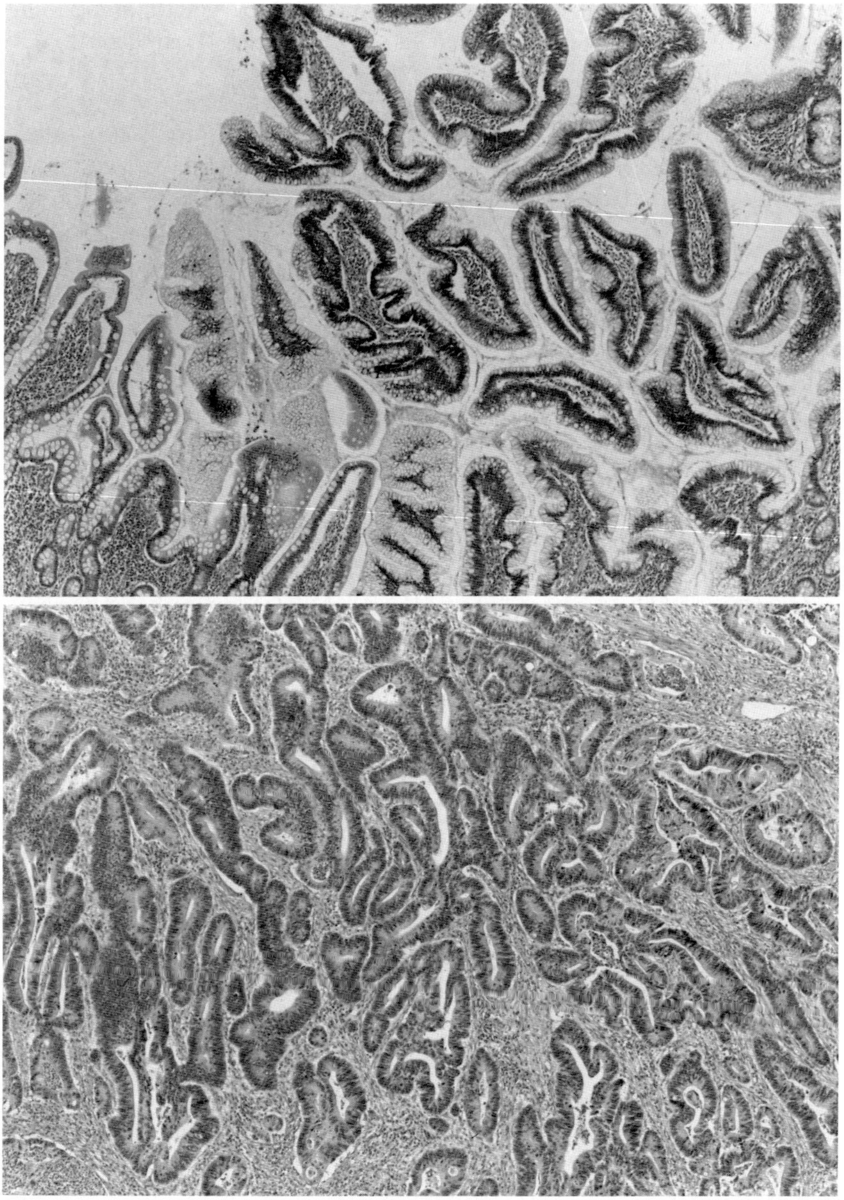

a

b

Fig. 7 a, b. Adenocarcinoma arising in villous adenoma of the duodenum. **a** Junction of normal and benign adenomatous epithelium. **b** Invasive adenomatous focus. HE: **a** × 50, **b** × 125

rovascular tissue lined by neoplastic tall columnar epithelium (Figs. 2, 7 a). Admixture of villous processes with tubules is not uncommon (Fig. 6 a). Variation in the pattern is frequent, with villi lined by a single layer of columnar and goblet cells in some areas and marked glandular budding with nuclear stratification, loss of mucin secretion (Fig. 5), nuclear hyperchromatism and atypia and plentiful mitoses in others. Paneth cells may be found. Their numbers vary and occasional tumours are rich in such cells. They are not confined to the bases of the crypts but are present at all levels of the neoplastic epithelium. Although nuclear atypia is frequent in the Paneth cells, mitoses are usually not found.

5 Development of Carcinoma

Evidence in the literature suggests that most duodenal carcinomas develop in pre-existing adenomas with an adenoma-cancer sequence similar to that accepted for colorectal carcinoma. The incidence of invasive carcinoma in adenomas of the colorectum is directly related to their size and the grade of dysplasia and carcinoma is commoner in villous adenomas than tubular adenomas (MUTO et al. 1975). Residual adenomatous tissue was found adjacent to 57% of early (submucosal) colorectal carinomas in one study (MUTO et al. 1975) and in 33% of all (KOZUKA 1975) in another. The same holds true for adenomas of the small bowel. In one study (PERZIN and BRIDGE 1981) two (22%) of nine tubular adenomas harboured an invasive carcinoma, as did three (60%) of five villous adenomas. Intramucosal carcinoma was present in another patient. SCHULTEN et al., in 1976, reviewed the literature and found 42 cases of duodenal villous adenomas and added one case of their own. Of these 43 cases, 15 (35%) had foci of carcinoma, including six with in situ carcinoma. In another study (KOMOROWSKI and COHEN 1981) four of the eight duodenal villous adenomas contained invasive carcinoma. A rare example of adenocarcinoma arising in a villous adenoma, in a bypassed duodenal stump 18 years after a Billroth II subtotal gastrecteomy, has been reported (LIPPER and GROVES 1985).

The risk of malignancy in ampullary and peri-ampullary adenomas is probably greater than elsewhere in the duodenum or the remaining small bowel (PERZIN and BRIDGE 1981). These workers found invasive adenocarcinoma in 10 (71%) of 14 tubular adenomas of the ampulla of Vater and in 12 (86%) of 14 ampullary villous adenomas. In another study (RYAN et al. 1986) carcinoma was present in 12 (75%) out of 16 villous adenomas of the ampulla. Earlier workers (BAGGENSTOSS 1938; CATTELL and PYRTEK 1950; OH and JEMERIN 1965) also identified adenomas of the ampulla of Vater as premalignant lesions.

A number of workers have examined adenocarcinomas of the small bowel and ampulla of Vater in an attempt to look for the presence of pre-existing adenomas. In the report by PERZIN and BRIDGE (1981), 25% of the carcinomas of the small bowel and 30% of carcinomas of ampulla of Vater showed histological evidence of residual adenomatous tissue. KOZUKA et al. (1981), in a similar study, examined surgical specimens from patients with carcinoma of ampulla of Vater and found evidence of pre-existing adenoma in 18 (82%) out of 22 cases. Another recent report (BACZAKO et al. 1985) found adenomatous elements adjacent to carcinoma of the ampulla of Vater in 53 (91%) out of 58 cases.

The size of small intestinal adenomas also has an important bearing on the eventual development of cancer. The larger the lesion, the greater the chance that carcinoma will be found on histological examination (PERZIN and BRIDGE 1985).

The evidence presented in the preceding paragraphs indicates that adenomas of the duodenum, including the ampulla, are premalignant lesions. Most, if not all, carcinomas of the duodenum and ampulla arise in pre-existing adenomas. PERZIN and BRIDGE (1981) have suggested that one of the reasons why primary adenocarcinoma of the small bowel is so uncommon is because the precancerous lesion, the adenoma, arises very rarely in the small intestine.

6 Diagnosis of Carcinoma

The detection of carcinoma in adenomas of the duodenum and ampulla is difficult on endoscopoic examination alone. Histological examination is necessary for a definite diagnosis. Larger lesions with ulceration, fixation or obstruction will usually show carcinomatous change on histological study. Small endoscopic biopsies may be diagnostic if the malignant focus is sampled but sampling errors with small biopsies are not uncommon. In one study (RYAN et al. 1986) the diagnosis of cancer by endoscopic biopsy was missed in five of the nine cases of adenocarcinoma arising in adenomas, a false-negative rate of 56%. If no cancer is found on multiple endoscopic biopsies, local excision should be the procedure of choice. If an invasive focus is present in the biopsy sample, then the histological diagnosis of carcinoma is usually not difficult. In addition to carcinomatous epithelium, desmoplastic reaction of the stromal elements is usually present. When there is severe dysplasia without unequivocal invasion associated with secondary gland formation, a back to back arrangement or glandular fusion, a diagnosis of in situ carcinoma is justified. Biopsy fragments displaying such changes are good indicators of coexistent invasive disease and justify surgical excision of the lesion to confirm invasive carcinoma.

In ampullary tumours, separation of well differentiated invasive adenocarcinoma from adenoma may at times be very difficult. Numerous small glands are normally present beneath the mucosa in the ampullary region, and when adenomatous epithelium extends into these glands there may be confusion with invasive disease. Care has to be exercised not to over-diagnose malignancy in such situations.

7 Management

The management of duodenal neoplasms should be based on the type of lesion, the location, the absence or presence of invasion, and patient risk. With widespread use of endoscopy and biopsy, adenomas of the duodenum and ampullary region are being recognised with increasing frequency. Small adenomas or those with a stalk are easily removed by polypectomy and the entire tumour studied histologically. If the tumour is large and cannot be removed endoscopically, then surgical resection becomes necessary. If the lesion is mobile, a local submucosal excision is the treatment of choice. This can easily be accomplished in the duodenum. If the ampulla of Vater is involved, local resection with ampullary reconstruction and duct implantation is recommended. Sphincteroplasty may be necessary if the ducts are small (ROSENBERG et al. 1986). If, following polypectomy or local excision, exhaustive histological examination fails to show invasive cancer, no further treatment is necessary.

If, at the time of surgery, the duodenal tumour appears ulcerated or is hard and fixed to surrounding structures, carcinoma should be suspected. An incisional biopsy should be obtained and submitted for frozen section diagnosis. When invasive carcinoma is diagnosed, either at the time of frozen section or following local excision, a pancreaticoduodenectomy may be indicated depending on patient risk and other factors.

8 Personal Experience

In our laboratory we have examined 16 duodenal or ampullary adenomas, from nine women and seven men with ages ranging from 30 to 87 years. The size of the tumours varied from 0.5 to 4 cm in maximum diameter. Five of the lesions were under 1.0 cm, five between 1.0 and 1.9 cm and six between 2.0 and 4.0 cm. Seven of the adenomas were located in the duodenum and nine involved the ampulla with or without involving the adjacent duodenal mucosa (Table 1). Five of the 16 tumours were tubular and 11 villous. All the villous lesions had an admixture of tubular and villous patterns, with the villous pattern being the dominant feature. Numerous Paneth cells were present in four villous adenomas. In six the dysplasia was mild, in six it was classed as moderate and in four the changes were consistent with severe dysplasia or intramucosal carcinoma. Invasive adenocarcinoma arose in 4 of the 16 adenomas, of which one was a tubular adenoma of the duodenum and the other three were villous adenomas of the ampulla.

Table 1. Duodenal and ampullary adenomas ($n = 16$)

Type of Lesion	Duodenum	Ampulla
Tubular Adenoma	3[a]	2
Villous Adenoma	4	7[b]

[a] One case associated with invasive carcinoma.
[b] Three cases associated with invasive carcinoma.

References

Baczako K, Buchler M, Beger HG, Kirkpatrick CJ, Haferkamp O (1985) Morphogenesis and possible precursor lesions of invasive carcinoma of the papilla of Vater: epithelial dysplasia and adenoma. Hum Pathol 16:305–310

Baggenstoss AH (1938) Major duodenal papilla. Variations of pathologic interest and lesions of the mucosa. Arch Pathol 26:853–868

Cattell RB, Pyrtek LJ (1950) Premalignant lesions of the ampulla of Vater. Surg Gynecol Obstet 90:21–30

Copperman M, Clausen KP, Hecht C, Lucas JG, Keith LM (1978) Villous adenomas of the duodenum. Gastroenterology 74:1295–1297

Dupas JL, Marti R, Capion JP, Delamarre J (1977) Villous adenoma of the duodenum. Endoscopy 9:245–247

Everett GD, Shirazi SS, Mitros FA (1981) Villous tumours of the duodenum. Report of two cases. Am J Gastroenterol 75:376–379

Golden R (1928) Non-malignant tumours of the duodenum. Am J Roentgenol Radium Ther Nucl Med 20:405–413

Hancock RJ (1970) An 11 year review of primary tumours of the small bowel including the duodenum. Can Med Assoc J 103:1177–1179

Hasleton PS, Shah S, Budkley CH, Tweedie DEF (1980) Ampullary carcinoma associated with multiple duodenal villous adenomas. Am J Gastroenterol 73:418–422

Haubrich WS, Johnson RB, Foroozan P (1973) Endoscopic removal of a duodenal adenoma. Gastrointest Endosc 19:201–203

Komorowski RA, Cohen EB (1981) Villous tumours of the duodenum: a clinicopathologic study. Cancer 47:1377–1386

Kozuka S (1975) Premalignancy of the mucosal polyp in the large intestine. 1. Histologic gradation of the polyp on the basis of epithelial pseudostratification and glandular branching. Dis Colon Rectum 18:483–493

Kozuka S, Tsubone M, Yamaguchi A, Hachisuka K (1981) Adenomatous residue in cancerous papilla of Vater. Gut 22:1031–1034

Leese T, Neoptolemos JP, West KP, Talbot IC, Carr-Locke DL (1986) Tumours and pseudotumours of the region of the ampulla of Vater: an endoscopic, clinical and pathological study. Gut 27:1186–1192

Lipper S, Groves GV (1985) Villous adenocarcinoma arising in the bypassed duodenum 18 years after Billroth II subtotal gastrectomy: report of a case and review of the literature. Am J Gastroenterol 80:174–176

Muto T, Bussey HJR, Morson BC (1975) The evolution of cancer of the colon and rectum. Cancer 36:2251–2270

Oh C, Jemerin EE (1965) Benign adenomatous polyps of the papilla of Vater. Surgery 57:495–503

Ohmori K, Konoshita H, Shiraha Y, Satake K (1976) Pancreatic duct obstruction by a benign polypoid adenoma of the ampulla of Vater. Am J Surg 132:662–663

Perzin KH, Bridge MF (1981) Adenomas of the small intestine: a clinicopathologic review of 51 cases and a study of their relationship to carcinoma. Cancer 48:799–819

Qizilbash AH (1984) Epithelial neoplasms of the duodenum and periampullary region. In: Appelman HD (ed) Pathology of the esophagus, stomach and duodenum, Contemporary issues in surgical pathology, vol 4. Churchill Livingstone, New York, pp 145–173

Reddy RR, Schuman BM, Priest RJ (1981) Duodenal polyps: diagnosis and management. J Clin Gastroenterol 3:139–145

Rosenberg J, Welch JP, Pyrtex LJ, Walker M, Trowbridge P (1986) Benign villous adenomas of the ampulla of Vater. Cancer 58:1563–1568

Ryan DP, Schapiro RH, Warshaw AL (1986) Villous tumours of the duodenum. Ann Surg 203:301–306

Schulten MF, Oyasu R, Beal JM (1976) Villous adenoma of the duodenum. A case report and review of the literature. Am J Surg 132:90–96

Sobol S, Cooperman AM (1978) Villous adenoma of the ampulla of Vater: an unusual cause of biliary colic and obstructive jaundice. Gastroenterology 75:107–109

Spira IA, Wolff WI (1977) Villous tumours of the duodenum. Am J Gastroenterol 67:63–68

Starling JR, Turner JH (1982) Villous adenoma involving the ampulla of Vater. Am Surg 48:188–190

Taxier M, Sivak MV, Cooperman A (1979) Villous adenoma of the ampulla of Vater. Gastrointest Endosc 25:155–156

Uppaputhangkule V, Maas LC, Gilzayjd EA (1976) Endoscopic diagnosis of villous adenoma of the duodenum. Gastrointest Endosc 23:97–98

Warshaw AL, Berry J, Gang DL (1987) Villous adenoma of the duct of Wirsung. Dig Dis Sci 32:1311–1313

Weiss JB, Semerdjian GG (1986) Recurrent villous adenoma of the duodenum. Gastroenterology 90:440–442

Wilson JM, Melvin DB, Gray GF, Thorbjarnarson B (1974) Primary malignancies of the small bowel: a report of 96 cases and review of the literature. Ann Surg 180:175–179

D Intra-epithelial Neoplasia in the Anal Canal and Peri-anal Area

C. FENGER

Intra-epithelial neoplasia in the anal canal and peri-anal area has been the subject of considerable interest in recent years and the number of cases reported is increasing. Much evidence has linked anal and genital neoplasia to venereal infections, particularly human papilloma virus (HPV), and a few cases of squamous carcinoma have been reported among patients with AIDS. Symptoms may be vague or absent and the diagnosis therefore rests on careful pathological examination.

1 Definitions and Nomenclature

1.1 Intra-epithelial Neoplasia

The term *intra-epithelial neoplasia*, originally introduced for changes in the squamous epithelium of the uterine cervix (RICHART 1973), can be defined as "a spectrum of intra-epithelial changes, that begins as a generally well differentiated intra-epithelial neoplasm, which has traditionally been classified as very mild dysplasia, and ends with invasive carcinoma". The terms CIN (cervical intra-epithelial neoplasia) and VIN (vulvar intra-epithelial neoplasia) are now commonly accepted, and the term ACIN (anal canal intra-epithelial neoplasia) has been proposed for similar changes in the anal canal (FENGER and NIELSEN 1986b). Precancerous changes in the peri-anal skin are normally called Bowen's disease, but will be referred to here for brevity as peri-anal skin intra-epithelial neoplasia (PSIN).

1.2 Anatomy and Histology

The (surgical) anal canal extends from the level of the pelvic floor to the anal opening or from the upper to the lower border of the internal sphincter (Fig. 1). It has a length of 3–4 cm and shows a characteristic surface relief. A little below the middle a line can be seen composed of the anal valves and sinuses and the bases of the anal columns. This line has been given at least ten different names, of which the term *dentate line* (DL) is preferable (FENGER 1987). This is the most important macroscopic landmark.

The mucosa can be divided into three zones according to the epithelial lining (FENGER 1988). The upper, *colorectal zone* roughly covers the first centimetre and is lined by colorectal type mucosa. The middle, *transitional zone* normally extends upwards for about 1 cm from the DL and shows a mixture of epithelial types. The lower, *squamous zone* is located below the DL and is lined by squamous epithelium, which at the lower border of the anal canal gradually becomes keratinised. The extent of the zones varies considerably (FENGER 1979).

The anal transitional zone (ATZ) is defined as "the zone interposed between uninterrupted colorectal type mucosa above and uninterrupted squamous epithelium below, irrespective of the type of epithelium present in the zone itself" (FENGER 1988). Many epithelial variants can be found in the ATZ, the most prominent being the so-called ATZ-epithelium. This consists of four to nine cell layers and the surface cells may be columnar, cuboidal, umbrella shaped or flattened (Fig. 2). Other areas may be covered by squamous or simple columnar epithelium and crypts of colorectal type may be present. The anal glands open into the ATZ.

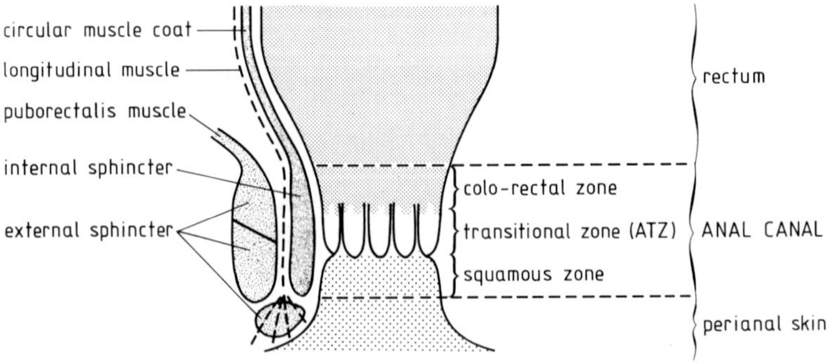

Fig. 1. Schematic drawing of the anal canal showing the three zones. (FENGER 1987b) (With permission from Raven Press)

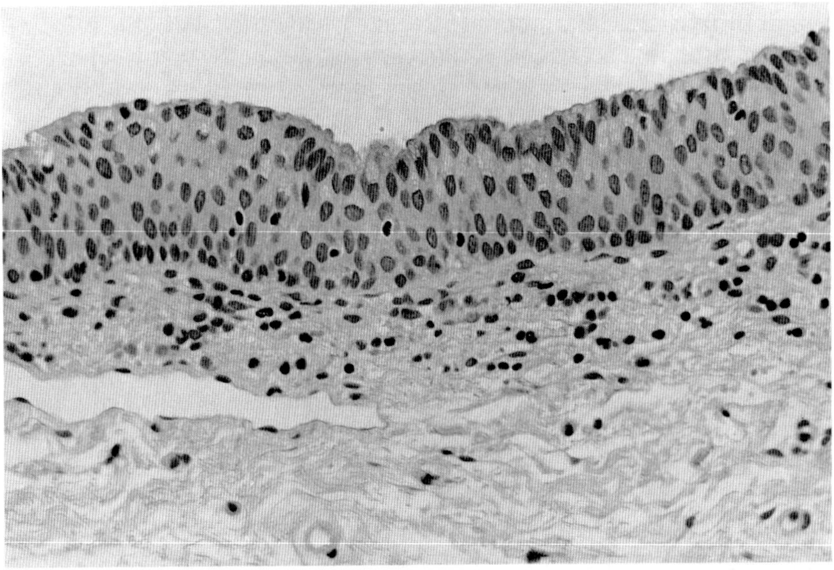

Fig. 2. Normal appearance of ATZ epithelium. The surface cells are polygonal to the *left* and columnar to the *right*, with slight mucin production. HE, × 400

The exact nature of the ATZ epithelium is not yet established. It has been likened to urothelium, but histochemical (FENGER and FILIPE 1981; FENGER and LYON 1982), ultrastructural (FENGER and KNOTH 1981) and DNA-flow cytometric studies (FENGER and BICHEL 1981) have not confirmed this hypothesis. It can be recognised in foetal life (FENGER 1988).

2 Aetiology

The aetiology of ACIN and PSIN is still unknown, but a venereal factor seems to be implicated, considering the many reports of concomitant vulvar, cervical and anal neoplasia (CHOO and MORLEY 1980; FENGER and NIELSEN 1986b; KAPLAN et al. 1981; SCHLAERTH et al. 1984 and many others), the epidemiology of cervical, vaginal, vulvar, penile and anal cancer (PETERS et al. 1984) and the increased risk of anal carcinoma among single males (DALING et al. 1982; PETERS and MACK 1983) and divorced or separate persons (PETERS et al. 1984). A history of syphilis is also common among patients with ACIN (FENGER and NIELSEN 1986b). Male patients with admitted homosexuality, bisexuality or a history of anal condylomas seem to represent a risk group (WEXNER et al. 1987).

Considerable evidence has now been collected indicating a relationship between infection with HPV and anogenital cancers, but the findings are not unequivocal. HPV DNA has been reported to be present in the cervical mucosa in a great proportion of women with CIN, but also in many histologically normal cervices. Koilocytosis is not consistently related to HPV infection and this is not necessarily followed by CIN (JENKINS et al. 1987; WICKENDEN et al. 1987). In only 13 of 21 women with VIN III and micro-invasive carcinoma of the vulva could HPV infection be confirmed by in situ hybridisation (GUPTA et al. 1987) and six cases of verrucous carcinoma were all negative (PILOTTI et al. 1984). On the other hand, bowenoid papulosis, a condition probably without malignant potential (PATTERSON et al. 1986), was found to contain HPV-16 DNA in eight of ten cases (IKENBERG et al. 1983). Differences in technique, subtyping and the stage of the lesions may, in part, be responsible for such variations.

There are comparatively few observations regarding anal carcinoma and its precursors. ACIN, PSIN and anal carcinoma have repeatedly been observed among male homosexuals and several of these have had condylomas (COOPER et al. 1979; CROXSON et al. 1984; EJECKAM et al. 1983; LI et al. 1982; NASH et al. 1986; WEXNER et al. 1986). It has been proposed that condylomas, giant condylomas and verrucous squamous carcinoma represent a continuous precancerous spectrum (BOGOMOLETZ et al. 1985). In a series of 7 males and 12 females with ACIN none showed positive reaction for HPV (FENGER and NIELSEN 1986b); a few cases of PSIN have been positive (IKENBERG et al. 1983). HPV 6 and/or 11, 16, and 18 DNA has been variably demonstrated in anal condylomas, intraepithelial neoplasia and carcinomas, with a tendency for HPV 16 to be associated with neoplastic changes (BECKMANN et al. 1985; DUGGAN et al. 1989; LÖNING et al. 1988; SCHEURLEN et al. 1986; WELLS et al. 1988).

Other factors may be of importance. A few cases of ACIN, PSIN and squamous carcinoma have been reported in male homosexuals with antibodies to HIV or AIDS and some of these have had signs of HPV infection (CROXSON et al. 1984; HOWARD et al. 1986; WEXNER et al. 1986). PSIN has been reported in association with Crohn's colitis (BECK et al. 1989).

3 Incidence

The incidence of ACIN and PSIN is unknown. Population screening programmes have not been carried out and would be difficult to design, as the only reliable diagnosis is histological. The only available figures are from a few series of minor surgical specimens from clinically benign anal diseases and from the accumulated data in tumour registers. Such reports only occasionally make a distinction between ACIN and PSIN.

Earlier series of minor surgical specimens from New York and San Francisco have shown that 0.2%–0.3% harboured ACIN or PSIN (GORDON 1956; GRODSKY 1967), but in a recent study from Los Angeles the percentage has been as high as 4, with a considerable excess among male homosexuals (NASH et al. 1986). The corresponding figures are 1.9% in

North-eastern Brazil (LEAO and FERREIRA 1979) and 0.3% in a rural district in Denmark (FENGER and NIELSEN 1981).

The annual incidence in Los Angeles for the period 1972–1981 was $0.2-0.3/10^5$ for anal carcinoma in situ and $0.8-1.2/10^5$ for invasive carcinoma (males-females) (PETERS et al. 1984). In Denmark the incidence in the period 1979–1980 was $0.2/10^5$ for ACIN and $0.7/10^5$ for carcinomas (FENGER and NIELSEN 1986b).

The figures are undoubtedly heavily biased with regard to age, sex, anal and venereal diseases and sexual behaviour. However, the experience of the extensively studied CIN-carcinoma sequence would predict that the incidence of ACIN and PSIN should be considerably higher than that of anal canal and peri-anal skin carcinomas.

4 Clinical Diagnosis

Bowen's disease or PSIN usually presents as slowly progressive, irregular, scaly, erythematous, raised, eventually fissured patches, and is often accompanied by discomfort, pruritus or pain (RAMOS et al. 1983; BECK et al. 1988). ACIN, on the other hand, does not seem to produce any special symptoms, and the extent of mucosal changes into the anal canal may be difficult to estimate (CHOO and MORLEY 1980; NASH et al. 1986; SCHLAERTH et al. 1984). Many cases have been found on clinical examination of females with genital dysplasia, but most have been incidental findings at routine microscopy of haemorrhoids, fibrous polyps, condylomas/papillomas, fissures, fistulas etc. There are no reports on the use of cytology for the diagnosis of ACIN.

As risk groups seem to exist, careful examination of the whole anogenital area should be carried out in all patients with venereal disease, and particularly in females with dysplasia of the cervix and vulva and in homosexual men. Biopsics should be taken from all mucosal and skin changes. The colposcope can eventually be used in the lower anal canal, where the lesion may present as well demarcated, greysish-white areas, while signs of changed vascularity are less pronounced. Induration may indicate micro-invasion (FENGER and NIELSEN 1986b).

5 Pathology

5.1 Handling of Specimens

As many cases of PSIN and ACIN are clinically unsuspected, all minor operative specimens from the area should be examined histologically. It is often possible macroscopically to identify the smooth grey-brown squa-

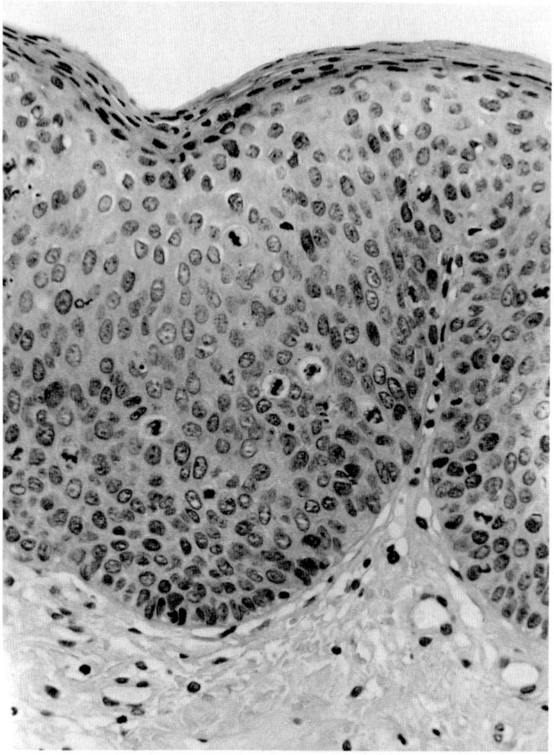

Fig. 3. PSIN or Bowen's disease in the peri-anal skin. HE, × 400

mous zone from the grey-blue more glistening anal mucosa and the specimens should be embedded and cut along the longitudinal axis. Only in this way will it be possible to correlate the findings to the three zones of the anal canal. Further it should be remembered that the ATZ, including areas of squamous epithelium, may be found as high as 2 cm above the DL (FENGER 1979) and that koilocytotic and dysplastic changes may involve this whole area (BOGOMOLETZ et al. 1985; FENGER and NIELSEN 1986a, b; FENGER 1989). Signs of HPV or herpetic changes should be noted and confirmed by immunocytochemistry or in situ hybridisation. The margins of larger resections should be investigated completely. Frozen sections may be used peroperatively to ensure complete excision of ACIN as well as for Paget's disease (STACY et al. 1986).

Only a few authors distinguish between PSIN and ACIN, and this may often be difficult. Many patients show a combination of these lesions. It is most important for the pathologist to assess carefully whether invasion has occurred, the relation of the lesion to the DL and whether local excision is complete. The morphology in both PSIN and ACIN may be modified by signs of infection with HPV or herpes virus (CROXSON et al. 1984; NASH et al. 1986).

5.2 Peri-anal Skin Intra-epithelial Neoplasia

The peri-anal lesions show the histological picture of Bowen's disease. The squamous epithelium is hyperplastic, with loss of stratification, variation in nuclear size, hyperchromasia, increased nuclear-cytoplasmic ratio, presence of mitoses (often atypical) in all layers and multinucleated cells. The surface may show keratosis or parakeratosis (Fig. 3).

Most cases reported in the literature have been non-invasive (RAMOS et al. 1983; STRAUSS and FAZIO 1979), but anal margin carcinoma may subsequently develop (QUAN 1980). The intra-epithelial changes may extend up into the anal canal above the DL, where they may present as ACIN (FENGER and NIELSEN 1986b; STRAUSS and FAZIO 1979). The anal lesion can often be treated by local excision (SCHLAERTH et al. 1984; BECK et al. 1988). PSIN is often associated with neoplasia of the vulva or cervix in females (CHOO and MORLEY 1980; QUAN 1980; RAMOS et al. 1983; SCHLAERTH et al. 1984; STRAUSS and FAZIO 1979); there are case reports of males having concomitant lymphoma (STRAUSS and FAZIO 1979) or Kaposi's sarcoma (CROXSON et al. 1984).

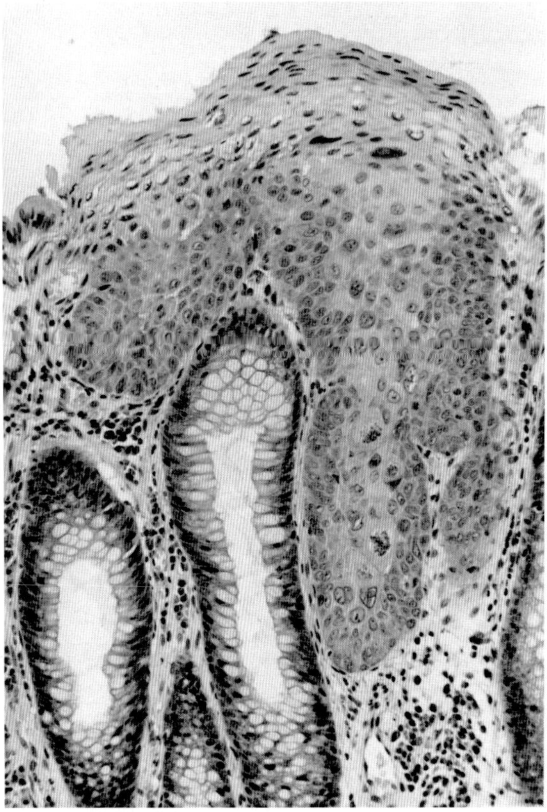

Fig. 4. ACIN in the ATZ. Extension into crypts of colorectal type. HE, × 400

5.3 Anal Canal Intra-epithelial Neoplasia

ACIN is defined as intra-epithelial neoplasia in the form of mild to severe dysplasia or carcinoma in situ (ACIN I-III), located in the anal canal, in the ATZ as well as below the DL. Histologically it resembles the corresponding CIN lesion and may extend into anal glands and rectal crypts present in the ATZ (Fig. 4) (FENGER and NIELSEN 1981, 1986a, b). Like CIN, the histological appearance may be modified by signs of virus infection.

ACIN has been found in minor surgical specimens from patients without anal canal carcinoma or genital neoplasia (FENGER and NIELSEN 1981) as well as in females with vulvar and cervical neoplasia (FENGER and NIELSEN 1986b). The average age for ACIN is a little lower than for anal canal carcinoma and the sex distribution is the same. ACIN is located in the area typical for anal canal carcinoma, there is a strong tendency to recurrence and ACIN eventually exhibits foci of micro-invasion (FENGER and NIELSEN 1986b). ACIN is present in most anal canals harbouring variants of squamous carcinoma (pure squamous, basaloid or muco-epider-

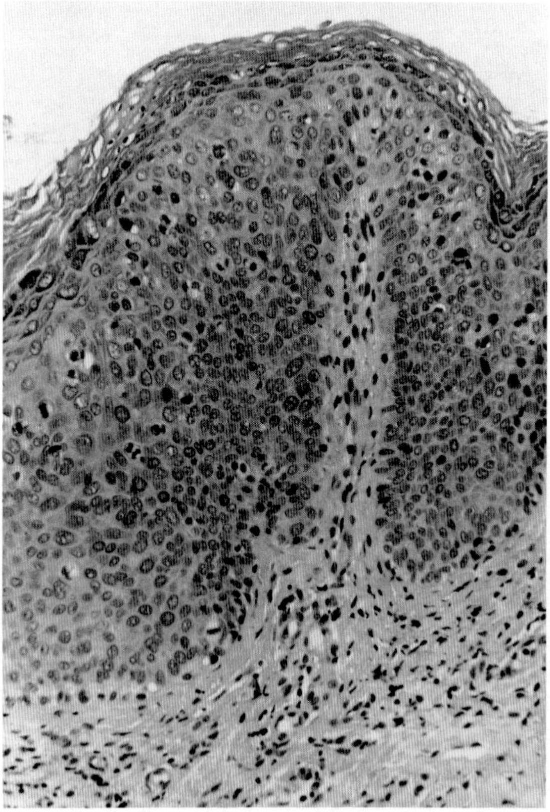

Fig. 5. Bowenoid papulosis in the peri-anal skin. HE, × 400

moid patterns), at the borders of the tumors as well as in isolated areas, and most often in the ATZ (FENGER and NIELSEN 1986a). Thus, there is considerable evidence that ACIN is the precursor for anal canal carcinoma, and possibly has a more aggressive behaviour than PSIN.

6 Differential Diagnosis

The pathologist must be familiar with the normal epithelial variants in the ATZ (FENGER 1987b) as these do not show the maturation characteristic of squamous epithelium in other mucosal surfaces. The uniform size of the nuclei, the lack of hyperchromasia and the tendency to a slight mucin production in the surface cells may be of help. Inflammatory changes show enlarged nuclei with prominent nucleoli but no hyperchromasia, and the nuclear-cytoplasmic ratio is relatively unchanged. Vacuolated cytoplasm is often observed in the anal canal epithelium and is not necessarily due to HPV infection (FENGER 1988).

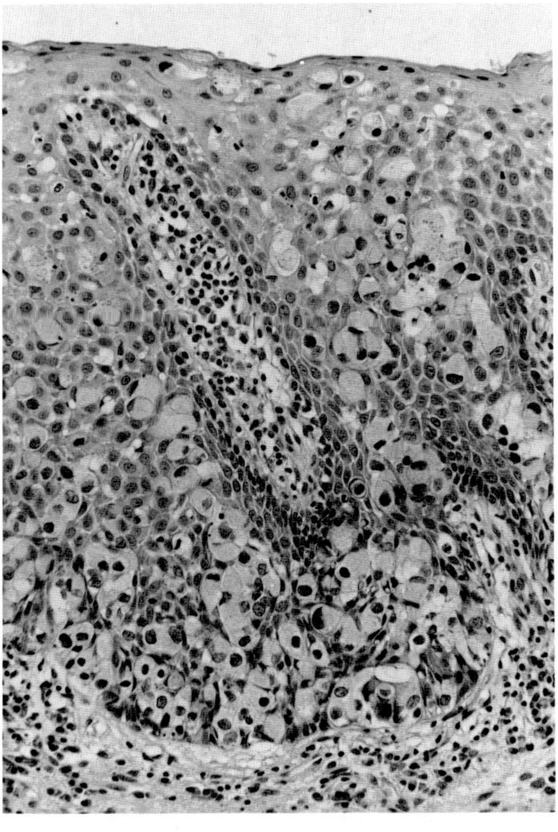

Fig. 6. Paget's disease of the peri-anal skin. HE, × 400

Bowenoid papulosis is characterised by hyperkeratosis, parakeratosis, hypergranulosis, vacuolated keratinocytes, irregular acanthosis, papillomatosis and inflammation. Dysplastic cells and mitoses are found scattered on a background of relatively orderly maturation, resulting in the characteristic "salt and pepper" appearance (Fig. 5). The cells may contain HPV-16 (IKENBERG et al. 1983). Some report that the condition is self-limiting and does not seem to have a malignant potential (PATTERSON et al. 1986). However, occasionally the lesion may show full thickness dysplasia and thus be histologically indistinguishable from PSIN, and invasion has recently been reported in a HPV 35-positive anogenital lesion. Follow-up may therefore be indicated for these patients also (RÜDLINGER et al. 1989).

Paget's disease presents with single or small groups of mucin-containing cells, located in the basal or all layers of the epidermis. It is normally located outside the anal canal but may extend up to the level of the DL (Fig. 6). The Paget's cells may contain carcino-embryonic antigen (ORDONEZ et al. 1987). There are several reports of peri-anal Paget's disease apparently unassociated with an underlying malignancy (FENGER 1989), but close observation of such cases is necessary, as a carcinoma may develop up to 10 years after the initial diagnosis (BECK and FAZIO 1987).

Basal cell carcinoma arises in the peri-anal skin but may involve the anal canal even above the DL (NIELSEN and JENSEN 1981). The histological picture is similar to basal cell carcinoma occurring elsewhere, so that ACIN or PSIN does not usually enter the differential diagnosis. However, distinction must be made from variants of squamous carcinoma, notably so-called basaloid (cloacogenic) carcinoma.

Acknowledgement. This publication has been supported by the Danish Medical Research Council.

References

Beck DE, Fazio VW (1987) Perianal Paget's disease. Dis Colon Rectum 30:263–266

Beck DE, Fazio VW, Jagelman DG, Lavery IC (1988) Perianal Bowen's disease. Dis Colon Rectum 31:419–422

Beck DE, Harford FJ, Roettger RH (1989) Perianal Bowen's disease associated with Crohn's colitis. Report of a case. Dis Colon Rectum 32:252–255

Beckmann AM, Daling JR, McDougall JK (1985) Human papillomavirus DNA in anogenital carcinomas. J Cell Biochem 9 C:68

Bogomoletz WV, Potet F, Molas G (1985) Condylomata acuminata, giant condyloma acuminatum (Buschke-Loewenstein tumour) and verrucous squamous carcinoma of the perianal and anorectal region: a continuous precancerous spectrum? Histopathology 9:1155–1169

Choo YC, Morley GW (1980) Multiple primary neoplasms of the anogenital region. Obstet Gynecol 56:365–369

Cooper HS, Patchefsky AS, Marks G (1979) Cloacogenic carcinoma of the anorectum in homosexual men: An observation of four cases. Dis Colon Rectum 22:557–558

Croxson T, Chabon AB, Rorat E, Barash IM (1984) Intraepithelial carcinoma of the anus in homosexual men. Dis Colon Rectum 27:325–330

Daling JR, Weiss NS, Klopfenstein LL, et al. (1982) Correlates of homosexual behavior and the incidence of anal cancer. JAMA 247:1988–1990

Duggan MA, Boras VF, Inoue et al. (1989) Human papillomavirus DNA determination of anal condylomata, dysplasias, and squamous carcinomas with in situ hybridization. Am J Clin Pathol 92:16–21

Ejeckam GC, Idikio HA, Nayak V, Gardiner JP (1983) Malignant transformation in an anal condyloma acuminatum. Can J Surg 26:170–173

Fenger C (1979) The anal transitional zone. Location and extent. Acta Pathol Microbiol Scand [A]87:379–386

Fenger C (1987) The anal transitional zone (thesis). Acta Pathol Microbiol Immunol Scand [A], Suppl 289, 95:1–42

Fenger C (1988) Histology of the anal canal. Am J Surg Path 12:41–55

Fenger C (1989) Surgical pathology of the anal canal. A review of recent literature on anatomy and pathology. Progress in Surgical Pathology 10

Fenger C, Bichel P (1981) Flow cytometric DNA analysis of anal canal epithelium and anorectal tumours. Acta Pathol Microbiol Scand [A]89:351–355

Fenger C, Filipe MI (1981) Mucin histochemistry of the anal canal epithelium. Studies of normal mucosa and mucosa adjacent to carcinoma. Histochem J 13:921–930

Fenger C, Knoth M (1981) The anal transitional zone. A scanning and transmission electron microscopic investigation of the surface epithelium. Ultrastruct Pathol 2:163–173

Fenger C, Lyon H (1982) Endocrine cells and melanin-containing cells in the anal canal epithelium. Histochem J 14:631–639

Fenger C, Nielsen VT (1981) Dysplastic changes in the anal canal epithelium in minor surgical specimens. Acta Pathol Microbiol Scand [A]89:463–465

Fenger C, Nielsen VT (1986 a) Precancerous changes in the anal canal epithelium in resection specimens. Acta Pathol Microbiol Immunol Scand [A] 94:63–69

Fenger C, Nielsen VT (1986 b) Intraepithelial neoplasia in the anal canal. The appearance and relation to genital neoplasia. Acta Pathol Microbiol Immunol Scand [A]94:343–349

Gordon BS (1956) Unsuspected lesions in anal tissue removed for minor conditions. Arch Surg 73:741–746

Grodsky L (1967) Unsuspected anal cancer discovered after minor anorectal surgery. Dis Colon Rectum 10:471–478

Gupta J, Pilotti S, Shah KV et al. (1987) Human papillomavirus-associated early vulvar neoplasia investigated by in situ hybridization. Am J Surg Pathol 11:430–434

Howard LC, Paterson-Brown S, Weber JN et al. (1986) Squamous carcinoma of the anus in young homosexual men with T-helper cell depletion. Genitourin Med 62:393–395

Ikenberg H, Gissmann L, Gross G et al. (1983) Human papillomavirus type-16-related DNA in genital Bowen's disease and in Bowenoid papulosis. Int J Cancer 32:563–565

Jenkins D, Tay SK, Maddox PH (1987) Routine papillomavirus antigen staining of cervical punch biopsy specimens. J Clin Pathol 40:1212–1216

Kaplan AL, Kaufman RH, Birken RA, Simkin S (1981) Intraepithelial carcinoma of the vulva with extension to the anal canal. Obstet Gynecol 58:368–371

Leao PHS, Ferreira FV (1979) Histologic similarities between dysplasia in the anorectal junction and in the cervix uteri. Ceara Medico 1/2:8–13

Li FP, Osborn D, Cronin CM (1982) Anorectal squamous carcinoma in two homosexual men. Lancet 14:391

Löning T, Riviere A, Henke RP et al. (1988) Penile/anal condylomas and squamous cell cancer. A HPV DNA hybridization study. Virchows Archiv [A]413:491–498

Nash G, Allen W, Nash S (1986) Atypical lesions of the anal mucosa in homosexual men. JAMA 256:873–876

Nielsen OV, Jensen SL (1981) Basal cell carcinoma of the anus – a clinical study of 34 cases. Br J Surg 68:856–857

Ordonez NG, Awalt H, Mackay B (1987) Mammary and extramammary Paget's disease. Cancer 59:1173–1183

Patterson JW, Kao GF, Graham JH, Helwig EB (1986) Bowenoid papulosis. A clinicopathologic study with ultrastructural observations. Cancer 57:823–836

Peters RK, Mack TM (1983) Patterns of anal carcinoma by gender and marital status in Los Angeles County. Br J Cancer 48:629–636
Peters RK, Mack TM, Bernstein L (1984) Parallels in the epidemiology of selected anogenital carcinomas. J Natl Cancer Inst 72:609–613
Pilotti S, Rilke F, Shah KV, et al. (1984) Immunohistochemical and ultrastructural evidence of papiloma virus infection associated with in situ and microinvasive squamous cell carcinoma of the vulva. Am J Surg Pathol 8:751–761
Quan SH (1980) Malignant anal and perianal tumors. Pract Gastroenterol 4:46–51
Ramos R, Salinas H, Tucker L (1983) Conservative approach to the treatment of Bowen's disease of the anus. Dis Colon Rectum 26:712–715
Richart RM (1973) Cervical intraepithelial neoplasia. Pathol Ann 163:301–328
Rüdlinger R, Grob R, Yu YX, Schnyder UW (1989) Human papillomavirus-35-positive Bowenoid papulosis of the anogenital area and concurrent human papillomavirus-35-positive verruca with Bowenoid dysplasia of the periungual area. Arch Derm 125:655–659
Scheurlen W, Stremlau A, Gissmann L et al. (1986) Rearranged HPV 16 molecules in an anal and in a laryngeal carcinoma. Int J Cancer 38:671–676
Schlaerth JB, Morrow CP, Nalick RH, Gaddis O (1984) Anal involvement by carcinoma in situ of the perineum in women. Obstet Gynecol 64:406–411
Stacy D, Burrell MO, Franklin EW (1986) Extramammary Paget's disease of the vulva and anus: use of intraoperative frozen-section margins. Am J Obstet Gynecol 155:519–523
Strauss RJ, Fazio VW (1979) Bowen's disease of the anal and perianal area. a report and analysis of twelve cases. Am J Surg 137:231–234
Wells M, Robertson S, Lewis F, Dixon MF (1988) Squamous carcinoma arising in a giant perianal condyloma associated with human papillomavirus types 6 and 11. Histopathology 12:319–323
Wexner SD, Smithy WB, Milsom JW, Dailey TH (1986) The surgical management of anorectal diseases in AIDS and pre-AIDS patients. Dis Colon Rectum 29:719–723
Wexner SD, Milsom JW, Dailey TH (1987) The demographics of anal cancers are changing. Identification of a high-risk population. Dis Colon Rectum 30:942–946
Wickenden C, Malcolm ADB, Byrne M et al. (1987) Prevalence of HPV DNA and viral copy numbers in cervical scrapes from women with normal and abnormal cervices. J Pathol 153:127–135

Gastrointestinal Biopsy Diagnosis in the Tropics

M. M. MATHAN and V. I. MATHAN

1 Introduction

A variety of infections and infestations of the gastrointestinal tract pose a diagnostic challenge for pathologists and gastroenterologists in the tropics. The interpretation of intestinal mucosal biopsies is complicated by the effect of the tropical, usually contaminated, environment and widespread malnutrition, which may influence gut mucosal morphology in even apparently healthy individuals. This chapter will concentrate on mucosal biopsy alterations that are widely prevalent in the healthy population in the small and large intestine and also on the specific bacterial and parasitic infections that can be diagnosed by gastrointestinal mucosal biopsy. It must be emphasised that the gastrointestinal pathologist working in the tropics should be fully familiar with the biopsy diagnosis of neoplastic conditions. This is particularly important since regional differences in the prevalence of malignancies are now becoming apparent (RAMAKRISHNA et al. 1988).

A particularly important concern is the response of the gastrointestinal mucosa as an immunological organ (PARROT 1976). In many tropical countries the lumen of the gastrointestinal tract, including the small intestine, is colonised by a variety of microbes, both anaerobes and aerobes (BHAT et al. 1972). An autochthonous flora, predominantly anaerobic, has also been shown to be present in the small intestine (BHAT et al. 1980). In addition a variety of bacterial enteric pathogens also colonise the gut lumen without apparent ill effect, as they can be recovered from faecal samples from healthy individuals (MATHAN and RAJAN 1986). The prevalence of enterovirus and adenovirus infections and enteric parasites is also high in this population (PATEL et al. 1983). The response of the gut-associated immune system to this antigenic challenge in the tropics has not been fully understood. Increases in small intestinal mucosal epithelial lymphocytes and total immunoglobulin fractions in the serum have been documented in such populations (ROSS and MATHAN 1981). The response of the gut mucosa to this challenge may be of considerable importance. For example, it has been documented that in the population of southern India the response to oral polio vaccine in children is not as appropriate as it is in the temperate climate, and these children may require up to nine doses before being adequately immunised (JOHN 1976). These findings suggest that a detailed study of the responses of the gut as an immunological organ in the tropics is likely to contribute significantly to public health measures to control enteric infection.

2 Stomach

2.1 Gastritis

A higher prevalence of gastritis and gastric atrophy has been documented in tropical populations (VAISH et al. 1967; DESAI et al. 1977). The reasons for this are not known, but the recent documentation of *Campylobacter pylori* in gastric biopsies (NAIR et al. 1986) (see page 1) and the high prevalence of other enteric *Campylobacter* species in tropical populations (RAJAN and MATHAN 1981), suggests that this organism, which has been implicated in the pathogenesis of gastritis and duodenal ulcer (MARSHALL and WARREN 1984), may be important in tropical countries. The presence of *C. pylori* is easily demonstrated in endoscopic biopsies (Fig. 1), especially if silver stains are used. Prospective epidemiological studies backed up by culture and histological examination of endoscopic gastric biopsies are needed to define the role of this organism in tropical regions.

2.2 Tuberculosis

Tuberculosis of the stomach is a rare entity (PALMER 1950). At gastroscopy the lesion may present as an ulcer in the antrum or lesser curvature of the stomach. These ulcers have characteristic undermined edges, serpiginous outline and pale nodules in the adjacent mucosa, and must be differentiated from malignant lesions. Occasionally tuberculosis of the stomach may present as an infiltrative and hypertrophic lesion which may closely mimic neoplastic growths. Biopsies, particularly if they are taken repeatedly at the same spot to obtain submucosal tissue or at the edge of

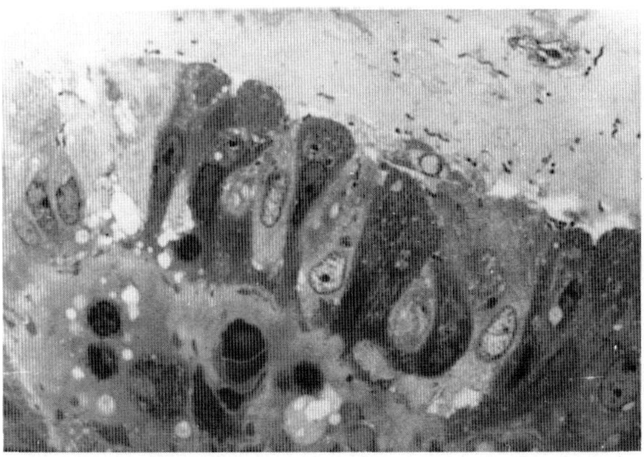

Fig. 1. Surface cells of gastric mucosa with many spiral organisms adherent to the luminal border and in the surface mucus. × 900

the ulcers, can be diagnostic with characteristic granulomatous inflammation, caseation and giant cells. Acid-fast organisms may be demonstrable in appropriately stained tissues.

3 Small Intestine

3.1 Tropical Enteropathy

Long, slender finger- or tongue-shaped villus structures are seldom present in jejunal mucosal biopsies from residents in many tropical countries (BAKER et al. 1962; LINDENBAUM et al. 1966; BAKER and MATHAN 1972; BAKER 1973). Broader leaf-shaped villi and ridges, which on occasion may be in a convoluted pattern, are found in the majority, changes which are termed tropical enteropathy. These architectural abnormalities are reflected on examination of histological sections by an increase in the thickness of the crypts and increased cellularity of the lamina propria and the epithelial layer (Fig. 2). The foetal intestine in tropical southern India is not different from that in temperate climates, but changes begin shortly after birth (CHACKO et al. 1968). It has been shown in experimental animals that exposure to the luminal contents is necessary for the changes to occur and that when the mucosa is isolated from gut continuity, in Thiry-Vella fistulae, the changes revert to normal or their progression is pre-

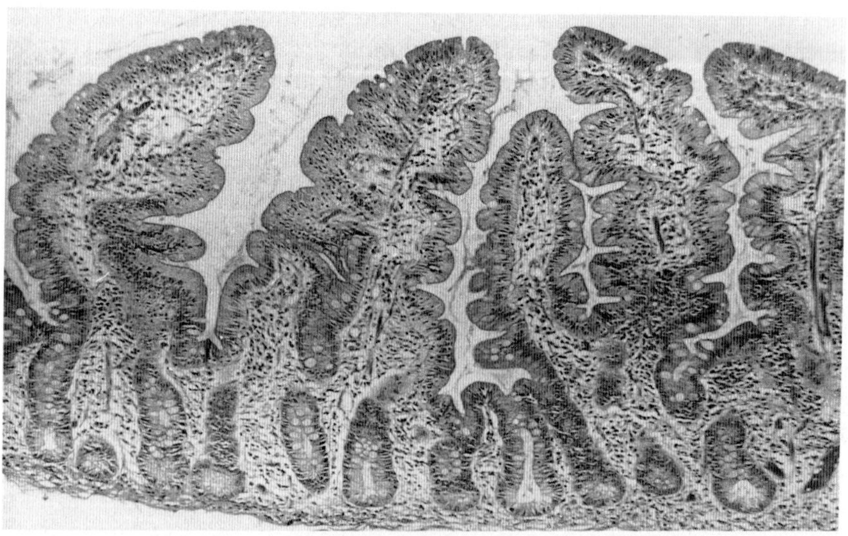

Fig. 2. Jejunal mucosa from a healthy control subject with changes of tropical enteropathy: increase in crypt thickness, shortening of villi and increased cellularity of lamina propria. × 100

vented (CHACKO et al. 1969). The morphological abnormalities are associated with functional alterations (BAKER and MATHAN 1972) and there is preliminary evidence to suggest that impaired intestinal absorption as a result of tropical enteropathy may lead to the loss of 5%–8% of ingested food energy in populations which can scarcely afford such a loss (CHACKO et al. 1984). Tropical enteropathy appears to be an adaptive response to a variety of environmental factors. There is increased turnover of enterocytes probably as a response to enterocyte loss from the villus compartment secondary to minimal damage (MATHAN et al. 1982). In addition to its possible contribution to malnutrition in tropical areas, tropical enteropathy makes it essential that the pathologist defines the range of "normality" in each region, especially when the subtle changes in the small intestinal epithelium associated with some of the malabsorption syndromes have to be interpreted.

3.2 Malnutrition

The elegant studies of DEO and RAMALINGASWAMY (1965) showed that it was possible to produce a gastrointestinal lesion in severely protein-depleted monkeys. However, whether a lesion results from protein or other malnutrition in humans is not yet established. Studies on children with protein energy malnutrition have shown that in marasmic children the morphology of the gut is apparently normal while in children who were clinically diagnosed as suffering from kwashiorkor there was a gut lesion with shortening of villi, hypertrophy of the crypt and marked infiltration of the lamina propria (BRUNSER et al. 1968). Whether this lesion was secondary to malnutrition or consequent upon infections of the gastrointestinal tract due to altered immunity in malnourished children is not yet clear.

3.3 Bacterial Infections

3.3.1 Cholera

Infection by *Vibrio cholerae* is the classical prototype of toxigenic diarrhoeas. Jejunal mucosal biopsies in patients studied in temperate countries showed an intact epithelium with degenerative lesions and subjacent mononuclear infiltrate (FRESH et al. 1964; SHEEHY et al. 1966; PASTORE et al. 1976). However, in several studies from tropical countries the abnormalities noted (GANGAROSA et al. 1960; SPRINZ et al. 1962; ASAKURA et al. 1974) are probably not specific to cholera but reflect the wide prevalence of tropical enteropathy.

3.3.2 Tuberculosis

Intestinal tuberculosis primarily affects the distal small intestine and is unlikely to be a common diagnosis in peroral mucosal biopsies of the small intestine. Duodenal tuberculosis is a rare entity and the characteristic features of tuberculosis may be occasionally seen with submucosal caseating tubercles (CHUTTANI 1970).

3.4 Parasitic Diseases

3.4.1 Hook Worm Infestation

Hook worm infestation due to *Ankylostoma duodenale or Necator americanus* is common in many warm moist parts of the world. The infective stage of the parasite develops in faecally contaminated soil, penetrates exposed skin surfaces and ultimately resides in the upper small intestine. The primary pathology resulting from hook worm infestation is iron deficiency anaemia due to blood loss caused by the parasite (MAHAMOOD 1966). There is some controversy as to whether there is an upper small intestinal mucosal lesion due to hook worm infestation. Experimental studies showed that in dogs a severe inflammatory lesion may develop in

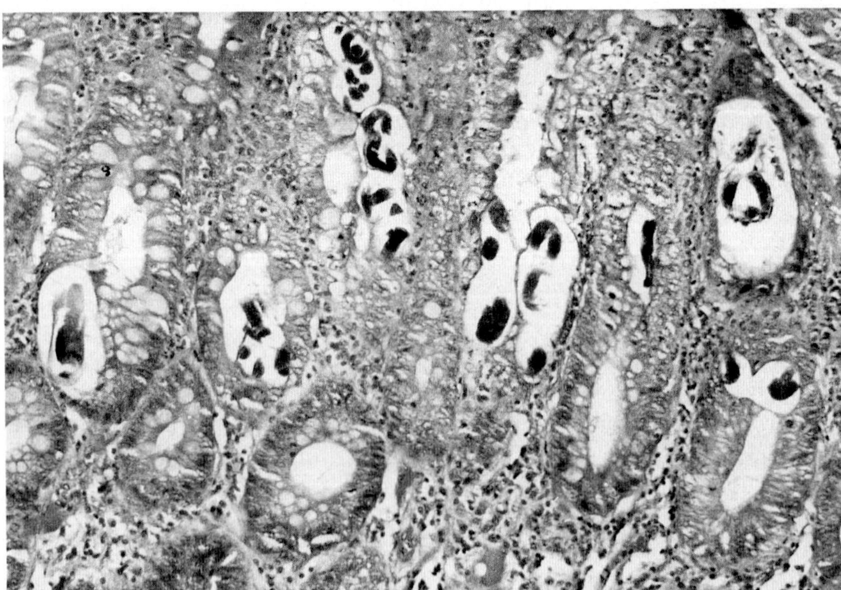

Fig. 3. Jejunal mucosa with many *Strongyloides* larvae, eggs and part of an adult female worm in the crypt region. × 100

the jejunum with marked surface ulceration and infiltration of the epithelium with neutrophils (KALKOFEN 1974). In contrast, several reports of jejunal biopsies from different tropical countries (BANWELL et al. 1967; CHUTTANI et al. 1967; TANDON et al. 1969) have suggested that there are no major histopathological changes in the upper small intestinal mucosa associated with hook worm infestation in the human.

3.4.2 *Strongyloidiasis*

Asymptomatic infestation of the small intestine by the nematode *Strongyloides stercoralis* is prevalent in many tropical countries. The parasite is found in about 8% of jejunal luminal fluid samples at Vellore. It lives mainly in the lumina of crypts and can give rise to chronic diarrhoea and malabsorption. In immunocompromised individuals a fatal hyperinfection may occur (MARCIAL-ROJAS 1975; IGRA-SIEGMAN 1981). The adult female worm penetrates the epithelium and many segmented eggs or larvae may be found in the crypt epithelium and lamina propria in duodenal and jejunal biopsies (Fig. 3). Eosinophils and mononuclear cells constitute the cellular reaction around such worms.

3.4.3 *Capillariasis*

Infestation of the intestine by the nematode, *Capillaria philippinensis* has been reported primarily from Philippines and Thailand. This infestation can also occur in an epidemic form with high mortality. The patients develop diarrhoea and malabsorption with protein losing enteropathy. Jejunal biopsies (WHALEN et al. 1969) show worms penetrating the mucosa but there is no diffuse lesion significantly different from the background tropical enteropathy. In patients who had died, autopsy showed atrophy of the jejunal mucosa with flattened villi, denudation of the epithelium and infiltration of the lamina propria with plasma cells, lymphocytes, macrophages, eosinophils and neutrophil polymorphs (CROSS and BHAIBULAYA 1983). Although these lesions were maximal in the jejunum it is difficult to know whether they represent primary damage caused by the worm or changes consequent upon events of the terminal illness.

3.4.4 *Cryptosporidium*

A monoxenous coccidian parasite of warm-blooded vertebrates, *Cryptosporidium*, is a zoonotic agent found in temperate zones primarily as an opportunistic infection in immuno-incompetent individuals, particularly patients suffering from acquired immune deficiency syndrome (AIDS) (ANGUS 1983; TZIPORI 1983; CURRENT 1984). This parasite has a wide prevalence, both in asymptomatic individuals and in people with acute diar-

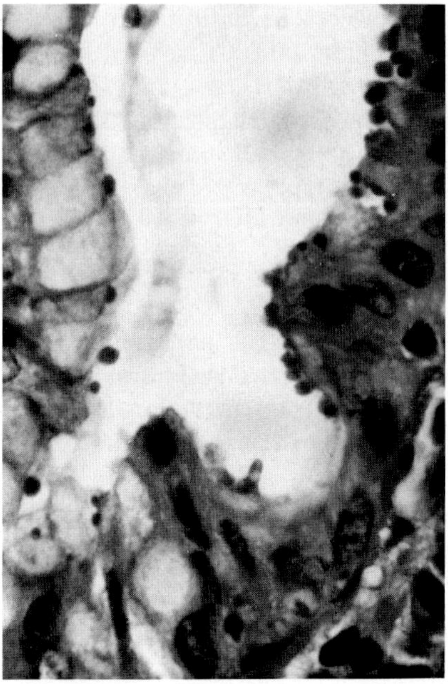
a

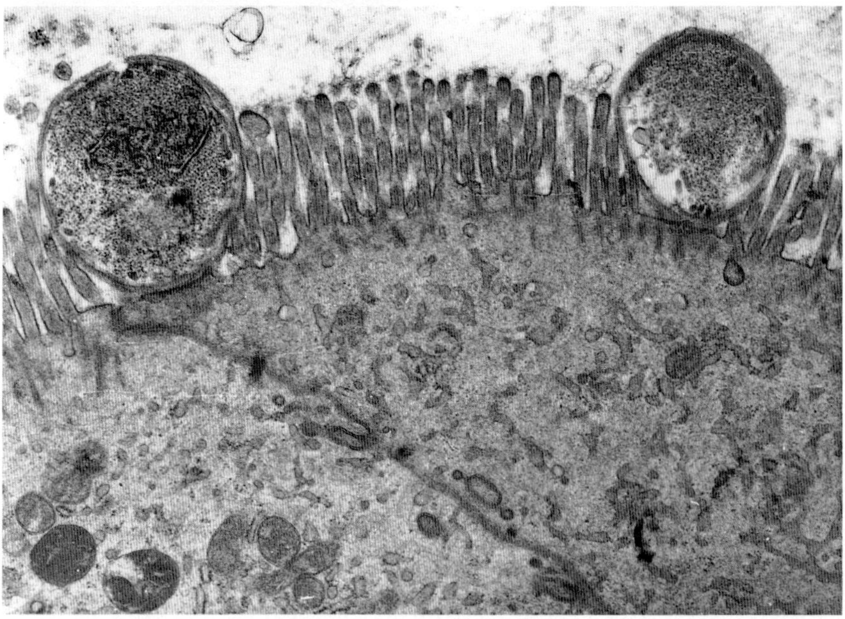
b

Fig. 4. **a** Gastric mucosa with many spherical *Cryptosporidium* attached to the luminal border. × 900. **b** Electron micrograph of jejunal enterocytes with 2 trophozoites of *Cryptosporidium* attached to the luminal border. × 15 000

rhoea, in several tropical countries (MATHAN et al. 1985). *Cryptosporidium* has been found throughout the gastrointestinal tract from the pharynx to the rectum. In severely infested patients at post-mortem the jejunum was most affected. In jejunal biopsies, the histological changes

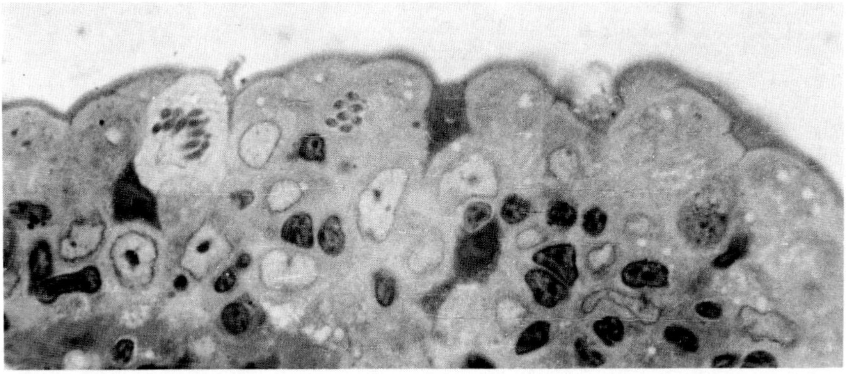

Fig. 5. Jejunal mucosa from a patient with diarrhoea with meronts of Microsporidia supranuclearly. Epon-embedded 1-μm section, toluidine blue. × 1000

are non-specific but the characteristic spherical basophilic structures attached to the microvillus border of the enterocytes are easily recognised (Fig. 4). Electron microscopic examination of jejunal biopsies shows all stages of schizogony and gametogony. The organism is enclosed in a modified epithelial surface membrane and is thus located intracellularly but extracytoplasmically. Adaptive and degenerative changes may be present in the enterocytes (LEFKOWITCH et al. 1984). There may be mild to moderate shortening of villi with increased crypt height and mononuclear infiltration of the lamina propria (CASEMORE et al. 1985).

3.4.5 Microsporidia

The Microsporidia are primitive coccidian parasites, primarily of invertebrates and fish, but are now being recognised in mammals. There are a large number of species of this parasite and one species, *Enterocytozoon bieneusi*, has now been reported from AIDS patients (CANNING and HOLLISTER 1987). It is an obligatory intracellular parasite and structures morphologically resembling these may occasionally be found within enterocytes in jejunal biopsies in the tropics (Fig. 5).

3.4.6 Kala Azar

Visceral leishmaniasis is widely prevalent in South America, the Mediterranean basin and large parts of Asia and Africa. Endemic for many years in India, kala azar has now assumed epidemic proportions in the Gangetic plain. The illness usually presents with prolonged pyrexia and marked splenomegaly and is primarily an infection of the reticulo-endothelial system. Leishman-Donovan (LD) bodies (the leishmanial form of the parasite) may be present in lamina propria histiocytes in gastric and jejunal

a

b

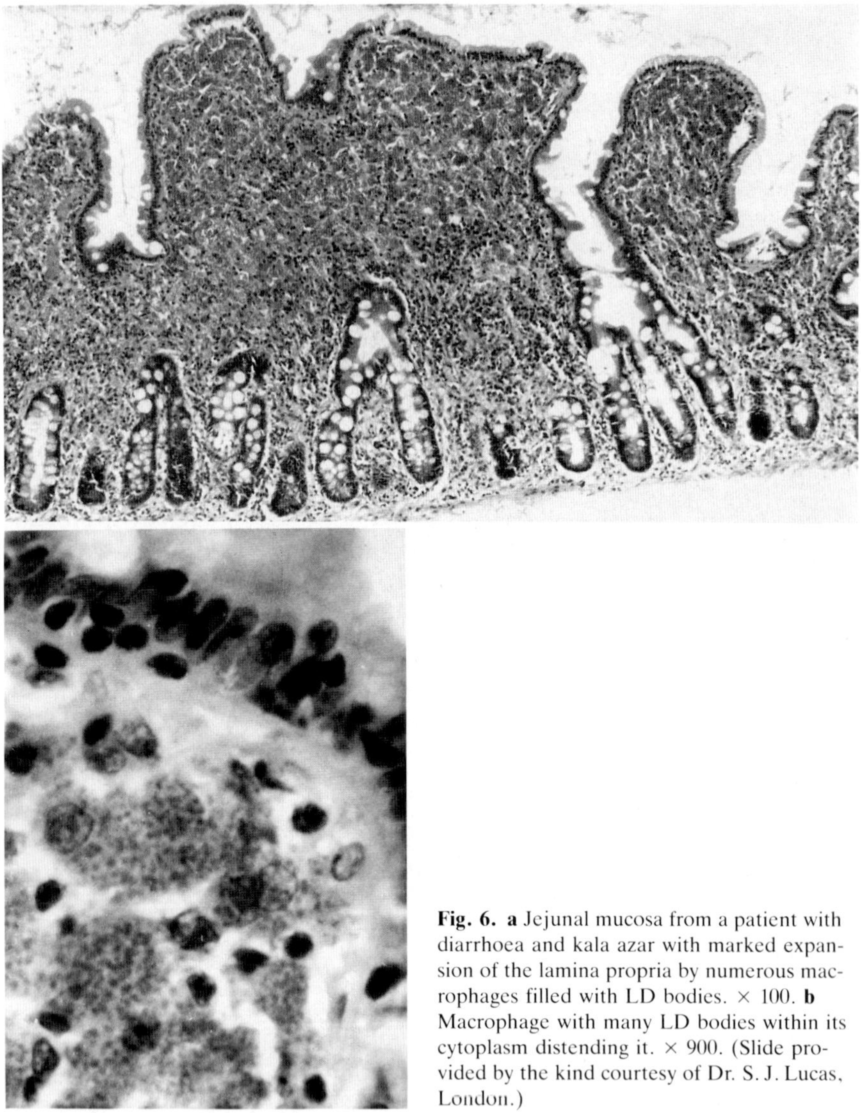

Fig. 6. **a** Jejunal mucosa from a patient with diarrhoea and kala azar with marked expansion of the lamina propria by numerous macrophages filled with LD bodies. × 100. **b** Macrophage with many LD bodies within its cytoplasm distending it. × 900. (Slide provided by the kind courtesy of Dr. S. J. Lucas, London.)

biopsies (Fig. 6). The LD bodies are 2–4.5 μm by 1–2.5 μm, oval or round structures with oval nuclei applied to the more convex ventral border. In severe cases diarrhoea may be present and enlarged villi with focal ulceration are scattered in the mucosa (EDDINGTON and GILLES 1969).

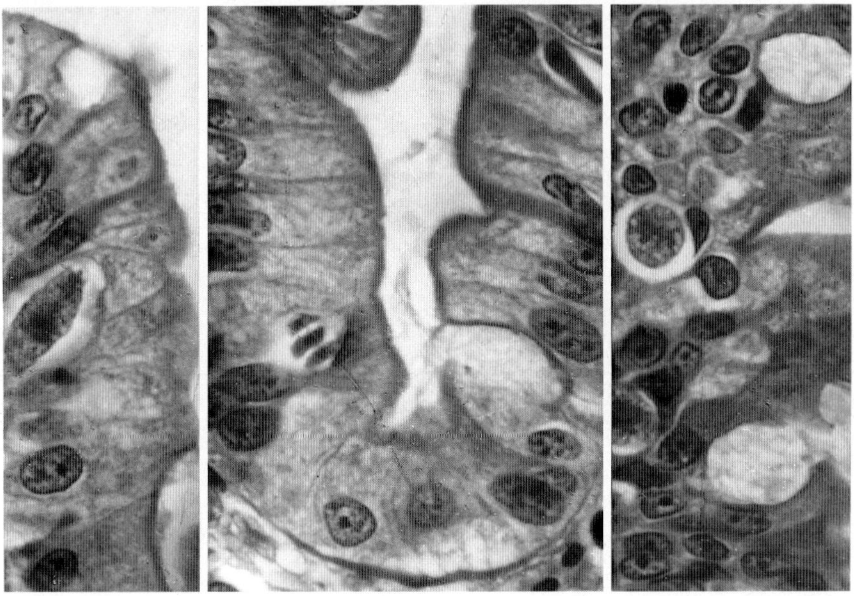

a b c

Fig. 7 a–c. Stages of development of *Isospora* in jejunal mucosa of a patient with malabsorption. **a** Immature schizont. **b** Mature schizont with merozoites. **c** Oocyst in parasitophorous vacuole. × 900

3.4.7 Coccidiosis

Gastrointestinal infection with two species of coccidia, *Isospora belli* and *I. hominis*, primarily parasites of the small intestinal epithelium in humans, is a cause of chronic diarrhoea and malabsorption in tropical and temperate climates. The parasite is present within or just below the villous epithelium and can be better identified with overstained Giemsa or haematoxylin-eosin-alcian blue stains (Brandborg et al. 1979). All stages of schizogony and gametogony (Fig. 7), including trophozoites, schizonts, merozoites, micro- and macrogametes and unsporulated oocysts, may be recognised in biopsies (Trier et al. 1974) and oocysts in duodenal luminal fluid.

3.4.8 Sarcosporidiosis

Human intestinal sarcosporidiosis has been reported from Thailand, particularly among people who eat undercooked beef (Bunyaratvej et al. 1982). The patients usually present with fever and acute abdominal pain as well as leucocytosis. Severe cases are characterised by necrotising enteritis of the jejunum and ileum with heavy eosinophilic infiltration. The sexual forms of Sarcosporidia are found in the epithelium (Fig. 8).

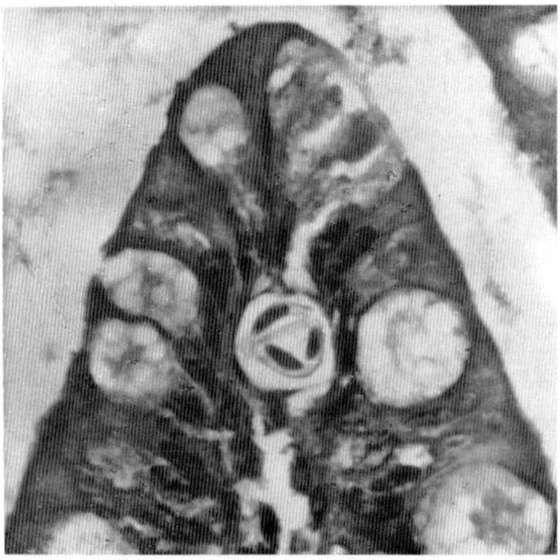

Fig. 8. Jejunal mucosa from a patient with segmental enteritis due to sarcosporidiosis with subepithelial sporocyst containing sporozoites. × 900. (Slide provided by kind courtesy of Dr. S. Bunyaratvej, Bangkok.)

3.4.9 Giardiasis

The protozoan parasite *Giardia lamblia* is worldwide in its distribution and it has been suggested that it may be the most frequent intestinal pathogen associated with diarrhoea in industrialised countries (SMITH and WOLFE 1980). In many tropical areas it is widely prevalent (30%–40%) in asymptomatic individuals (GILMAN et al. 1985). Giemsa-stained smears of the intestinal luminal fluid or the mucus associated with jejunal biopsies are particularly useful for detecting these parasites, which are pear shaped with the broad rounded anterior end containing two nuclei. Phosphotungstic acid or Giemsa stains demonstrate the organisms in the intervillus space in sections better than do haematoxylin and eosin stains. The jejunal mucosa of asymptomatic individuals harbouring the parasite may not show any significant abnormality although damage to microvilli, felt to be caused by the suction disc of the parasite, has been documented (TANDON et al. 1974) (Fig. 9). The most consistent abnormality in symptomatic individuals is an increase in epithelial lymphocytes (WRIGHT and TOMKINS 1977; ROSEKRANS et al. 1981). *G. lamblia* is frequently associated with immunoglobulin deficiency and nodular lymphoid hyperplasia in the upper small intestine. Jejunal biopsies from such individuals show marked abnormalities which are probably related to the underlying disease (ROSS and MATHAN 1987).

3.5 Tropical Sprue

Tropical sprue is a primary malabsorption syndrome which affects residents of and visitors to several tropical regions (MATHAN 1988). While it has not yet been fully documented from subsaharan Africa it is widely prevalent in India and Southeast Asia as well as in many of the Caribbean

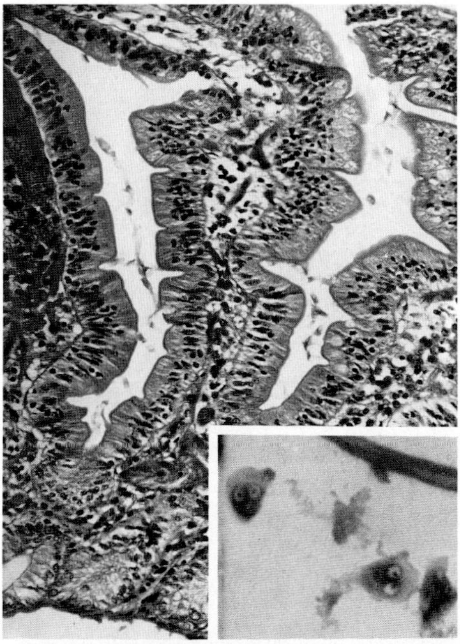

a

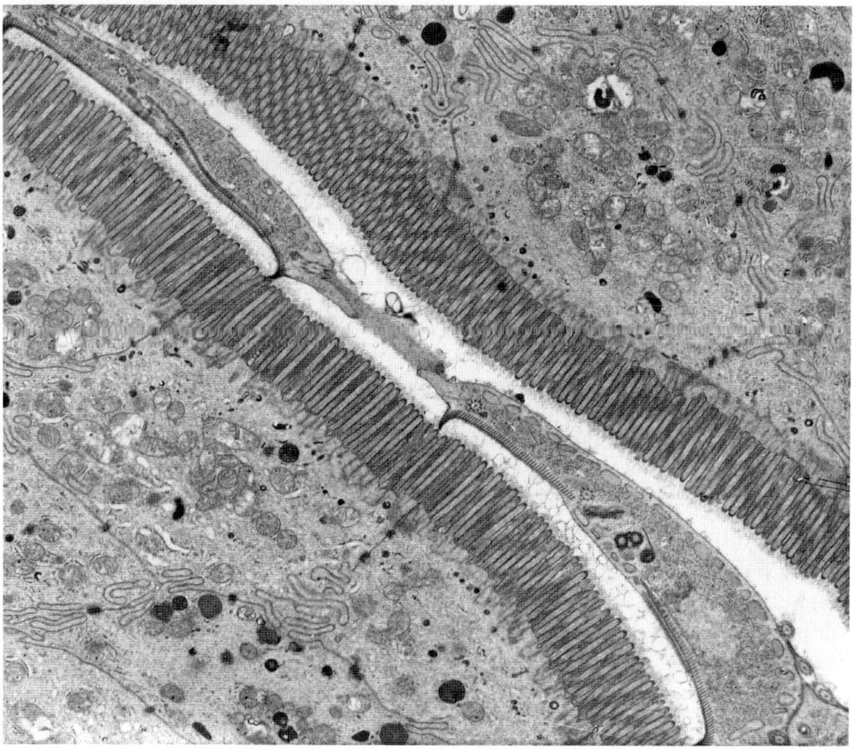

b

Fig. 9. a Jejunal mucosa with many giardial trophozoites in the intervillous space, × 150. *Inset* shows giardia with characteristic pear shape and two prominent nuclei in its anterior end, × 900. **b** Electron micrograph of giardial trophozoites adherent to each other and anchored on the microvilli by their suction discs. × 7050

a

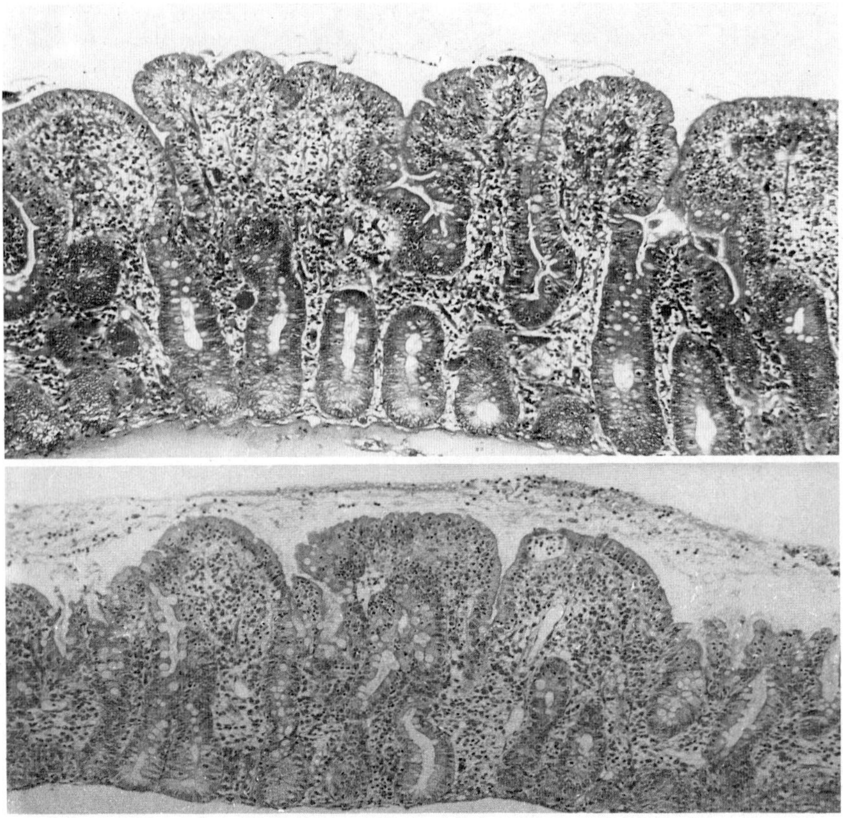

b

Fig. 10. **a** Jejunal mucosa from a patient with tropical sprue with moderate change showing increase in crypt height and shortening of villi. The cellularity of the epithelium and lamina propria is increased. × 100. **b** Jejunal mucosa from a sprue patient with severe change showing decrease in total height with more prominent decrease in villous height and increased cellularity of lamina propria. × 100

islands. As early as 1914 it was suggested, by examination of autopsy material, that the primary lesion in tropical sprue involved the small intestinal mucosa. Subsequent to the availability of peroral intestinal biopsy instruments, the morphological alterations in the jejunal mucosa in tropical sprue have been described extensively (SCHENK et al. 1965; SWANSON and THOMASSEN 1965). However, even now tropical sprue is a diagnosis of exclusion in a patient with malabsorption syndrome, where the many conditions which give rise to secondary malabsorption have been ruled out (MATHAN 1988).

Sections of jejunal biopsies show varying degrees of increase in the thickness of the crypts and shortening and distortion of villi (Fig. 10). Partial villous atrophy has been the term used to describe these changes but since the morphogenesis of the lesion occurs by primary damage to the

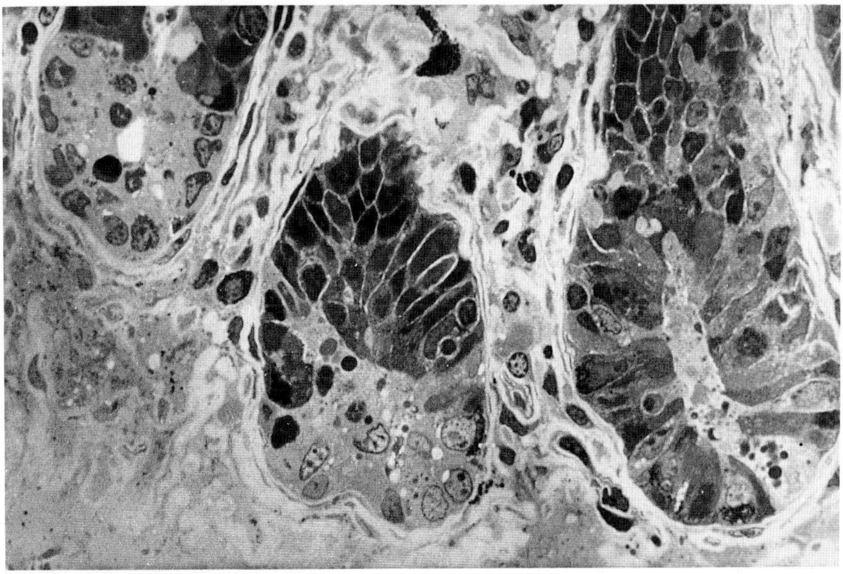

Fig. 11. Resin-embedded 1-μm section of jejunal mucosa of a patient from an epidemic of tropical sprue. Base of crypt shows focal degeneration of cells. × 750

crypt it is better to avoid this term, which implies a primary lesion in villi (MATHAN et al. 1986).

Details of enterocyte damage are more apparent when 1-μm sections of plastic-embedded tissue are examined by light microscopy or thin sections are studied in the electron microscope. Damaged enterocytes, with altered brush border, dilated rough endoplasmic reticulum, loss of mitochondrial cristae and marked increase in lysosomes, are scattered throughout the epithelium of the crypt-villus unit. Extrusion of damaged enterocytes, some with poor staining characteristics and others condensed and with pyknotic nuclei, takes place all along the crypt-villus unit and not only at the zone of extrusion at the villus tips (MATHAN et al. 1975). Epithelial lymphocytes are clustered around these damaged cells. Epithelial lymphocytes are increased both in the villus and in the crypt (ROSS and MATHAN 1981). The initial enterocyte lesion in patients with short duration was not associated with an increase in epithelial lymphocytes, which occurred 3–4 weeks later. The increase in epithelial lymphocytes appears to be secondary to the loss of barrier function consequent to enterocyte damage (MARSH et al. 1983). The basement membrane is thick and fat droplets are present in enterocytes, the basement membrane and superficial layers of the lamina propria, even after a 10-h fast, indicating a defect of fat transport. The cellular infiltrate in the lamina propria, lymphocytes and plasma cells is also increased.

It has been possible to examine jejunal biopsies from patients with very short duration of diarrhoea, affected in epidemics of tropical sprue in southern India (MATHAN and BAKER 1971). The first lesion, detectable within 48 h of onset of diarrhoea, was damage to crypt enterocytes (Fig. 11). At that time surface enterocytes were apparently morphologically intact although the patient had malabsorption. In vitro culture of jejunal biopsies, pulse labelled with ^{3}H-thymidine, with follow-up of migration of the label up the villus for up to 48 h, suggested that increased stem cell turnover and more rapid migration of enterocytes to and loss from the functional compartment, the villus, were characteristic of the established lesion of tropical sprue (MATHAN et al. 1986). These data suggest that the initial lesion, caused by an as yet unidentified agent, occurs in crypt enterocytes. The damaged crypt enterocytes (stem cells) give rise to damaged progeny which migrate and are extruded rapidly from the functional layer in the villi, leading to shortening of the villi. The balance between the extent of the enterocyte stem cell damage, damaged progeny enterocyte loss from the functional compartment, and compensatory increase in proliferation of the stem cells explains the short villi and hypertrophy of the crypts. It is not yet possible, based on published reports from other parts of the world, to say whether the crypt lesion which has been described in tropical sprue in southern India occurs elsewhere.

3.6 Immunoproliferative Small Intestinal Disease

Originally known as the Mediterranean type of lymphoma, and later alpha heavy chain disease, because of the abnormal monoclonal gammopathy which many of these patients develop, this disease is now recognised as an abnormality of the gut-associated lymphoid tissue (ISAACSON 1985) (see also page 143). In addition to the Mediterranean region and the Middle East, immunoproliferative small intestinal disease (IPSID) has been reported from several other tropical regions. Histologically three stages in the evolution of the lymphoma have been described. Infiltration of the lamina propria by plasma cells without invasion of the crypts occurs in stage A. In stage B the appearance of a band-like or nodular lymphoid infiltrate composed of a mixture of lymphocytes, centrocytes and centroblasts in the lower part of the lamina propria is the characteristic finding. Cells from this lymphoid infiltrate may invade and destroy the jejunal crypts, forming typical lympho-epithelial lesions (ISAACSON and SPENCER 1987). Plasma cells are still the predominant cell in the lamina propria, although they are few in the infiltrating nodules, which may resemble lymphoid follicles. A malignant lymphomatous infiltrate involving the submucosa is characteristic of stage C and plasma cells at this stage are much less evident. The histological picture can be quite pleomorphic in these lymphomas, with a predominance of follicle centre-like cells. Since IPSID affects the upper small intestine diffusely, per oral jejunal biopsies may be diagnostic (Fig. 12). The demonstration of alpha heavy chains, without light chains, in tissue sections by immunocytochemistry helps to confirm

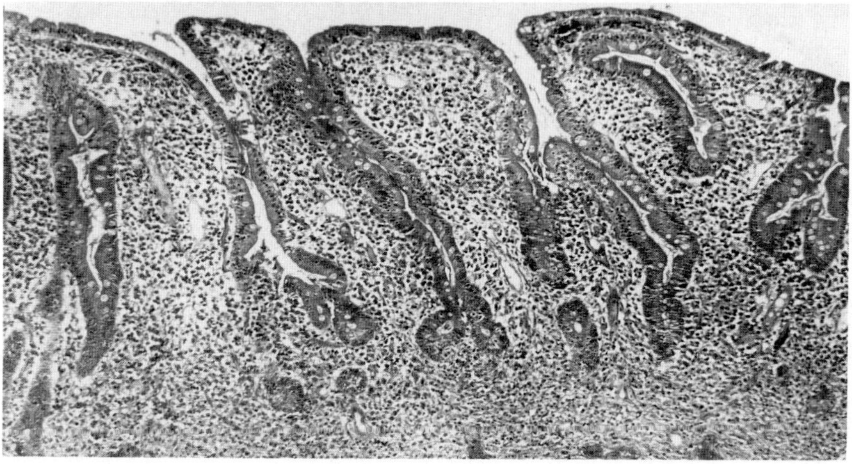

Fig. 12. Jejunal mucosa from a patient with malabsorption. The lamina propria is diffusely infiltrated with mature plasma cells effacing the crypt architecture. Stage A in IPSID. × 100

the diagnosis in stage A. This is particularly useful as long-term antibiotic therapy can arrest or revert the disease at this stage.

4 Large Intestine

4.1 Tropical Colonopathy

Conventional histological examination of rectal mucosal biopsies from residents of tropical countries does not show striking changes similar to those of tropical enteropathy in the jejunum. However, a detailed study of the ultrastructural morphology of rectal biopsies at Vellore showed an increase in lysosomes, electron dense bodies and vesicles in both crypt and surface colonocytes (Fig. 13). In comparison with biopsies from volunteers in temperate climates the surface colonocytes were shorter, with short, irregularly grouped microvilli and poor plication of lateral cell membranes indicating immaturity. There were also alterations in goblet cell mucus granules, a reticulohistiocytic response in the subluminal lamina propria and evidence of vascular damage. These changes in biopsies from "normal" subjects in the tropics suggested a response to non-specific damage (MATHAN and MATHAN 1985 a).

Another striking finding was the wide prevalence of spiral organisms attached to the apical border of luminal colonocytes (spirochaetosis). In contrast to temperate zones (see page 249), where spiral organisms are found in about 2%–3% of biopsies from controls, similar bacteria were present in 66% of asymptomatic individuals in southern India.

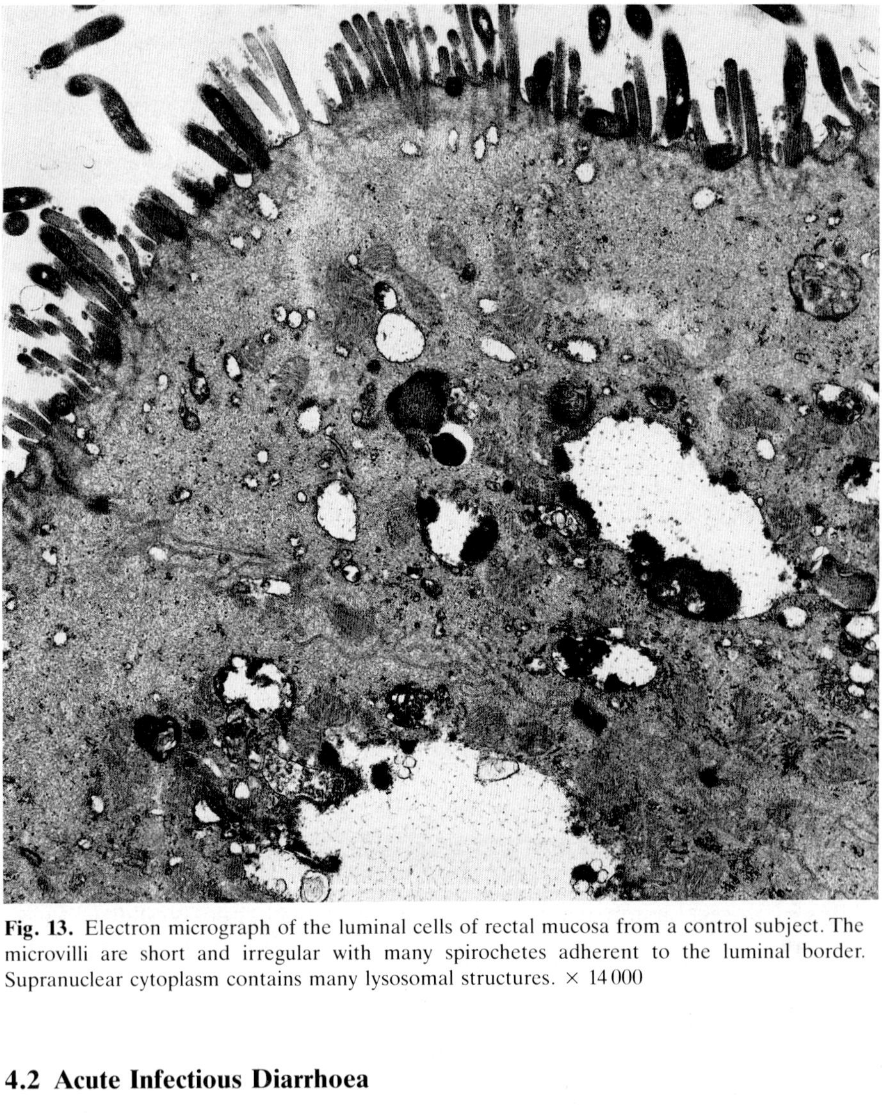

Fig. 13. Electron micrograph of the luminal cells of rectal mucosa from a control subject. The microvilli are short and irregular with many spirochetes adherent to the luminal border. Supranuclear cytoplasm contains many lysosomal structures. × 14000

4.2 Acute Infectious Diarrhoea

Intestinal mucosal biopsies are not part of the regular work-up of acute infectious diarrhoea. The majority of patients can be diagnosed on clinical grounds associated with appropriate microbiological investigation. Two recent developments, the recognition of acute self-limited colitis and the increasing frequency with which idiopathic inflammatory bowel disease (IBD) is being diagnosed in tropical countries, make it necessary to define clearly the rectal mucosal histopathological features of a variety of acute diarrhoeal diseases.

4.2.1 Watery Diarrhoea

Infection by enterotoxigenic bacteria [*V. cholera*, heat labile (LT) and heat stable (ST) toxin-producing coliforms, entero-adhesive *E. coli* etc.] is the classical example of infectious diarrhoea with large watery stools. The primary site of action of the enterotoxins is in the small intestine and the large volume of fluid secreted overwhelms the absorptive capacity of the colon, giving rise to diarrhoea. The architecture of colonocytes is preserved in these conditions although evidence of increased water absorption with oedema of the lamina propria may be present. A lamina propria vascular lesion (see below) may also occur (MATHAN and MATHAN 1985 b).

4.2.2 The Dysenteries

It is particularly important to differentiate IBD from the dysenteries, the result of invasive damage of the colonic mucosa by bacteria and parasites.

4.2.2.1 Bacterial Dysenteries

Histological examination of rectal mucosal biopsies from 37 patients from whom a pure culture of *Shigella* was obtained (ANAND et al. 1986) showed a mixed round cell and polymorphonuclear, or a predominantly round cell,

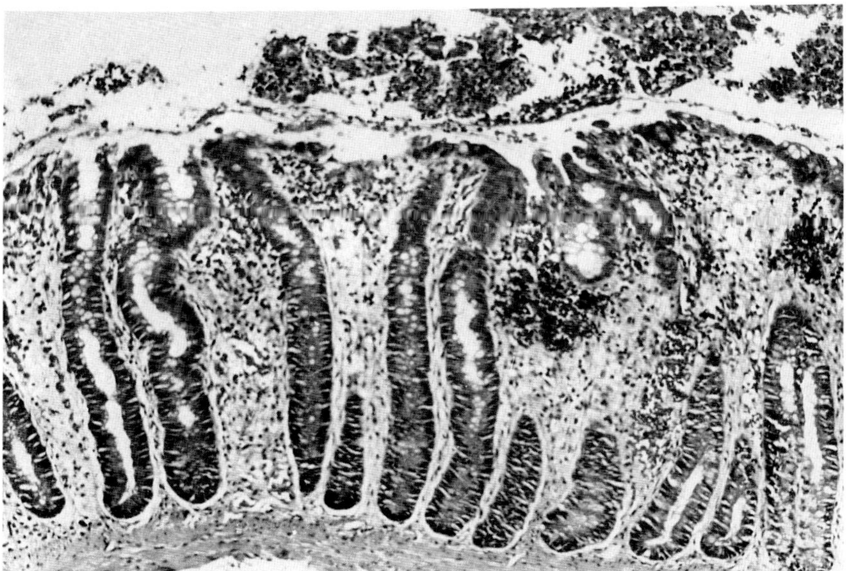

Fig. 14. Patient with acute colitis due to *Shigella* infection. There is marked mucus depletion and focal ulceration with a luminal inflammatory exudate. The lamina propria shows oedema, multiple focal haemorrhages and increased neutrophil polymorphs, plasma cells and lymphocytes. × 100

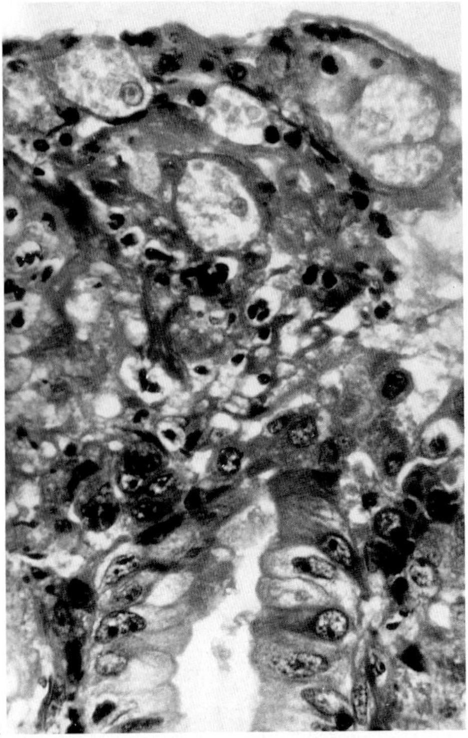

a

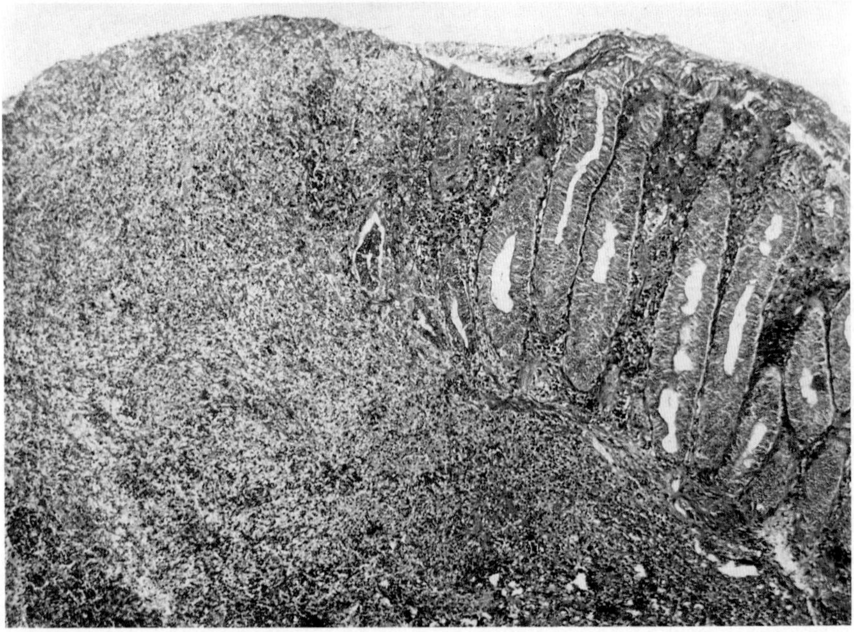

b

Fig. 15. **a** Rectal mucosal biopsy from a patient with amoebic colitis. The superficial mucosa shows cell necrosis and is covered by an exudate with many neutrophils and trophozoites of *Entamoeba histolytica*. × 650. **b** Rectal mucosal biopsy from the edge of an undermined ulcer in amoebic colitis with edges covered by necrotic tissue and acute inflammatory exudate. A few scattered amoebae are present at the junction of necrotic tissue and mucosa. The adjacent mucosa shows marked mucus depletion. × 100

infiltrate extending into the muscularis mucosae and submucosa, oedema of the muscularis mucosa and submucosa, and mild disorganisation of the crypts. The mucosal abnormalities were maximal in patients from whom *S. dysenteriae* was isolated and milder in patients with non-bloody diarrhoea (Fig. 14). At colonoscopy the lesions mainly affect the distal colon (SPEELMAN et al. 1984). Ultrastructural studies (MATHAN and MATHAN 1986) showed colonocyte damage and ulceration due to invasion by shigellae, as well as a lamina propria vascular lesion (see below). Longer duration of symptoms was associated with features suggesting relative vascular insufficiency, lymphocyte activation, eosinophil and mast cell degranulation and the possibility of antibody-mediated colonocyte damage.

Similar features are present in dysentery associated with *Salmonella* and *Campylobacter* infection, but to a lesser extent.

4.2.2.2 Parasitic Dysenteries

Amoebic dysentery is the prototype of the parasitic dysenteries and can produce lesions in the entire colon and terminal ileum, commonly in the caecum, rectosigmoid and hepatic flexure (HARRIES 1982). Several types of gross pathological changes have been described but the histological diagnosis is facilitated by the detection of *Entamoeba histolytica* (EH), which can be differentiated from other amoebae and macrophages by the characteristic erythrophagocytosis and the round nucleus with a central karyosome (GILMAN and PRATHAP 1971). In tissue sections PAS and iron stains help to distinguish EH from tissue macrophages. In early lesions, which appear as minute superficial ulcers at sigmoidoscopy, many EH may be present and small superficial ulcers with subjacent acute inflammation can be seen in tissue sections. The more established lesions are associated with flask-shaped ulcers with undermined edges and submucosal extension (Fig. 15). EH are fewer in such lesions (PRATHAP and GILMAN 1970). Amoebic granulomas may mimic carcinoma of the colon but can be distinguished in colonoscopic biopsies (KAUSHIK et al. 1973).

Other parasitic disorders that may give rise to dysenteries are associated with schistosomiasis and infection by *Balantidium coli*. Concentric fibrosis around degenerated schistosome eggs in the submucosa, with eosinophils, lymphocytes and macrophages, is diagnostic of *S. mansoni* and *S. japonicum* (Fig. 16) (GAMBESCIA et al. 1976; NASH et al. 1982). *B. coli* dysentery is rare. Superficial ulcers covered by large saccular trophozoites, containing red blood cells and other ingested debris with large kidney-shaped nucleus and numerous cilia, is diagnostic (CASTRO et al. 1983).

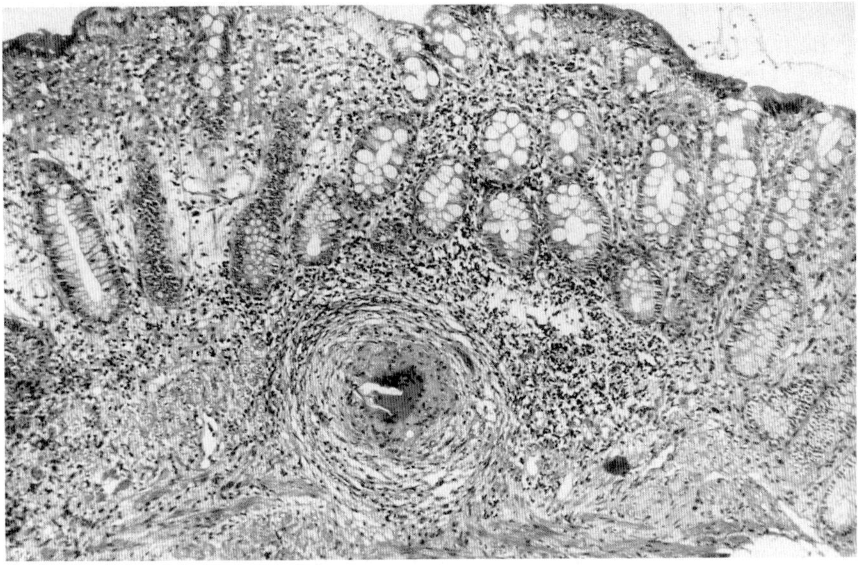

Fig. 16. Rectal mucosal biopsy from a patient with a rectal stricture. The submucosa shows a granuloma with concentric fibrosis around degenerating schistosome eggs. × 100

4.2.3 Differentiation of Idiopathic Inflammatory Bowel Disease from Acute Self-limited Colitis

Acute self-limited colitis is a transient, presumably infectious, colonic inflammation presenting usually with the sudden onset of bloody diarrhoea and recovering in under 1 month. A proportion of patients with *Salmonella* and *Shigella* colitis in tropical countries have symptoms persistent for up to a month (MATHAN et al. 1984). In the last 10 years IBD has been diagnosed in over 150 patients in this centre and the frequency of detection of new patients is increasing.

Studies from temperate climates suggest that crypt atrophy, distorted crypt architecture, increased number of round cells and neutrophils in the lamina propria, a villus surface epithelium, basal lymphoid aggregations, granulomas and isolated giant cells are helpful in distinguishing IBD from infective self-limited colitis (DICKINSON et al. 1979; MANDAL et al. 1982; KUMAR et al. 1982; SURAWICZ and BELIC 1984). Plasmacytosis in the lamina propria extending to the mucosal base with distortion of the crypt architecture is also suggested as diagnostic of ulcerative colitis (NOSTRAND et al. 1987).

In evaluating biopsies from tropical countries these features are useful but the presence of a mixed infiltrate in the lamina propria even in *S. dysenteriae* infections (ANAND et al. 1986) and the altered immune response in such populations, with many plasma cells in the lamina propria, has to be kept in mind (CHOUDARI et al. 1985). The extent and severity of

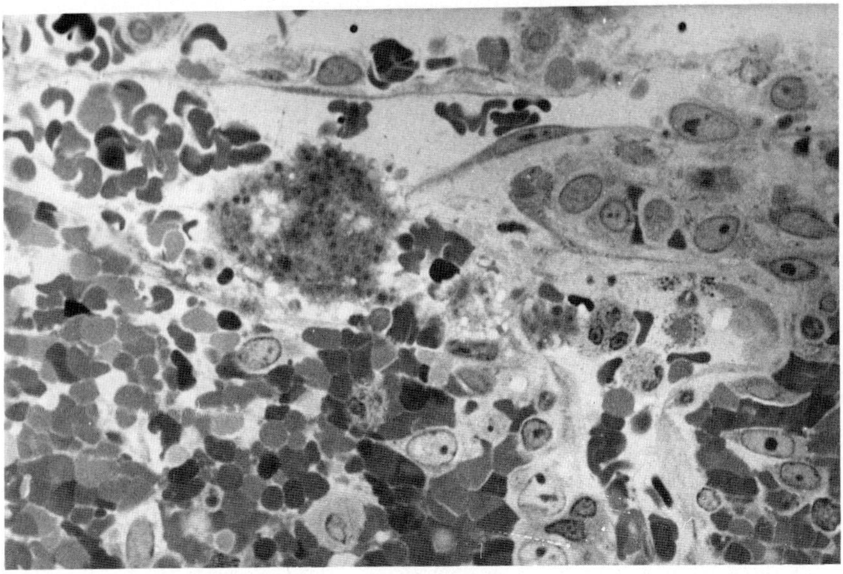

Fig. 17. Resin-embedded tissue of rectal mucosa from *Shigella* colitis. The lamina propria blood vessel shows total denudation of endothelium in the upper part while the remaining endothelial cells show swelling. The vascular lumen contains platelet thrombi and many polymorphs. Marked haemorrhage into the lamina propria is seen with distorted and de-haemoglobinised red blood cells. Toluidine blue, × 950

the changes associated with acute infective colitis depend on the duration of illness. Some of the features that help in the differentiation are the minimal amount of architectural distortion and disproportionately increased oedema and haemorrhage in the lamina propria compared to the extent of the inflammatory exudate. Epithelial cell regeneration is more rapid, with increased mitosis and signs of cellular immaturity, than in patients with ulcerative colitis.

4.2.4 *Lamina Propria Vascular Lesion*

Focal deep or pericryptal haemorrhage was a striking feature in rectal mucosal biopsies of an unselected group of adults with acute undifferentiated diarrhoea in southern India (CHOUDARI et al. 1985). The prevalence of these haemorrhages was unrelated to the pathogen isolated from the patient but was associated with a vascular lesion with endothelial damage (Fig. 17). Ultrastructural studies showed that a lesion resembling a local Shwartzman reaction was present in many of the lamina propria blood vessels (MATHAN and MATHAN 1985 b). The prevalence of this lesion correlated well with the clinical severity of illness and not with any aetiological agent. These findings suggest that bacterial lipopolysaccharide (endotoxin) may also play a role in the pathogenesis of acute diarrhoea in tropical countries.

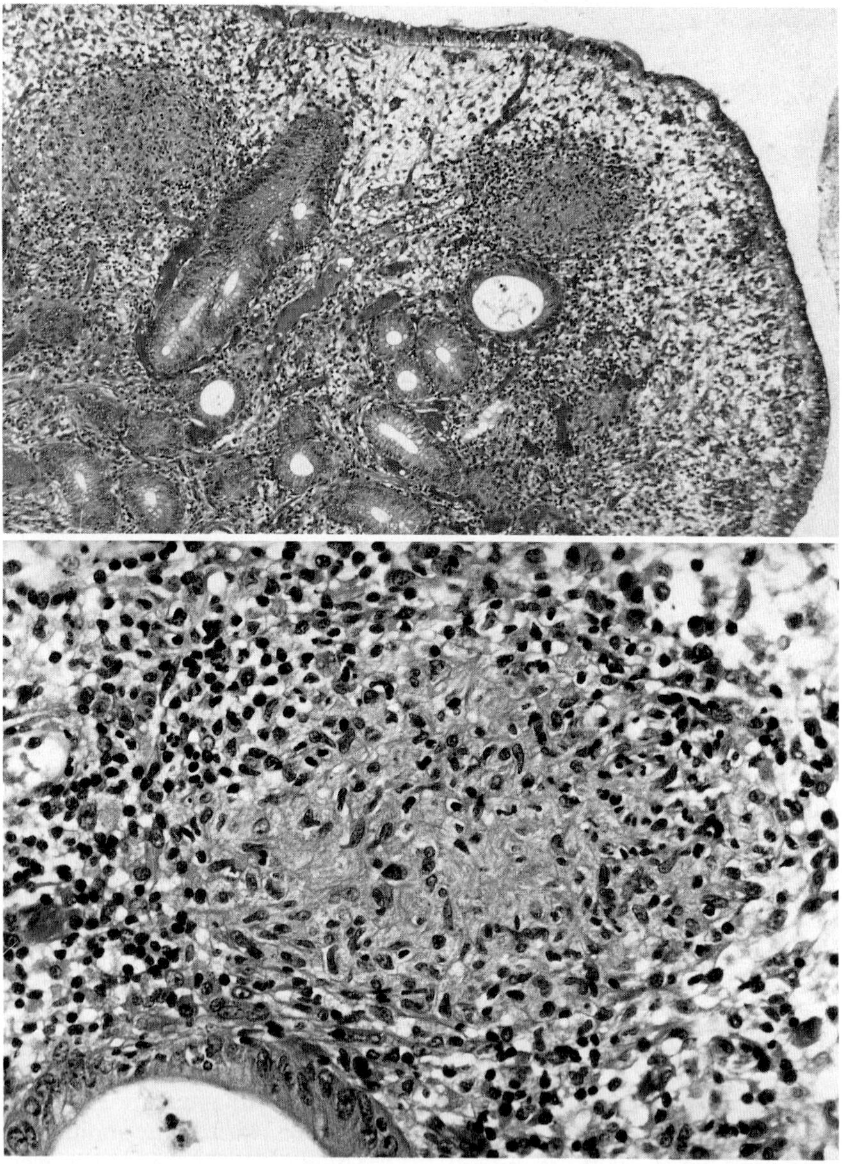

a

b

Fig. 18. **a** Colonic mucosal biopsy from a patient with segmental colonic tuberculosis. Lamina propria shows multiple granulomas. × 80. **b** Granuloma composed of epithelioid cells surrounded by lymphocytes. × 370

4.3 Tuberculosis

The facility with which mucosal samples of the colon, caecum and even the terminal ileum can be obtained by colonoscopy has made biopsies from ulceroconstrictive lesions of the colon and hypertrophic lesions of the caecum and terminal ileum an important diagnostic aid. The colonoscopic biopsy diagnosis of a tuberculous lesion helps the early institution of appropriate therapy and avoids unnecessary laparotomies and resections. The majority of available literature on the pathology of colonic and ileocaecal tuberculosis is based on the study of resected specimens (CHAWLA et al. 1971; VAIDYA and SODHI 1978; TANDON and PRAKASH 1972). Although there are isolated reports of cases of colonic tuberculosis diagnosed at colonoscopy (FRANKLIN et al. 1979; EHSANNULLAH et al. 1984), diagnosis is still often made after resection (KNUTSON and AROSENIUS 1984).

In 11 proven cases of ileocaecal tuberculosis, colonoscopy showed deformed ileocaecal valves in all and a contracted caecal lumen in ten (BHARGAVA et al. 1985). Typical granulomas were found in biopsies from only three and *M. tuberculosis* was isolated on culture from a further four patients. However, a non-specific infiltration of the mucosa by inflammatory cells was found in all the patients. Biopsies from a total of 31 patients with colonic tuberculosis were studied at Vellore between 1980 and 1986. Nine of these had isolated colonic tuberculosis and 22 ileocaecal tuberculosis. The disease was confined to the ileocaecal region alone in only 8 of these 22 patients; in the others it extended to the ascending colon (9 patients) or was associated with segmental involvement in the transverse or sigmoid colon. Granulomas with or without Langhans type giant cells were present in biopsies from 21 of the 31 patients while the others had chronic inflammatory infiltrate without granulomas or caseation (Fig. 18). Colonoscopic biopsies are small and seldom obtain tissue deep within the submucosa. A higher yield can be expected if repeated biopsies are done at the same site to obtain deeper tissue. This technique enabled confirmation of the diagnosis in nearly two-thirds of suspected cases at Vellore.

5 Conclusion

The availability of peroral biopsy instruments for the small intestine and endoscopic biopsy of stomach, duodenum, colon, caecum and terminal ileum has made a variety of gastrointestinal mucosal samples available for histopathological examination. In the tropics interpretation of such biopsies has to be done in the light of the prevalence of tropical enteropathy and colonopathy. In addition to enabling the diagnosis of a variety of infective and parasitic conditions the examination of such biopsies by the electron microscope provides valuable clues to the pathogenesis of the diseases.

Acknowledgment. The authors' work is supported by the Wellcome Trust, London.

References

Anand BS, Malhotra V, Bhattacharya SK et al. (1986) Rectal histology in acute bacillary dysentery. Gastroenterology 90:654–660

Angus KW (1983) Cryptosporidiosis in man, domestic animals and birds: a review. J R Soc Med 76:62–70

Asakura H, Tsuchiya M, Watanabe Y et al. (1974) Electron microscopic study on the jejunal mucosa in human cholera. Gut 15:531–544

Baker SJ (1973) Geographical variations in the morphology of the small intestinal mucosa in apparently healthy individuals. Pathol Microbiol 39:222–237

Baker SJ, Mathan VI (1972) Tropical enteropathy and tropical sprue. Am J Clin Nutr 25:1047–1050

Baker SJ, Ignatius M, Mathan VI, Vaish SK, Chacko CJG (1962) Intestinal biopsy in tropical sprue. In: Wolstenhome GEW, Cameron MP (eds) Intestinal Biopsy. Ciba Foundation Study Group No. 14. Little Brown, Boston, pp 84–99

Banwell JG, Marsden PD, Blackman V, Leonard PJ, Hutt MSR (1967) Hookworm infection and intestinal absorption amongst Africans in Uganda. Am J trop Med Hyg 16:304–308

Bhargava DK, Tandon HD, Chawla TC, Shriniwas, Tandon BN, Kapur BML (1985) Diagnosis of ileocecal and colonic tuberculosis by colonoscopy. Gastrointest Endosc 31:68–70

Bhat P, Shanthakumari S, Rajan D, Mathan VI, Kapadia CR, Swarnabai C, Baker SJ (1972) Bacterial flora of the gastrointestinal tract in southern Indian control subjects and patients with tropical sprue. Gastroenterology 62:11–21

Bhat P, Albert MJ, Rajan D, Ponniah J, Mathan VI, Baker SJ (1980) Bacterial flora of the jejunum: a comparison of luminal aspirate and mucosal biopsy. J Med Microbiol 13:247–256

Brandborg LL, Goldberg SB, Breidenbach WC (1979) Human coccidiosis – a possible cause of malabsorption. The life cycle in small bowel mucosal biopsies as a diagnostic feature. N Engl Med J 283:1306–1313

Brunser O, Reid A, Monckeberg F, Maccioni A, Contreras I (1968) Jejunal mucosa in infant malnutrition. Am J Clin Nutr 21:976–983

Bunyaratvej S, Bunyawongwiroj P, Nitiyanant P (1982) Human intestinal sarcosporidiosis: report of six cases. Am J Trop Med Hyg 31:36–41

Canning EU, Hollister WS (1987) Microsporidia of mammals – widespread pathogens or opportunistic curiosities? Parasitol Today 3:267–273

Casemore DP, Sands RL, Curry A (1985) *Cryptosporidium* species: a "new" human pathogen. J Clin Pathol 38:1321–1336

Castro J, Vazquez-Iglesias JL, Arnal-Monreal F (1983) Dysentery caused by *Balantidium coli* – report of two cases. Endoscopy 15: 272–274

Chacko CJG, Paulson KA, Mathan VI, Baker SJ (1968) The villus architecture of the small intestine in the tropics: a necropsy study. J Pathol 98:146–151

Chacko CJG, Mathan VI, Baker SJ (1969) Changes in the mucosal pattern of isolated loops of jejunum in Albino rats. Br J Exp Pathol XLIX: 40–43

Chacko A, Begum A, Mathan VI (1984) Absorption of nutrient energy in Southern indian control subjects and patients with tropical sprue. Am J Clin Nutr 40:771–775

Chawla S, Mukerjee P, Bery K (1971) Segmental tuberculosis of the colon. Clin Radiol 22:104–109

Choudari CP, Mathan M, Rajan DP, Raghavan R, Mathan VI (1985) A correlative study of etiology, clinical features and rectal mucosal pathology in adults with acute infectious diarrhea in southern India. Pathology 17:443–450

Chuttani HK (1970) Intestinal tuberculosis. In: Card WI, Creamer B (eds) Modern trends in gastroenterology, Butterworth, London, pp 308–327

Chuttani HK, Puri SK, Misra RC (1967) Small intestine in hookworm disease. Gastroenterology 53:381–388

Cross JH, Bhaibulaya M (1983) Intestinal capillariasis in the Philippines and Thailand. In:

Croll NA, Cross JA (eds) Human ecology and infectious diseases. Academic Press, Orlando, pp 103–136

Current WL (1984) *Cryptosporidium* and cryptosporidiosis. In: Acquired immune deficiency syndrome. Alan R. Liss, New York, pp 355–373

Deo MG, Ramalingaswamg (1965) Reaction of the small intestine to induced protein malnutrition in rhesus monkeys. A study of cell population kinetics in the jejunum. Gastroenterology 49:150–157

Desai HG, Chitale A, Purandare SM, Kumar A, Antia FP (1977) Histological and functional studies of the gastric mucosa in duodenal ulcer. Indian J Med Res 65:236–240

Dickinson RJ, Gilmour HM, McClelland DBL (1979) Rectal biopsy in patients presenting to an infectious disease unit with diarrhoeal disease. Gut 20:141–148

Eddington GM, Gilles GM (1969) Pathology in the tropics. Edward Arnold, London, pp 45–57

Ehsannulah M, Isaacs A, Filipe IM, Gazzard BG (1984) Tuberculosis presenting as inflammatory bowel disease. Report on two cases. Dis Colon Rectum 27:134–136

Franklin GO, Mohapatra M, Perrillo RP (1979) Colonic tuberculosis diagnosed by colonoscopic biopsy. Gastroenterology 76:362–364

Fresh JW, Versage P, Reyes V (1964) Intestinal morphology in human and experimental cholera. Arch Pathol 77:529–537

Gambesicia RA, Kaufman B, Noay J, Young J, Tedesco FJ (1976) *Schistosoma mansoni* infection of the colon: a case report and review of the late colonic manifestations. Dig Dis Sci 21:988–991

Gangarosa EJ, Beisel WR, Benyajati C, Sprinz H, Piyarian P (1960) The nature of the gastrointestinal lesion in Asiatic cholera and its relation to pathogenesis; a biopsy study. Am J Trop Med 9:125–135

Gilman RH, Prathap K (1971) Acute intestinal amoebiasis – proctoscopic appearances with histopathological correlation. Ann Trop Med Parasitol 65:359–365

Gilman RH, Brown KH, Visweswana GS, Mondal G, Greenberg B, Sack RB, Brandt F, Khan MU (1986) Epidemiology and serology of Giardia lamblia in a developing country; Bangladesh. Trans Roy Soc Trop Med Hyg 79:469–473

Harries J (1982) Amoebiasis: a review. J R Soc Med 75:190–197

Igra-Siegman Y, Kapila R, Sen P, Kaminski ZC, Louria DB (1981) Syndrome of hyperinfection with *Strongyloides stercoralis*. Rev Infect Dis 3:397–407

Isaacson PG (1985) Middle Eastern intestinal lymphoma. Semin Diagn Pathol 2:210–223

Isaacson PG, Spencer J (1987) Malignant lymphoma of mucosa-associated lymphoid tissue. Histopathology 11:445–462

John TJ (1976) Antibody response of infants in tropics to five doses of oral polio vaccine. Br Med J I:812

Kalkofen UP (1974) Intestinal trauma resulting from feeding activities of *Ancylostoma caninum*. Am J Trop Med Hyg 23:1046–1053

Kaushik SP, Perianayagam WJ, Budhraja SB (1973) Amebic granuloma of the large bowel. Int Surg 58: 715–720

Knutson L, Arosenius KE (1984) Tuberculosis of the large bowel. Report of two cases. Acta Chir Scand 150:345–348

Kumar NB, Nostrant TT, Appelman HD (1982) The histopathologic spectrum of acute self limited colitis (acute infectious-type colitis). Am J Surg Pathol 6:523–529

Lefkowitch JH, Krumholz S, Feng-Chen KC, Griffin P, Despommier D, Brasitus TA (1984) Cryptosporidiosis of the human small intestine. A light and electron microscopic study. Human Pathol 15:746–752

Lindenbaum J, Kent TH, Sprinz H (1966) Malabsorption and jejunitis in American Peace Corps volunteers in Pakistan. Ann Intern Med 65:1201–1207

Mahamood A (1966) Blood loss caused by helminthic infections. Trans R Soc Trop Med Hyg 60:766–769

Mandal BK, Schofield PF, Morson BC (1982) A clinicopathological study of acute colitis: the dilemma of transient colitis syndrome. Scand J Gastroenterol 17:865–869

Marcial-Rojas RA (1975) Strongyloidiasis. In: Marcial-Rojas RA (ed) Pathology of protozoal and helminthic diseases. Krieger, New York, pp 711–733

Marsh MN, Mathan M, Mathan VI (1983) Studies of intestinal lymphoid tissue. VII. The secondary nature of lymphoid cell "activation" in the jejunal lesion of tropical sprue. Am J Pathol 112:302–312

Marshall BH, Warren JR (1984) Unidentified curved bacilli in the stomach of patients with gastritis and peptic ulceration. Lancet I:1311–1315

Mathan M, Mathan VI (1985 a) Rectal mucosal morphologic abnormalities in normal subjects in southern India: a tropical colonopathy? Gut 26:710–717

Mathan M, Mathan VI (1985 b) Local Shwartzman reaction in the rectal mucosa in acute diarrhoea. J Pathol 146:179–187

Mathan M, Mathan VI (1986) Ultrastructural pathology of the rectal mucosa in *Shigella* dysentery. Am J Pathol 123:25–38

Mathan M, Mathan VI, Baker SJ (1975) An electron microscopic study of jejunal mucosal morphology in control subjects and in patients with tropical sprue in southern India. Gastroenterology 68:17–32

Mathan M, Venkatesan S, George R, Mathew M, Mathan VI (1985) *Cryptosporidium* and diarrhoea in southern Indian children. Lancet II:172–175

Mathan M, Ponniah J, Mathan VI (1986) Epithelial cell renewal and turnover and its relationship to morphologic abnormalities in the jejunal mucosa in tropical sprue. Dig Dis Sci 31:586–592

Mathan VI (1988) Tropical sprue in southern India. Trans R Soc Med Hyg (In Press)

Mathan VI, Baker SJ (1971) The epidemiology of tropical sprue. In: Tropical sprue and megaloblastic anaemia. The Wellcome Trust. Churchill Livingstone, Edinburgh, pp 159–188

Mathan VI, Rajan DP (1986) The prevalence of bacterial enteric pathogens in a healthy rural population in southern India. Med Microbiol 22:93–96

Mathan VI, Ponniah J, Mathan M (1982) Tropical enteropathy: an adaptation of the small intestine to accelerated cell loss in 'contaminated' environment. In: Robinson JWL, Dowling RH, Riecken EO (eds) Mechanisms of intestinal adaptation. Falk Symposium 30. MTP Press, Boston, pp 609–610

Mathan VI, Bhat P, Kapadia CR, Ponniah J, Baker SJ (1984) Epidemic dysentery caused by the Shiga bacillus in a southern Indian village. J Diar Dis Res 1:27–32

Nair GB, Bhattacharya SK, Dutta P et al. (1986) *Campylobacter pyloridis* in samples of endoscopic biopsy in patients with upper gastrointestinal tract disease. Indian J Med Res 84:574–576

Nash TE, Cheever AW, Ottesen EA, Cook JA (1982) Schistosome infections in humans: perspectives and recent findings. Ann Intern Med 97:740–754

Nostrand TT, Kumar NB, Appelman HD (1987) Histopathology differentiates acute self-limited colitis from ulcerative colitis. Gastroenterology 92:318–328

Palmer ED (1950) Tuberculosis of the stomach and the stomach in tuberculosis. A review with particular reference to gross pathology and gastroscopic diagnosis. Am J Tuberc 61:116–130

Parrot DMV (1976) The gut as a lymphoid organ. Clin Gastroenterol 5:761–770

Pastore G, Schiraldi G, Fera G, Sforzas E, Schiraldi O (1976) A bioptic study of gastrointestinal mucosa in cholera patients during an epidemic in southern Italy. Dig Dis Sci 21:613–617

Patel JR, Daniel J, Mathan M, Mathan VI (1983) Isolation and identification of enteroviruses from faecal samples in a differentiated epithelial cell line (HRT-18) derived from human rectal carcinoma. J Med Virol 14:255–261

Prathap K, Gilman R (1970) The histopathology of acute intestinal amebiasis. A rectal biopsy study. Am J Pathol 60:229–246

Rajan DP, Mathan VI (1981) Prevalence of *Campylobacter fetus* subsp. *jejuni* in healthy populations in Southern India. J Clin Microbiol 15:749–751

Ramakrishna B, Kurian S, Mathan MM, Bhaktaviziam A (1988) A morphologic study of gastric carcinoma in southern India. J Gastroent Hepat 3:565–571

Rosekrans PCM, Lindeman J, Meijer CJLM (1981) Quantitative histological and immunohistochemical findings in jejunal biopsy specimens in giardiasis. Virchows Archiv [A]393:145–151

Ross IN, Mathan VI (1981) Immunologic alterations in tropical sprue. Q J Med 50:435–449

Ross IN, Mathan VI (1987) Primary immunodeficiency presenting with gastrointestinal disease in the tropoics. J Gastroent Hepat 2:507–516

Schenk EA, Samloff IM, Klipstein FA (1965) Morphologic characteristics of jejunal biopsies in celiac disease and tropical sprue. Am J Pathol 47:765–780

Sheehy TW, Sprinz H, Augerson WS, Formal SB (1966) Laboratory vibrio cholera infection in the United States. JAM 197:321–326

Smith JW, Wolfe MS (1980) Giardiasis. Ann Rev Med 31:373–383

Speelman P, Kabir I, Islam M (1984) Distribution and spread of colonic lesions in shigellosis: a colonoscopic study. J Infect Dis 150:899–903

Sprinz H, Sribhibhadh R, Gangarosa EJ, Benyajati C, Kundel D, Halstead S (1962) Biopsy of small bowel in Thai people, with special reference to recovery from Asiatic cholera and to an itestinal malabsorption syndrome. Am J Clin Pathol 38:43–51

Surawicz CM, Belic L (1984) Rectal biopsy helps to distinguish acute self-limited colitis from idiopathic inflammatory bowel disease. Gastroenterology 86:104–113

Swanson VL, Thomassen RW (1965) Pathology of the jejunal mucosa in tropical sprue. Am J Pathol 46:511–551

Tandon HD, Prakash A (1972) Pathology of intestinal tuberculosis and its distinction from Crohn's disease. Gut 13:260–269

Tandon BN, Kohli RK, Saraya AK, Ramachandran K, Om Prakash (1969) Role of parasites in the pathogenesis of intestinal malabsorption in hookworm disease. Gut 10: 293–298

Tandon BN, Puri BK, Gandhi PC, Tewari SG (1974) Mucosal surface injury of jejunal mucosa in patients with giardiasis: an electron microscopic study. Indian J Med Res 62:1838–1842

Trier JS, Moxey PC, Schimmel EM, Robles E (1974) Chronic intestinal coccidiosis in man: intestinal morphology and response to treatment. Gastroenterology 66:923–935

Tzipori S (1983) Cryptosporidiosis in animals and humans. Microbiol Rev 47:84–96

Vaidya MG, Sodhi JS (1978) Gastrointestinal tract tuberculosis: a study of 102 cases including 55 hemicolectomies. Clin Radiol 29:189–195

Vaish SK, Sampathkumar J, Jacob R, Baker SJ (1967) The stomach in tropical sprue. Gut 6:458–465

Whalen GE, Rosenberg EB, Strickland GT et al. (1969) Intestinal capillariasis. A new disease in man. Lancet I:13–16

Wright SC, Tomkins AM (1977) Quantification of the lymphocytic infiltrate in jejunal epithelium in giardiasis. Clin Exp Immunol 29:408–412

The Gut-Associated Lymphoid Tissue and Its Tumours

D. A. Levison, P. A. Hall, and A. J. Blackshaw

1 Introduction

Our joint experience of primary gut lymphomas is based on studies performed on a series of over 250 cases culled from the files of the Departments of Histopathology of St. Bartholomew's and St. Mark's hospitals, London, England. We attempt, herein, to provide a practical account of present understanding of the pathology of gut lymphomas. This is a rapidly evolving subject and some of our views may be regarded as controversial at least. We intend our statements on classification to be regarded as tentative because of the incompleteness of understanding of the biology, pathology, clinical course and optimal treatment of these relatively rare tumours. However, we believe the line we have taken to be compatible with the emerging consensus view on a provisional classification of gut lymphomas.

2 Gut-Associated Lymphoid Tissue

Gut-associated lymphoid tissue, often referred to by the acronym GALT or MALT (mucosa-associated lymphoid tissue), consists of intra-epithelial lymphocytes, lymphocytes and plasma cells diffusely distributed in the lamina propria, and mucosal and submucosal lymphoid nodules distributed throughout the small and large intestine; the largest lymphoid nodules are the Peyer's patches of terminal ileum. In man the normal gastric mucosa is virtually devoid of lymphoid tissue in childhood and young adulthood, but mucosal lymphoid nodules develop with age in most individuals either as part of a natural process or due to chronic gastritis (ISAACSON and WRIGHT 1987). It is debatable whether Waldeyer's ring should be considered as part of MALT or part of the peripheral lymphoid tissue: lymphomas of Waldeyer's ring are associated with gastric lymphomas (REE et al. 1980), but Waldeyer's ring also shows features of peripheral lymphoid tissue (ISAACSON and WRIGHT 1987). In the large bowel and rectum of man, lymphoid aggregates in mucosa and submucosa almost invariably have an intimate relationship with the surface epithelium, which has led to their designation as lympho-epithelial or lymphoglandular complexes (O'LEARY and SWEENEY 1986). In the normal colon the frequency of lymphoglandular complexes increases threefold from the caecum to the rectum and the volume of lymphoid tissue in the rectum led STRINDEL (1935) to coin the term "rectal tonsil".

Detailed morphological and immunohistochemical studies of normal human MALT have revealed similarities to and differences from peripheral lymphoid tissue (SPENCER et al. 1985a, 1986a). Some of the special features of normal MALT appear directly relevant to the understanding of gut lymphomas. Peyer's patches have been most intensively studied in humans, but are generally regarded as structurally representative of the other smaller lymphoid nodules in MALT. B cells predominate and are present from early in the second trimester of foetal development (SPENCER et al. 1986 b). The most obvious component of the human Peyer's patch is the B cell follicle consisting of a reactive follicle centre surrounded by a mantle of small lymphocytes. External to this is a further diffuse B cell zone variably admixed with macrophages and some T cells. The smaller distinct T zone containing high endothelial venules is situated between the B cell follicle and the muscularis mucosae.

The cells in the diffuse B cell zone may be related to nodal monocytoid B cells (PIRIS et al. 1986; SHEIBANI et al. 1986) but differ phenotypically from mantle zone cells and other cells of peripheral lymphoid tissue apart from the cells in the splenic marginal zone (SPENCER et al. 1985 b). Mantle zone B cells express both surface IgM and IgD while the surrounding B cells lack IgD but express IgM or IgA. These extrafollicular B cells are further distinguished by their size and nuclear morphology: they are larger than mantle zone cells and contain irregularly shaped heterochromatic nuclei resembling those of centrocytes and have thus been designated centrocyte-like cells (ISAACSON and SPENCER 1987).

These centrocyte-like cells selectively infiltrate the epithelium covering the Peyer's patches or other lymphoid nodules (so-called dome epithelium) at the sites of M cells (OWEN and JONES 1974; OWEN 1977; BOCKMAN et al. 1983). M cells are flattened epithelial cells through which antigens, macromolecules and particulate material pass from the lumen of the gut into the Peyer's patch, and which contain the centrocyte-like cells in "hollows" in the cytoplasm, separated from the gut lumen by a thin bridge of cytoplasm containing electron-lucent vesicles. This intra-epithelial population of B cells is not found in the epithelium outside the dome area and must be distinguished from intra-epithelial T cells, which form the majority of intra-epithelial lymphocytes in the gut (FERGUSON 1977). Intra-epithelial T cells are distributed throughout the small intestine and, in smaller numbers, the large intestine. Their numbers increase in certain conditions such as coeliac disease and lymphocytic gastritis (DIXON et al. 1988). They are mostly T suppressor cells. Lamina propria T cells are principally of T helper/inducer phenotype and in the T zones of Peyer's patches the T helper/inducer to T suppressor ratio is about 4:1. There is some evidence (ELSTON et al. 1979) for a homing population of gut-associated T cells.

The precise role of centrocyte-like cells in mucosal immunity is not known, nor is their place in B cell ontogeny. However, their identical phenotype and morphological similarity to splenic marginal zone cells (SPENCER et al. 1985 b) could be significant. Little is known about these splenic cells in man, but in rodents they are known to mount T-independent antibody responses and to be particularly effective in dealing with bacterial carbohydrate (capsular) antigens (KUMARARATNE et al. 1981; MACLENNAN et al. 1982). These cells appear to belong to a distinct B cell lineage which, though derived from a circulating precursor, does not recirculate itself. The possibility that centrocyte-like cells and splenic marginal zone cells in man are indeed part of the same lineage could account for many of the peculiarities of lymphomas arising in the gut mucosa, particularly the tendency to remain localised to the primary site for a long period.

Another explanation offered previously for this prolonged localisation of gut lymphomas is the known circulating pattern of MALT lymphocytes which "home" back to the mucosa (GOUDIE et al. 1974; HALL et al. 1977). It was suggested that circulating neoplastic gut lymphomatous cells would "home" to the lymphoma. However, even using sensitive and specific immunoglobulin (Ig) gene rearrangement studies on peripheral lymphocytes, ISAACSON could not find circulating neoplastic cells in patients with gastric lymphoma (ISAACSON and SPENCER 1987). Also, there is now good evidence that mucosal B cells do not necessarily "home" to their site of origin (HUSBAND and GOWENS 1978; HUSBAND 1982) and therefore one would expect tumours of MALT to be multiple. As this is not usually the case, apart from malignant lymphomatous polyposis (see below), the "homing" of neoplastic recirculating lymphocytes to the gut is not a good explanation for the prolonged localisation of gut lymphomas.

Most knowledge on the migratory pathways of intestinal lymphoid cells is based on animal studies and interspecies differences do occur. For example in rodents there is evidence that lymphoid cells migrate between different types of mucosa (BIENENSTOCK et al. 1978; MONTGOMERY et al. 1983), while in sheep there is evidence against such a mechanism (SPENCER and HALL 1984). It is important to bear these differences in mind when extrapolating from animals to man. It has been shown in animals and seems likely in man that different intestinal lymphoid cell populations are interrelated through the migration of cells from one site to another. Accordingly, lymphoid cells from Peyer's patches migrate to the lamina propria and intra-epithelial region of the small intestine. A subset of B lymphocytes in Peyer's patches are the precursors of the lamina propria IgA-producing cells (KAGNOFF 1981). T lymphocytes from Peyer's patches have been reported to populate the lamina propria and the intra-epithelial region (KAGNOFF 1981).

After antigen stimulation, lymphocytes in Peyer's patches divide and migrate. B and T lymphocytes, activated as a result of antigenic challenge, leave the Peyer's patches by efferent lymphatics, pass to the mesenteric lymph nodes and thence via the thoracic duct to the bloodstream before returning to the lamina propria and intra-epithelial regions. Most of the returning lymphoid cells in the lamina propria appear as plasma cells (GRISCELLI et al. 1969; HALL et al. 1972). The majority of these plasma cells synthesise dimeric IgA (CRABBE et al. 1968). Some of the IgA enters the mucosal lymphatics and from there the bloodstream (VAERMAN et al. 1973). The intravascular dimeric IgA is available for uptake and transport by cells synthesising secretory component at other mucosal sites and in this way the mucosal surfaces of the body are united by a common immune system.

3 Criteria for Diagnosis of a Primary Gut Lymphoma

Lymphomas of the gut are most commonly found in association with systemic malignant lymphoma (HERRMANN et al. 1980). The standard minimum criteria for acceptance of a gut lymphoma as a primary are laid out in Table 1. These criteria have been widely accepted and are therefore very useful when it comes to comparing series in the literature since 1961. However, newer investigative techniques and improved understanding of the biology of gut lymphomas may make modificatons of these criteria necessary. Nowadays, a stricter definition of a primary gut lymphoma would include, in addition, a normal mediastinal CAT scan and normal bone marrow examination, but it would seem sensible to us to retain the standard five criteria as the minimum requirements for inclusion of a case as a primary. However, not all authors are prepared to be even as strict as this and include as primary gut lymphomas, any lymhoma which appears to involve the gut predominantly. Thus, in a histological and immunohistochemical study of 36 cases of primary gastric lymphoma (MOORE and WRIGHT 1984), eight of the cases had presented with lymphoma elsewhere (all at other sites of MALT, e.g. lung), but appeared principally to involve the stomach.

4 Incidence of Primary Gut Lymphomas

As different series use different criteria for the diagnosis of primary gut lymphomas, it is difficult to compare accurately the incidences of primary gut lymphoma and secondary involvement of the gut in systemic lymphoma. One study indicates that clinically apparent gastrointestinal lymphomatous involvement in systemic lymphoma may be present in as many as 32% of cases and even up to 43% at autopsy (HERRMANN et al. 1980) In comparison, the same authors found that primary gut lymphoma accounted for only 9% of all cases of lymphoma. Therefore, although this group used less rigid criteria for the definition of primary gut lymphoma than we suggest, primary gut lymphoma probably accounts for less than 30% of all cases of gut involvement by lymphoma.

Table 1. Criteria for diagnosis of a primary gut lymphoma (Dawson et al. 1961)

1. No palpable superficial lymphadenopathy at presentation
2. Chest X-rays show no enlargement of mediastinal nodes
3. Normal white cell count (total and differential)
4. At laparotomy the bowel lesion predominates, the only obviously affected nodes being those immediately related
5. The liver and spleen appear free of tumour

The problem of failure to follow proper criteria in distinguishing primary from secondary gut lymphoma, coupled with terminological differences and diagnostic difficulties, makes it impossible to determine the true incidence of gut lymphoma nationwide and worldwide. Calculations of the incidence of gut lymphoma in Western populations have varied from 3% to 15% of all non-Hodgkin's lymphomas (SUGARBAKER and CRAVER 1940; GALL and MALLORY 1942; FREEMAN et al. 1972; BROWN et al. 1975; FULLER et al. 1975; RUDDERS et al. 1978; GREEN et al. 1979).

That there are geographical and ethnic variations in incidence of primary gut lymphoma is widely recognised. For example, a higher incidence is said to exist in Middle Eastern countries and in Sephardic Jews than in European countires and Ashkenazic Jews. In these examples the differences refer principally to primary lymphoma of the small intestine. However, it is interesting to compare the incidence of gut lymphoma in Israel and in the UK. The former is supposed to be a high incidence area and the latter a low incidence area. In Israel the incidence of lymphoma at all sites in the gut is approximately 1/100 000 per annum (SHANI et al. 1969). In the Grampian area of Scotland the incidence is approximately 1.6/100 000 per annum (GREEN et al. 1979). Unfortunately no other figures are available for the indicence of gut lymphoma in the UK, so that it is not known whether the fairly high frequency in Scotland is representative of the country as a whole.

Most authors from the Middle East state that the small bowel is the commonest site within the gut for lymphoma, while in Western populations the stomach is the commonest site. On this basis lymphoma of the small bowel may be slighly commoner in the Middle East than elsewhere. The differences in incidence are not marked and it is probable that the Middle East is the focus of attention on the part of the medical profession because of immunoproliferative small intenstinal disease (IPSID, alpha chain disease, Mediterranean lymphoma) (KHOJASTEH et al. 1983), rather than because of a particularly high incidence of gut lymphoma. The different incidences at different sites are further commented on below.

If the estimates for the incidence of gut lymphoma in the UK are of the order of 1.6/100 000 (GREEN et al. 1979), then a district general hospital in the UK will see roughly four new cases of gut lymphoma every year. Approximate figures can be given for the average numbers of cases of gut lymphoma per year seen in large hospitals on the North American continent, and these are comparable to the above UK estimates. In North America such hospitals report between 1.7 and 2.8 cases per year when all sites in the gut are included. Primary gastric lymphoma occurs at a frequency of between 1 and 2.5 per year, small bowel lymphoma at a frequency between 0.6 and 1.1 per year, and large bowel lymphoma at a frequency between 0.3 and 0.9 per year (ALLEN et al. 1954; NICOLOFF et al. 1963; KAY 1964; WELBORN et al. 1965; JOSEPH and LATTES 1966; STOBBE et al. 1966; WYCHULIS et al. 1966; BUSH and ASH 1969; LOEHR et al. 1969; FU and PERZIN 1972; HOERR et al. 1973).

5 Sites of Origin in the Gut

5.1 Stomach

There is no doubt that the stomach is the most favoured site for primary gut lymphomas in Western populations. Estimates range from 50%–60% of all primary gut lymphomas (AZZOPARDI and MENZIES 1960; LOEHR et al. 1969; LEWIN et al. 1978). A series from South Africa (KAHN et al. 1972) has only 33% of gastric lymphomas in the total. In that part of the world the small bowel is the most favoured site within the gut and the distribution of lymphomas here may be closer to that found in the Middle East. By combining a large number of cases from different reported series an overall figure of 61% is reached for the proportion of primary Western gut lymphoma found in the stomach. A similar calculation from Middle Eastern populations shows that 38% of primary lymphomas in these countries are gastric.

As regards the distribution of lymphoma within the stomach, most authors agree that the pyloric antrum is the commonest site, followed by the body then the cardia (FRIEDMAN 1959; CONNORS and WISE 1974; LIM et al. 1977). Some authors have found a higher incidence in the body than in the antrum (THORBJARNARSON et al. 1956; SALMELA 1968). FRIEDMAN (1959) found lymphoma to be more common on the greater curve than on the lesser.

Estimates of the proportion of all gastric malignancy which is formed by lymphoma have varied from 0.4% in Denmark (JENSEN 1967) and 0.9% in Finland (SALMELA 1968) up to 9% in the USA (HERTZER and HOERR 1976) and 11.5% in Italy (RILKE et al. 1978; RUSSO et al. 1978). Most analyses of Western populations give figures in the range of 2%–5% (THORBJARNARSON et al. 1956; Friedman 1959; KAY 1964; BERG 1969; LOEHR et al. 1969; CONNORS and WISE 1974).

5.2 Small Bowel

In Western populations the small bowel is the second commonest site for primary gut lymphomas; most authors give figures in the region of 30% for the proportion located here. In the Middle East, by way of contrast, small bowel is the most favoured site of origin, accounting for at least half of all gut lymphomas in Israel (SHANI et al. 1969), in Iraq (AL-BAHRANI and BAKIR 1971), in Iran (HAGHIGHI et al. 1971) and in Lebanon (SHAHID et al. 1975). This increased incidence of small bowel lymphoma may be the explanation for the supposedly higher overall incidence of gut lymphoma in these regions. Because other forms of malignancy in the small bowel are uncommon, lymphoma constitutes between 19% and 50% of all malignancy at this site in Western populations and over 95% of all malignancy at this site in the Middle East (AL-BAHRANI and BAKIR 1971; HAGHIGHI et al. 1971).

The distribution of tumours within the small bowel shows some interesting variations. In Western populations the tumours predominate in the distal small bowel (LEWIN et al. 1978). Combining figures from several reported series gives the following distribution: duodenum 8%, jejunum 33%, ileum 59%. Distal predominance is found also in adults in South Africa (LEWIN et al.1976) and in Israel (SELZER et al. 1979 b) when the tumours are unassociated with malabsorption.

In Middle Eastern countries the ileal predominance is lost in those cases with a background of malabsorption related to IPSID. Such "Mediterranean lymphomas" show the following distribution: duodenum 3%, jejunum 31%, ileum 34%, more than one site 32% (NASR et al. 1970; AL-BAHRANI and BAKIR 1971; AL-SALEEM and AL-BAHRANI 1973; SHAHID et al. 1975; SELZER et al. 1979 a). In the West there is also a definite tendency to a more proximal distribution of lymphomas associated with malabsorption: jejunum 38%, ileum 29%, unspecified site 33% (BRUNT et al. 1969; HOLMES et al. 1976; BRANDT et al. 1978; SELBY and GALLAGHER 1979; ISAACSON and WRIGHT 1980).

5.3 Appendix

Since proper criteria for diagnosing primary gut lymphomas were established (DAWSON et al. 1961) there have been remarkably few reports of primary lymphoma of the appendix and none stands up to critical scrutiny. The three purported cases in the series of GLICK and SOULE (1966) also showed tumour in caecum which could have been the primary site. Older reports, reviewed by CLARKE and SIMONDS (1951), suggested a mean age of 25 years for appendiceal lymphomas (cf. mean of 55 years for other gut lymphomas), and mostly follicular lymphomas (a rare type anywhere in the gut). This makes us think that most older reports of follicular lymphoma of the appendix are cases of misdiagnosed reactive hyperplasia.

The rarity of appendiceal lymphoma is perhaps surprising in view of the high concentration of lymphoid tissure in the normal appendix.

5.4 Large Bowel

This is the least common of the three major sites in the gut for the development of lymphoma. Only 9%–16% of primary gut lymphomas originate here, both in Western populations (BERG 1969; LOEHR et al. 1969; NAQVI et al. 1969; CAMILLERI and DIEBOLD 1972; GREEN et al. 1979) and in Middle Eastern and South African populations (SHANI et al. 1969; KAHN et al. 1972). Of all colorectal malignancy, lymphoma constitutes between 0.1% and 1% (ALLEN et al. 1954).

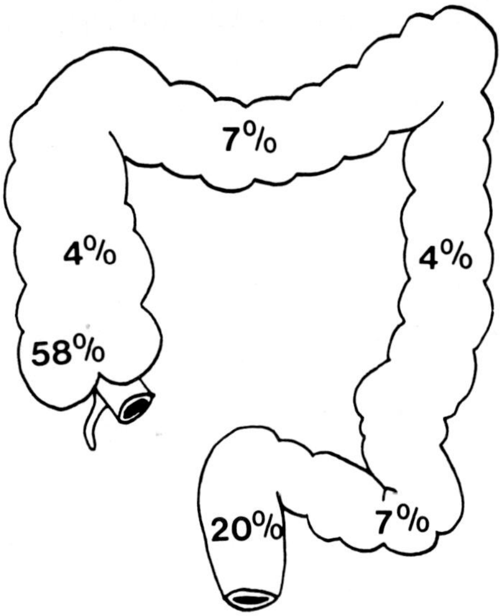

Fig. 1. Overall incidence related to site of colorectal lymphomas from review of literature

The subsite distribution of colonic lymphoma is shown in Fig. 1. The apparent caecal predominance may in part be spurious, since in the literature the ileocaecal region is often considered as part of the large bowel. Some, at least, of the tumours in this category are likely to be intussuscepting bulky tumours originating in the terminal ileum. After the caecum the rectum is the next commonest site.

6 Age Incidence and Sex Ratio

If all the histological types of primary gut lymphoma and all the sites in the gut are considered together, the age distribution shows a peak incidence in the sixth decade. There are possibly minor subsidiary peaks in the third and first decades. In general terms one may state that no age is exempt from lymphoma of the gut, although it is very rare under the age of 2 years.

If gut lymphomas are considered by site, the age incidence distributions are similar for the stomach, small bowel and large bowel in Western populations. The minor peak of incidence in the first decade is only really distinguishable in small bowel cases. This is because lymphoma of the gut in children is very largely confined to the ileum.

In our series and in the literature as a whole the sex ratio of primary gut lymphomas taken together as a group shows a male predominance (M:F = 2:1). This overall male predominance in gut lymphomas is matched by the sex ratios of non-Hodgkin's lymphomas arising in nodes. The ratio given above is for adults; in children male predominance is even more striking (M:F = 9:1). The reason for the male predominance in lymphomas of both gut and of nodes is entirely unexplained.

7 Aetiology and Predisposing Factors

The aetiology and predisposing factors for the vast majority of gut lymphomas are quite unknown. The incidence of primary gut lymphomas does not relate proportionally to the amount of lymphoid tissue normally present in the mucosa: the stomach, the commonest site of primary gut lymphoma in the West, is normally virtually devoid of lymphoid tissue.

Conditions for which there is good evidence that they predispose to primary gut lymphomas are coeliac disease, IPSID (alpha chain disease), ulcerative colitis and to a lesser extent Crohn's disease, AIDS and other immunosuppressed states. The topic of pseudolymphoma and its possible relationship to lymphoma is discussed in Sect. 8.

7.1 Coeliac Disease

Coeliac disease is now accepted as a predisposing factor for several malignancies, but most commonly a lymphoma of the small bowel (SWINSON et al. 1983). Most such lymphomas are pleomorphic T cell lymphomas (see Sects. 9.7 and 9.8) currently usally referred to as "enteropathy-associated T cell lymphomas" (ISAACSON et al. 1985; LOUGHRAN et al. 1986; SALTER et al. 1986). Until 1985 such lymphomas were widely thought to be of true histiocytic origin and called malignant histiocytosis of the intestine (ISAACSON and WRIGHT 1978), a term which should now be abandoned. So-called "ulcerative jejunitis" is now regarded as an early manifestation of enteropathy-associated lymphoma (ISAACSON and WRIGHT 1980), in which the inflammatory reaction to the ulceration and the deceptively benign appearance of the neoplastic cells combine to make the microscopic diagnosis of malignancy very difficult. Areas of "ulcerative jejunitis" are commonly seen adjacent to more obvious lymphoma. Enteropathy-associated lymphoma is further discussed below in Sects. 9.7 and 9.8. Malignant lymphoma with eosinophilia (SHEPHERD et al. 1987) is a variant of T cell lymphoma which shows an association with coeliac disease; it is also discussed in detail below (Sect. 9.9). Not all lymphomas with associated enteropathy have been reported to be of T cell phenotype and in one series B cell tumours predominated (MORGAN et al. 1985).

Though it is now established that coeliac disease and malabsorption usually precede the development of gut lymphoma by a number of years (SWINSON et al. 1983), this is not always so. Coeliac disease may be subclinical and may not present until symptoms appear due to the development of lymphoma. However, the usual clinical setting heralding the development of lymphoma is for a previously controlled coeliac patient to relapse despite strict adherence to a gluten-free diet.

It is also valid to consider the possibility that lymphoma per se can cause malabsorption. This is most likely if there is extensive mediastinal node involvement with blockage of the lymphatics. It is interesting that the first reported association between malabsorption and lymphoma (FAIRLEY and MACKIE 1937) noted the presence of retroperitoneal nodes at the base of the mesentery, but did not mention lymphoma in the bowel! The likely mechanism of malabsorption in this oft misquoted case was thus lymphatic obstruction.

7.2 Immunoproliferative Small Intestinal Disease

This is the currently preferred term for the condition which used to be known as alpha chain disease. It occurs predominantly but not exclusively in the Middle East, South Africa being another high incidence area. Its clinical features are diarrhoea, weight loss, abdominal pain and finger clubbing. Pathologically it is characterised by a heavy plasmacytic or lymphoplasmacytic infiltrate in the mucosa of the upper small intestine and related mesenteric nodes. In most, if not all, cases these plasma cells synthesise, without necessarily secreting an abnormal alpha immunoglobulin heavy chain (RAMBAUD et al. 1980). A frankly malignant lymphoma, so-called Mediterranean lymphoma, often arises in the setting of IPSID and there has been much debate over whether IPSID is a malignant proliferation ab initio or whether the onset of Mediterranean lymphoma represents a complication of a benign disorder (KHOJASTEH et al. 1983; GALIAN et al. 1977). The benign view is supported by the excellent response of some cases of uncomplicated IPSID to broad spectrum antibiotics (KHOJASTEH et al. 1983; GALIAN et al. 1977; ASSELAH et al. 1983), while frank Mediterranean lymphoma requires more radical treatment. A recent study set out to settle this issue by looking for immunoglobulin gene rearrangements in cases of uncomplicated IPSID and in established Mediterranean lymphoma; light and heavy chain Ig gene rearrangements were found in both (SMITH WJ et al. 1987). The authors interpret these results as indicating that IPSID is neoplastic even in its early stages, but that the neoplastic cells respond to normal stimuli. The epidemiology of IPSID, together with reports of specific HLA association (NOVIS 1979; NIKBIN et al. 1979), points to a genetic predisposition in this disease, which when combined with one or more environmental factors leads to abnormal IgA synthesis and lymphoma.

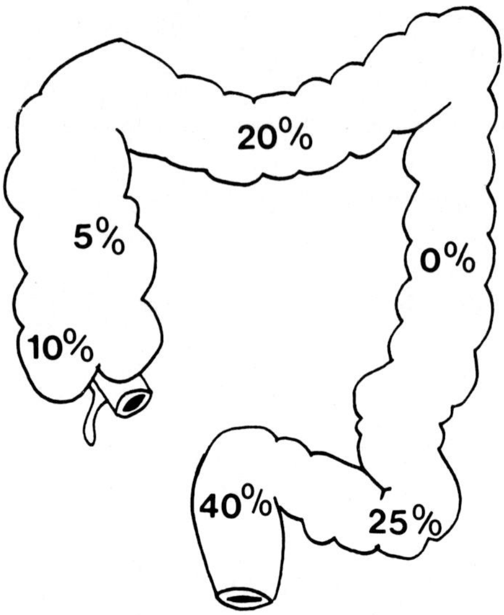

Fig. 2. Incidence related to site of colorectal lymphomas complicating ulcerative colitis from review of literature

7.3 Ulcerative Colitis and Crohn's Disease

Lymphoma is a rare complication of ulcerative colitis. As with adenocarcinoma, such lymphoma tends to occur in patients with extensive disease and a long history. Both types of malignancy are more frequently multifocal when occurring in the context of ulcerative colitis. Approximately one lymphoma of the large bowel will be seen for every ten carcinomas complicating ulcerative colitis (RENTON and BLACKSHAW 1976). The distribution of lymphomas in the large bowel in ulcerative colitis is shown in Fig. 2. This is obviously different from the distribution of lymphoma in general in the large bowel (Fig. 1), but similar to the distribution of adenocarcinoma in ulcerative colitis, which also shows rectal predominance (RIDDELL et al. 1978). Most ulcerative colitis related lymphomas in the literature appear to be high grade (RENTON and BLACKSHAW 1976) and our recent morphological and immunohistochemical studies on seven cases confirm this and show all seven to be of B cell phenotype (SHEPHERD et al. 1989).

There are even fewer reports of lymphoma complicating Crohn's disease and all are single case reports. One describes two "reticulum cell sarcomas" in the small intestine of a patient with a 15-year history of Crohn's disease (HUGHES 1955). In two series of small bowel lymphomas, one patient in each also had Crohn's disease but details of these two cases are scanty (NAQVI et al. 1969; BLACKLEDGE et al. 1979). The best documented case pathologically is that of a malignant lymphoma, immunoblastic with plasmacytic differentiation, of the colon complicating Crohn's disease (KWEE et al. 1985). We have recently studied three cases of lymphoma in

Crohn's disease. Immunohistochemical studies on paraffin sections showed one of these to be of T cell type while the other two were of uncertain lineage and included large bizarre cells (SHEPHERD et al. 1989). We presume, as with coeliac disease and ulcerative colitis, that the chronic inflammatory cell infiltrate in Crohn's disease forms the substrate for the development of lymphoa. However, all three of our patients had also been treated with immunomodifying agents such as steroids and azathioprine.

7.4 AIDS

Lymphomas are now well established as a manifestation of AIDS. Most such lymphomas appear to be of extranodal origin (ZIEGLER et al. 1984). The commonest sites appear to be the central nervous system, bone marrow, skin/mucosa and the gastrointestinal tract (ZIEGLER et al. 1984; LEVINE et al. 1985). Virtually all of the lymphomas appear to be of B cell origin and most are high grade. Virtually any site in the gastrointestinal tract appears to be vulnerable, but most reported cases are in the small bowel though anorectal lymphomas are being reported with increasing frequency (BURKES et al. 1986; IOACHIM et al. 1987). We are aware of one case report of Hodgkin's disease presenting with rectal symptoms in a homosexual male though it is not clear whether that patient had AIDS (COONLEY et al. 1984).

7.5 Other Immune Deficiency States

Lymphoma is a well recognised complication in immunosuppressed transplant patients. Although the brain has been the site of most of the lymphomas following renal transplantation (SCHNECK and PENN 1971), other primary sites including the colon are reported (PINKUS et al. 1974, COGGON et al. 1981). The lymphomas developing in this context are usually high grade.

There are a few reports of localised high grade lymphoma in the bowel in patients with chronic lymphatic leukaemia (BURMAN and VAN WYK 1956; GIVLER 1968; ARMITAGE et al. 1978). The development of the high grade tumour in this situation could either represent a second malignancy in a patient whose immune incompetence predisposes to the development of further tumours, or represent dedifferentiation of a low grade tumour into a high grade. In patients with treated Hodgkin's disease there certainly is an increased incidence of second malignancies (DORREEN et al. 1986; HENRY et al. 1987). We have seen several cases of primary gut lymphoma in patients previously treated for nodal Hodgkin's disease.

8 Pseudolymphomas

8.1 Stomach

The term gastric pseudolymphoma in most standard texts is used to describe a lesion which is considered in the final analysis to be reactive rather than neoplastic, but which, because of its size, the density of the lymphocytic infiltrate and the extent of that infiltrate, has caused a careful initial consideration of the possibility of neoplasia. The histological feature which was said to be the most reliable indicator of benignity was the presence of typical reactive follicles (JACOBS 1963; FARIS and SALTZSTEIN 1964; VAN DEN HEULE et al. 1979) with germinal centres containing centrocytes, centroblasts, dendritic reticulum cells and tingible body macrophages, and surrounded by obvious mantle zones. A good reason for regarding gastric pseudolymphomas as benign appreared to be that they virtually never recurred or gave further trouble, following removal.

This was the situation until various workers (EIMOTO et al. 1985; ISAACSON et al. 1986; MYHRE and ISAACSON 1987) by means of their very elegant immunohistochemical studies convincingly showed monotypic cell populations in gastric lesions containing obvious reactive follicles. ISAACSON et al. (1986) argued strongly that the term gastric pseudolymphoma should be dropped and that these lesions were essentially low grade B cell lymphomas. The reasons for lack of recurrence of such lesions are suggested to be (a) that they are usually excised in the specimen on which the diagnosis is based (b) that most unequivocal B cell lymphomas of the stomach characteristically remain localised for long periods and "pseudolymphomas" represent the most benign end of the spectrum, and (c) that the reason for this long localisation period is that these tumours are derived from "centrocyte-like cells" which are derived from a special subset of non-recirculating B lymphocytes (SPENCER et al. 1985 b).

Our opinion, based on the present evidence and our own experience, is that many of the cases diagnosed previously by us and reported in the literature as pseudolymphomas, are in fact probably low grade B cell lymphomas. However, a lymphoma does have to start somewhere and as there is virtually no lymphoid tissue present in the normal stomach it seems likely that most gastric lymphomas must evolve in the setting of a reactive lymphoid infiltrate. Lymphomas of the salivary glands and thyroid develop from such reactive infiltrates (SCHMID et al. 1982; ANSCOMBE and WRIGHT 1985). Any florid reactive lymphoid infiltrate in the gastric mucosa could on this basis be regarded as a potentially premalignant lesion. From a practical point of view, therefore, it would seem to us sensible to regard with suspicion all very dense gastric lymphoid infiltrates which fail to respond to medical treatment for chronic gastritis. Surgery, as for overt gastric lymphoma, should then be seriously considered.

8.2 Small Bowel

The term pseudolymphoma is much less often applied to lesions of the small bowel. Most of these were considered entirely benign, but recently some evidence has emerged to suggest that one type may predispose to malignancy (MATUCHANSKY et al. 1985). This is the generalised reactive hyperplasia of small bowel lymphoid tissue ("nodular lymphoid hyperplasia") resulting in benign lymphoid polyposis which may be associated with hypogammaglobulinaemia (HERMANS et al. 1966; ADJUKIEWICZ et al. 1972). The immediate differential diagnosis of benign lymphoid polyposis is from malignant lymphomatous polyposis (see below), but microscopically malignant lymphomatous polyposis is a diffuse infiltrate of centrocytic cells while benign lymphoid polyposis is a follicular hyperplasia. However, the report of MATUCHANSKY et al. (1985) in which three patients with benign lymphoid polyposis developed malignant lymphoma, suggests that there must be some increased expectation of lymphoma in such patients.

In children and young adults reactive hyperplasia of the lymphoid tissue of Peyer's patches can produce a localised tumefaction with the gross appearances of a malignant lymphoid tumour (MORSON and DAWSON 1979). Microscopically this shows a florid follicular hyperplasis, and does not apparently predispose to malignancy.

8.3 Large Bowel

The lesion referred to as a pseudolymphoma of the large bowel is also a localised hyperplastic tumefaction of lymphoid tissue, most often called a benign lymphoid polyp. Benign lymphoid polyps of the rectum are fairly common and several large series have been published, some with more than a hundred cases (HAYES and BURR 1952, CORNES et al. 1961). Histologically benign lymphoid polyps of the rectum consist of a mass of reactive lymphoid tissue showing follicular hyperplasia and covered by intact mucosa. They occupy an expanded submucosa but there is often a mucosal component in addition and sometimes deeper penetration into the muscularis propria is seen. Benign lymphoid polyps are not the precursors of malignant lymphomatous polyposis (LI 1948). Provided the whole polyp is removed there should be no possibility of confusing these two diagnoses, but if only a small superficial biopsy is taken then diagnosis is usually impossible; such a practice must be condemned as unhelpful.

9 Histopathological Classification

Whatever classification is used, it is now widely accepted that the incidences of the various types of lymphoma differ markedly in series of primary nodal and primary gut tumours. Hodgkin's disease constitutes about 45% of nodal lymphomas. The incidence of Hodgkin's disease amongst gastric lymphomas is quoted as being between 5% and 10% in the USA (LOEHR et al. 1969; NAQVI et al. 1969), Finland (SALMELA 1968), and Israel (SHANI et al. 1969). Amongst gut lymphomas as a whole LEWIN et al. (1978) found 1.7% to be Hodgkin's disease, while ISAACSON et al. (1979) found an incidence of 1%. Some series, including our own, contain no examples of Hodgkin's disease (FU and PERZIN 1972; HENRY and FARRER-BROWN 1977; Selzer et al. 1979 a). The reason why Hodgkin's disease of the gut should be so uncommon is not clear. There is still argument over the histogenesis of Hodgkin's disease, but currently a favoured view is that the cell of origin is an activated lymphocyte more often T cell than B cell (DREXLER et al. 1988). If Hodgkin's disease does usually evolve from a particular type of activated T cell, the very low incidence of primary Hodgkin's disease in the gut may partly reflect the low incidence of primary gut T cell lymphomas (see below).

There is still no generally accepted agreement on the subject of the classification of nodal non-Hodgkin's lymphomas, which have been much more intensively studied than gut tumours. This lack of agreement reflects our imperfect understanding of the precise histogenesis and biology of many of these tumours, and difficulties and differences in the interpretation of fine cytological and architectural detail in paraffin sections. Ideas on histogenesis based on technically improved and more widely applied immunohistochemical methods and the application of molecular biological techniques are currently evolving rapidly with regard to both nodal (STANSFELD et al. 1988) and gut lymphomas (GRODY et al. 1985; ISAACSON et al. 1985, 1986; MORGAN et al. 1985; MYHRE and ISAACSON 1987; MOUBAYED et al. 1987). Each new advance seems to emphasise differences in types and incidences of nodal and gut lymphomas. In nodes, although B cell tumours still predominate, T cell tumours are being recognised with increasing frequency and a logical and comprehensive scheme of classification of nodal T cell lymphomas has been recently proposed by the Kiel group (SUCHI et al. 1987) and related to an updated Kiel classification of B cell tumours (STANSFELD et al. 1988). In the gut, apart from the lymphomas complicating coeliac disease (ISAACSON et al. 1985; SHEPHERD et al. 1987), T cell lymphomas appear to be rare and the vast majority of gut lymphomas appear to be of B cell origin (GRODY et al. 1985; ISAACSON et al. 1986; ISAACSON and SPENCER 1987; MYHRE and ISAACSON 1987; SHEPHERD et al. 1988).

The majority of B cell tumours arising in the gut are currently suggested to be derived from non-recirculating centrocyte-like cells (vide supra) (SPENCER et al. 1985 b; ISAACSON et al. 1986, 1987; ISAACSON and

Table 2. Proposed classification of primary gut lymphomas

	B cell	T cell
Low grade	Polymorphic B cell[a] (predominantly small cell)	Small cell pleomorphic (+/− enteropathy)
	Mediterranean lymphoma (also known as IPSID[b])	
	Centrocytic lymphoma (also known as malignant lymphomatous polyposis)	
	Others including: Plasmacytoma[c] Centroblastic-centrocytic follicular[c]	Others including epitheliotropic
High grade	Polymorphic B cell[a] (with prominent large cell component)	Medium/large cell pleomorphic (+/− enteropathy −/− tissue eosinophilia)
	Burkitt-type lymphoma[d]	
	Others including: Pure centroblastic[c] Pure immunoblastic[c]	Others including: Pure immunoblastic[c] Large cell anaplastic[e]
	Unclassified	Unclassified

[a] "Polymorphic" as it is composed of a mixed population of small lymphocytes, centrocyte – like cells, lymphoplasmacytoid cells, plasma cells, centroblasts and immunoblasts in variable proportions. More than 20% blast type (large) cells indicates high grade.
[b] Immunoproliferative small intestinal disease.
[c] Such classical Kiel types appear to be rare in the gut.
[d] Formerly B lymphoblastic.
[e] Rarely the large cell anaplastic lymphoma may be of a B cell lineage.

Spencer 1987; Isaacson and Wright 1987; Myhre and Isaacson 1987). Such tumours have been variously labelled as tumours of centrocyte-like cells, maltomas, low grade B cell tumours of MALT, or simply primary gastric lymphomas. None of these names is ideal: most tumours are composed of a polymorphic population of cells many of which are morphologically unlike centrocytes; "maltoma" and "low grade B cell tumour of MALT" strictly embrace other distinct tumours of MALT, e.g. centrocytic lymphoma; and "primary gastric lymphoma" also embraces a number of types of tumour. Furthermore, knowledge of the physiology of centrocyte-like cells is based on animal studies and, as noted previously, there are interspecies differences. Though the idea is attractive, and the experimental work of Isaacson is very persuasive, we think it still premature to assume that all such tumours are centrocyte-like cell derived, and therefore opted in our most recent study, as explained below, for the less committal term of "polymorphic B cell lymphoma".

We have ourselves previously attempted to classify gut lymphomas according to conventional Kiel criteria (LEVISON and SHEPHERD 1986), as have others (ISAACSON et al. 1979; VAN DEN HEULE et al. 1979; MOORE and WRIGHT 1984; MORGAN et al. 1985). In 1987 in the course of a review of 45 primary colorectal lymphomas (SHEPHERD et al. 1988), three independent observers, including two of the presend authors (D.A.L. and P.A.H.) found that, apart from diffuse centrocytic lymphomas, there was no consistent interobserver agreement with regard to different Kiel classes. This was because of the marked polymorphism of the tumour cell population. There was consistent observer agreement on the grade of such tumours using 20% of blast cells as the cut-off point between high grade and low grade tumours. We therefore classified these tumours, which were all of B cell phenotype, into three main groups; centrocytic lymphomas (malignant lymphomatous polyposis), low grade polymorphic B cell lymphomas, and high grade polymorphic B cell lymphomas.

We believe from our experience at other sites in the gut that polymorphic B cell tumours are the predominant type of primary gut lymphoma, but that one does see occasional examples, other than Burkitt-type and centrocytic, of classic Kiel types of lymphoma. One also sees tumours which are very difficult to classify. In the light of this evolving experience, and of the evolving ideas in the literature based mainly on the work of ISAACSON and co-workers, we suggest that gut lymphomas might currently be most usefully classified according to the scheme outlined in Table 2. This scheme attempts to incorporate terms currently in use, and follows the pattern of the updated Kiel classification for nodal lymphomas with major divisions into B and T cell types and high and low grade (STANSFELD et al. 1988). Our polymorphic B cell tumours correspond closely to the tumours of centrocytic-like cells of ISAACSON and our reasons for preferring our terminology are explained above. The distinctive macroscopic, microscopic and behavioural characteristics of each of these tumours is now described.

9.1 Polymorphic B Cell Lymphoma

The reasons for adopting this terminology are outlined above. This entity corresponds closely to the tumour variously referred to by ISAACSON and co-workers as a "tumour of centrocytic-like cells", "maltoma" or "primary B cell gastric lymphoma" (ISAACSON et al. 1986; ISAACSON and SPENCER 1987; ISAACSON and WRIGHT 1987; MYHRE and ISAACSON 1987). It shows variable but often marked cytological polymorphism and is composed of a mixed population of B cells: small lymphocytes, centrocyte-like cells, plasma cells, plasmacytoid cells, centroblasts and immunoblasts (Fig. 3, 4). It exhibits a spectrum of grade in terms of the proportion of blast cells present (Fig. 3, 4). In our study of colorectal lymphomas we found that high grade tumours (with more than 20% blast cells) had a significantly

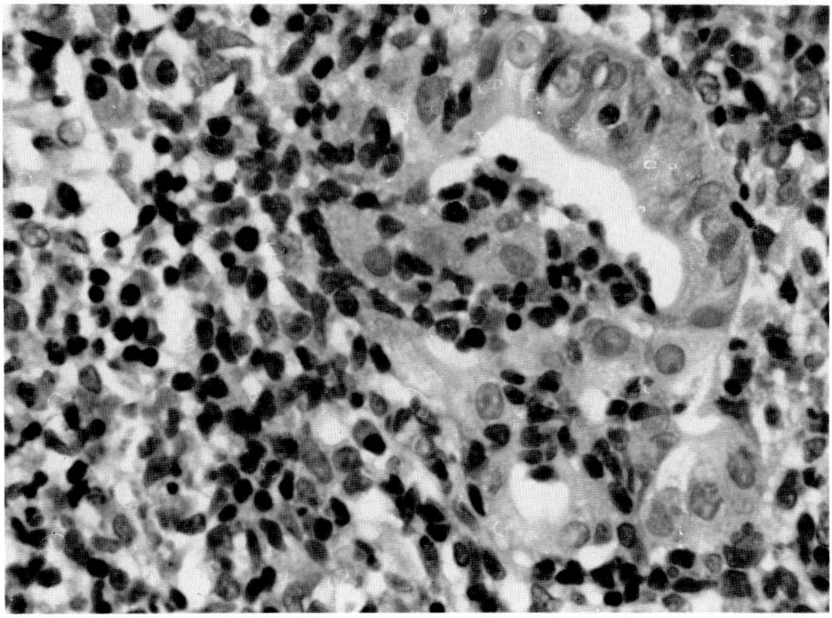

Fig. 3. Low grade polymorphic B cell lymphoma of stomach with partial destruction of a gland (lympho-epithelial lesion). The infiltrate is composed of small centrocytic-like cells and some plasma cells. HE, × 625

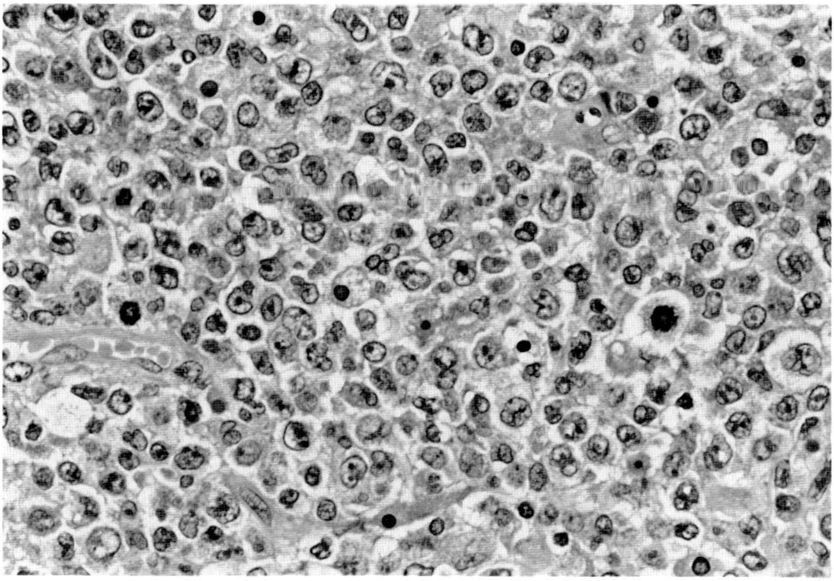

Fig. 4. High grade polymorphic B cell lymphoma of jejunum showing mainly blast-type cells and several mitoses. HE, × 625

poorer prognosis than low grade tumours (SHEPHERD et al. 1988). Low grade tumours also tend to contain more, and more obvious, follicles and most of these are clearly reactive on both morphological and immunohistochemical grounds. The presence of such reactive follicles has, in the past, been erroneously interpreted as indicating that the whole lesion was reactive and spawned the term pseudolymphoma (discussed above), but immunohistochemical evidence of monotypic B cells around such reactive follicles (ISAACSON and SPENCER 1987), and the gradual invasion and effacement of follicles by these monotypic B cells, proves that reactive follicles can be a component of B cell gut lymphomas. We are sure that we have underdiagnosed low grade polymorphic B cell lymphomas in the past (calling them simply reactive, or pseudolymphomas), but as the diagnosis was usually based on a surgically resected specimen, the patient had usually already had the appropriate treatment.

Another characteristic though not invariable microscopic feature of these tumours is the lympho-epithelial lesion in which centrocyte-like cells invade and damage crypt epithelium (Fig. 3). This lesion is not present in our experience in reactive infiltrates, nor in centrocytic lymphomas. It has to be distinguished from the ubiquitous normal presence of intra-epithlelial T lymphocytes, increased numbers of intra-epithelial T lymphocytes in coeliac disease and certain forms of chronic gastritis (DIXON et al. 1988), and very rare "epitheliotropic" T cell lymphomas of the gut, of which we have only seen a single example. These distinctions can be made most objectively by the use of B and T cell markers which work on paraffin sections (see below). The epitheliotropism of neoplastic centrocyte-like B cells seems to mimic the normal behaviour of centrocyte-like cells over Peyer's patches. Lympho-epithelial besions are more often seen with low grade than high grade polymorphic B cell tumours.

Plasma cells are a prominent feature of a proportion of polymorphic B cell lymphomas. Unless the plasma cells are cytologically atypical, their neoplastic nature can only be inferred by the immunohistochemical detection of light chain restriction in the cell cytoplasm. Characteristically, the plasma cell infiltrate is most prominent towards the luminal aspect of the mucosa and merges with the underlying more polymorphic infiltrate. The plasma cells do not take part in lympho-epithelial lesions, and they are usually scanty or absent in the invasive part of the tumour.

Low grade polymorphic B cell lymphomas tend to be well defined protuberant growths, but often show deep invasion of the bowel wall. Most are single growths; occasionally they are multiple, but with the tumours confined to the same or adjacent parts of the bowel (Fig. 5). High grade polymorphic B cell lymphomas are more often larger, strictured, ulcerating lesions with involvement of long segments of the bowel (Fig. 6). Fissuring ulceration is not uncommon in the high grade tumours and is the basis of the not insignificant incidence of associated perforation.

When low grade polymorphic B cell lymphomas metastasise to adjacent lymph nodes they initially produce a highly distinctive growth pattern

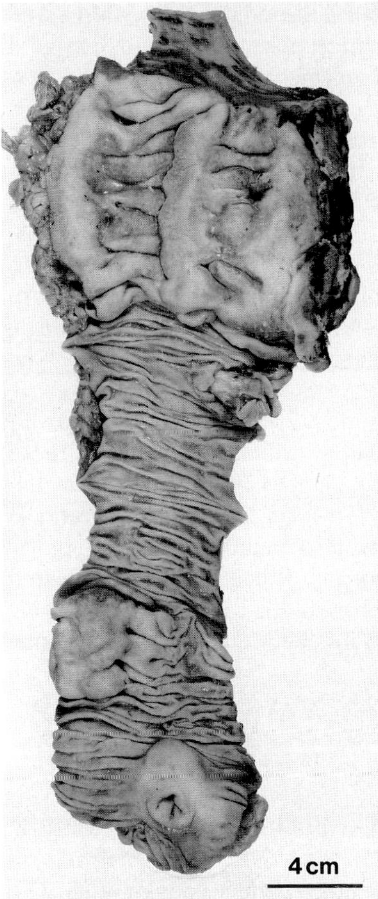

5

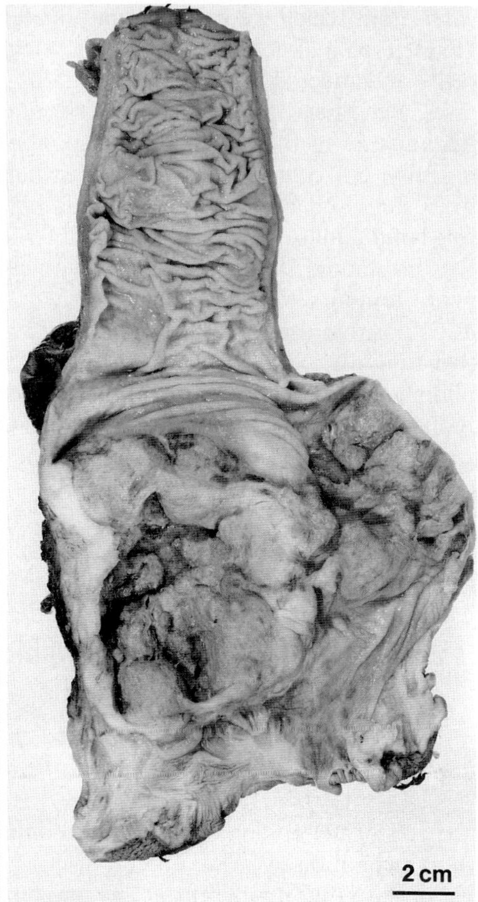

6

Fig. 5. Low grade polymorphic B cell lymphoma of ascending colon. Two well defined protuberant tumours

Fig. 6. High grade polymorphic B cell lymphoma of rectum. A typically large, ulcerated tumour

(ISAACSON and SPENCER 1987). The tumour cells form an interfollicular infiltrate external to the follicle mantle and this may suggest a T zone lymphoma to the inexperienced. As the follicles are replaced, a nodular or diffuse pattern of nodal involvement results. When high grade polymorphic B cell lymphomas metastasise to nodes they commonly produce discrete foci of tumour in the nodes in a similar manner to carcinomatous deposits (another potential pitfall for the unwary).

Immunohistichemically, provided a panel of B cell markers is used, the B cell nature of such polymorphic tumours can be confirmed in almost all cases in paraffin sections. We have found one or more of the currently available B cell markers to be positive in tumour cells in all suspected cases from which we hae adequate material. Antibodies such as MT1 and UCHL1 will almost invariably show the presence of admixed ractive T cells, and macrophage markers such as lysosyme and Mac 400 will show associated macrophages (SHEPHERD et al. 1988; HALL et al. 1988a). In frozen sections the tumour cells in polymorphic B cell lymphomas are CD5 negative (cf. centrocytic lymphoma where the cells are CD5 positive). We were surprised by the results of staining with MT2 in our polymorphic B cell lymphomas of colon and rectum. Most of our low grade polymorphic B cell tumours stained positively with this reagent while most of the high grade tumours were negative. Survival analysis showed that patients with MT2 positive tumours did significantly better than those with MT2 negative tumours. Similar observations have been made in nodal B cell lymphoma (HALL, unpublished observations).

The mainstay of treatment is surgical removal of the tumour. Adjuvant radiotherapy and chemotherapy have not been properly assessed for these tumours. We applied a modified Dukes' staging to these tumours in the colorectum and found trends towards better survival in stages A and B compared to C (SHEPHERD et al. 1988). We also found statistically significantly better survival for low grade polymorphic B cell tumours compared with high grade. The survival of patients with high grade polymorphic B cell lymphoma was similar to that of patients with malignant lymphomatous polyposis.

9.2 Mediterranean Lymphoma

Aspects of the epidemiology of this condition and its relationship to ISPID (alpha chain disease) have been discussed in Sect. 7.2. It is a small intestinal disease that may occur at any age but tends to affect young adults. The clinical presentation is usually that of malabsorption not due to gluten sensitivity. Abdominal pain, weight loss and finger clubbing are often additional features. Diarrhoea or signs of small bowel obstruction may then develop or may be the initial presenting features (ISAACSON 1985).

The macroscopic features are also variable. In most cases there is diffuse, even thickening of the upper small intestine together with enlarged mesenteric lymph nodes. Localised, sometimes multiple tumours may be present and gastric involvement is not uncommon. The histological features are characteristic and have been divided into three stages (ISAACSON 1985): stage A with diffuse plasma cell infiltration of the lamina propria but little or no invasion of crypt epithelium (Fig. 7a); stage B with a nodular or band-like infiltrate deep in the lamina propria below the plasma cells and composed of a mixture of B lymphocytes (morphologically small lymphocytes, centrocyte-like and centroblast-like cells) (lympho-epithelial lesions are present at this stage); and stage C with the mixed lymphomatous infiltrate predominating and less noticeable plasma cells dispersed through the tumour. Sometimes the infiltrate at stage C contains many immunob-

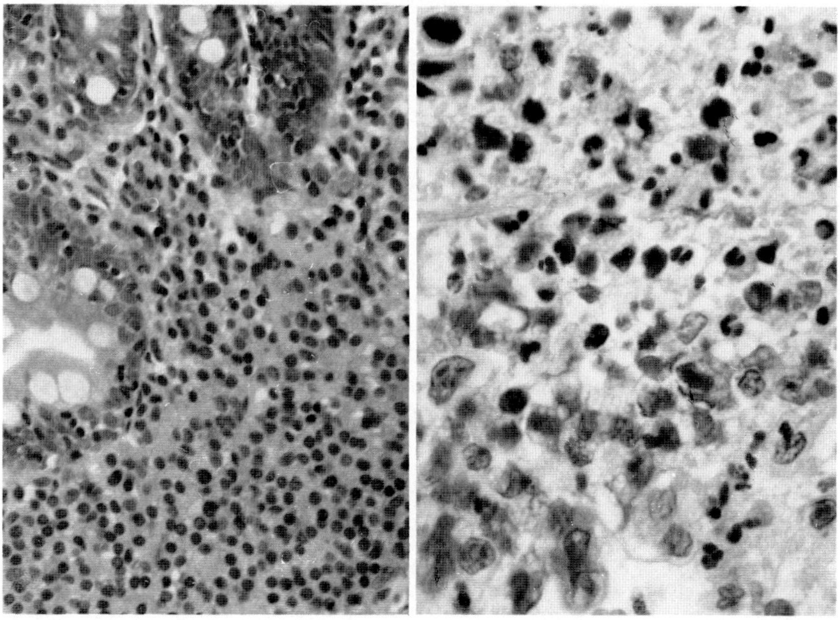

a b

Fig. 7a, b. Jejunal biopsies from a patient with IPSID. Biopsy (**a**), done 3 years before (**b**), shows a monotonous plasmacytic infiltrate in the lamina propria; **b** shows more obviously cytologically malignant b lymphoid cells in the base of an ulcer. HE, × 400 (**a**), × 625 (**b**)

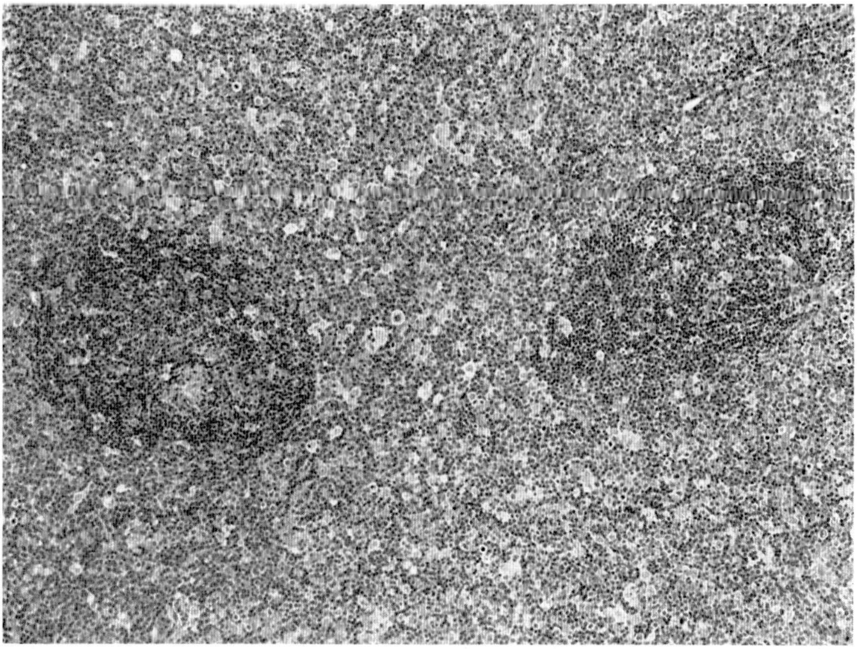

Fig. 8. Mediastinal node from a patient with IPSID at a frankly lymphomatous stage with a diffuse neoplastic interfollicular infiltrate surrounding two surviving follicles. HE, × 100

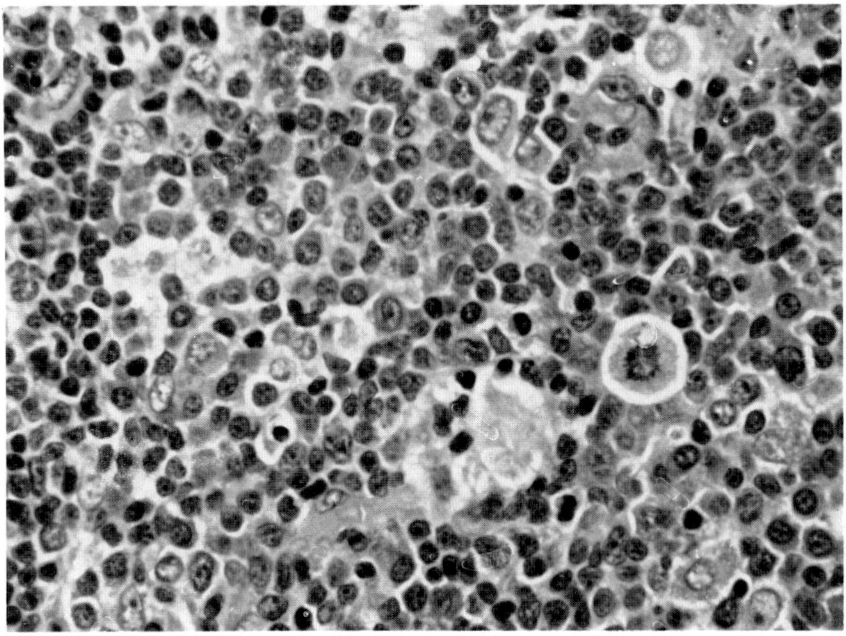

Fig. 9. Higher power of part of the field in Fig. 8 showing a polymorphic B cell infiltrate. The pattern of infiltration shown in Fig. 8 and the cytological components shown in Fig. 9 are typical of a low grade polymorphic B cell lymphoma, and suggest that IPSID is a variant of this neoplasm. HE, × 625

lasts and the histological picture is markedly polymorphic (Fig. 7b). Lympho-epithelial lesions are also present at this stage. The tumour is thus a polymorphic B cell lymphoma and when it involves nodes the pattern of involvement and cytological appearances are those of a polymorphic B cell lymphoma (see Sect. 9.1 and also Fig. 8 and 9). It seems most logical to regard Mediterranean lymphoma as a subgroup of polymorphic B cell lymphoma with a peculiar natural history, geographical and anatomical distribution.

Cytoplasmic alpha chain can be consistently demonstrated in the plasma cells in such tumours, but not in the more obvious tumour cells. Monotypic light chains were said to be present only in tumour cells and not in the plasma cells until ISAACSON and PRICE (1985) recently demonstrated the same monotypic light chains in both the plasma cells and other tumour cells of some cases. This evidence and the more recent gene rearrangement studies (SMITH WJ et al. 1987) have indicated that the plasma cells and the other tumour cells are of the same monoclonal origin. The absence of immunohistochemically detectable light chains from some cases means that in such cases monotypia is not demonstrable by this technique.

Spread of Mediterranean lymphoma outside the abdominal cavity is rare until the terminal stages of the disease, but surgery is not always effective because of the characteristically extensive involvement of the bowel.

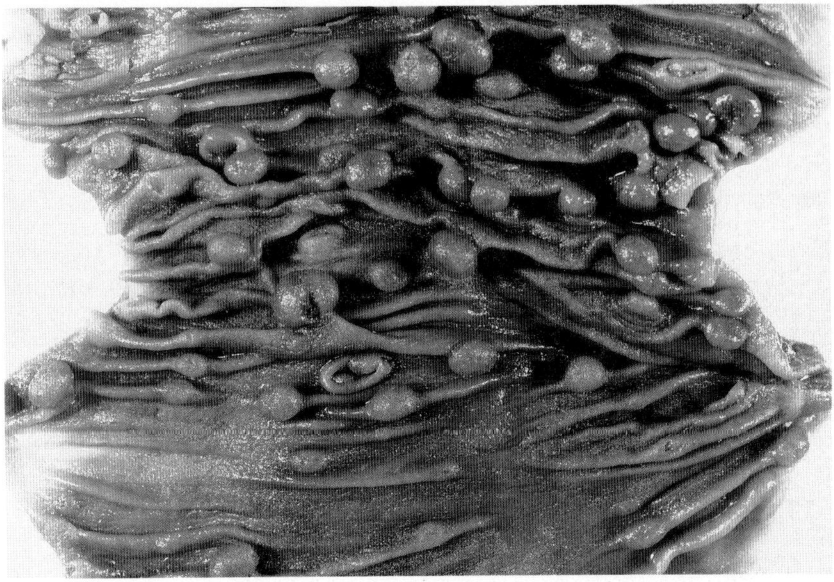

Fig. 10. Malignant lymphomatous polyposis (centrocytic lymphoma) of colon

Radiotherapy and chemotherapy have been tried. The unique feature of this disease is the long-term remissions which may be induced by broad spectrum antibiotics in its early stages.

9.3 Centrocytic Lymphoma

In our experience of primary gut lymphomas, this type is the basis of the lesion known in the literature as multiple or malignant lymphomatous polyposis (Blackshaw 1980; Isaacson et al. 1984). Most older reports suggest that any lymphoma, including Hodgkin's disease, may be the basis of malignant lymphomatous polyposis. This mistaken view arose for two reasons: first, centrocytic lymphomas were only recognised as a distinct entity in relatively recent times (Lennert 1978); secondly, multinuclear macrophages in this condition have sometimes been interpreted as Reed-Sternberg cells. The first decription of malignant lymphomatous polyposis is attributed to Briquet and appears, accompanied by illustrations in Cruveilhier's Atlas (1835–1842). Here it is entitled *"Maladies des follicles de l'eestomac, du duodenum, de l'intestin grele et du gros intestin"* – an informative but somewhat cumbersome terminology.

In our series, this lymphoma accounts for about 15% of all primary gut lymphomas. As with most lymphomas, it is a tumour of adults; our age range is 45–75, with a mean age of 55. It hardly ever presents with perforation (never in our series), due to the usually superficial infiltrate involving only mucosa and submucosa, often without ulceration. The sup-

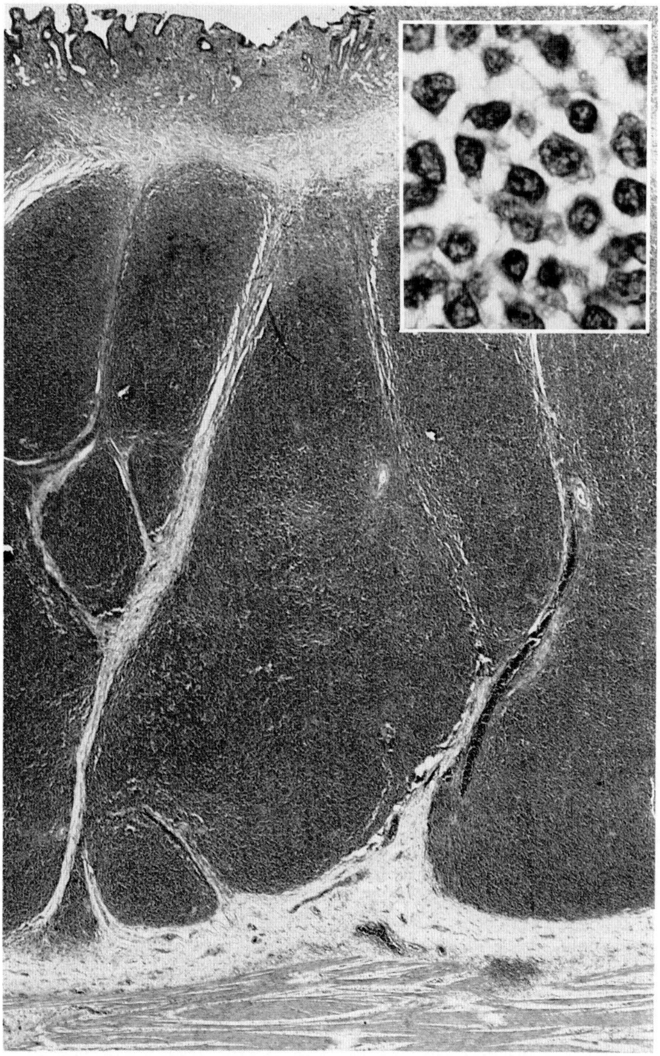

Fig. 11. Malignant lymphomatous polyposis (centrocytic lymphoma) of small bowel showing the dense infiltrate characteristically confined to mucosa and submucosa. The *insert* shows that the infiltrate is composed virtually entirely of centrocytes. HE, × 50. *Insert*, × 625

erficial location of the infiltrate also accounts for the polypoid (Fig. 10) or sometimes convoluted cerebriform appearance of the mucosa. In our experience virtually all purely centrocytic lymphomas are multiple, and apparently isolated involvement of a single part of the gut such as the colon or even a segment such as the rectum should be regarded with suspicion since there is usually more disease beyond the limits of clinical detection. Malignant lymphomatous polyposis therefore forms the exception to the rule that the principal treatment of gut lymphomas is surgical. The only hope of control of this disease lies with chemotherapy (Richards 1986).

Eventually in most cases, despite the contrary view expressed in earlier reports (CORNES 1961; SHEAHAN et al. 1971), a centrocytic leukaemia and peripheral lymphadenopathy develop (DAVIES et al. 1970; HALKIN et al. 1973; FROMKE and WEBER 1974; BLACKSHAW 1980). The lymph nodes show a characteristically diffuse infiltrate of centrocytes. The prognosis is generally poor; CORNES (1961) states that most patients with malignant lymphomatous polposis are dead within 2–3 years. BLACKSHAW (1980) found a median survival of the order of 18 months. Our 11 large bowel cases represent the largest published series to date and showed a median survival of 2 years (SHEPHERD et al. 1988).

Histologically, once the predominant cell has been identified as a centrocyte, the diagnosis of centrocytic lymphoma is relatively straightforward. The tumour is composed of a monomorphic infiltrate of small or large centrocytes (Fig. 11). These cells resemble the centrocytes (cleaved cells) of the germinal centre of the lymphoid follicle. An admixture of inflammatory cells, apart sometimes from large macrophages, is not usually seen in this lymphoma, as ulceration is a rare event. The infiltrate is usually strictly confined to submucosa and mucosa, is diffuse or nodular, but does not display a true follicular pattern (Fig. 11).

The tumour cells often show a very striking mitotic rate. As may be seen in nodal centrocytic lymphomas, bundles and strands of hyalinised collagen are a common feature. Lympho-epithelial lesions (see Sect. 9.1) are not a feature of pure centrocytic lymphomas. In paraffin sections the cells of centrocytic lymphomas react with most B cell paraffin markers. In frozen sections the cells of this tumour express Leu 1 (CD5) (ISAACSON et al. 1984) in contrast to the cells of polymorphic B cell lymphomas, which are negative for this marker (ISAACSON et al. 1986).

9.4 Follicular Centroblastic/Centrocytic Lymphoma

In most series of nodal lymphomas this is the commonest non-Hodgkin's lymphoma and that is certainly our experience. In the gut true primary centroblastic/centrocytic follicular lymphomas are very rare. They have to be carefully distinguished from low grade polymorphic B cell lymphomas with reactive and overrun follices (see above) and also from florid reactive hyperplasia. The criteria for distinguishing between reactive and neoplastic follicles in the gut are the same as in nodes and the distinction, though usually easy, can be very difficult. It is generally safe to assume that if there are reactive follicles present in a gut lesion, then it is not a follicular lymphoma.

The very few cases of probable primary follicular lymphomas of the gut which we have seen also had mediastinal node involvement. One could argue that even they represent secondary gut involvement by primary nodal lymphoma. The literature on primary follicular lymphomas of the gut is too confused to allow any firm conclusions to be drawn on treatment and prognosis.

9.5 Burkitt-Type Lymphoma

As a primary gastrointestinal lymphoma, Burkitt-type lymphoma, formerly B lymphoblastic lymphoma, is classically seen in the ileocaecal region in children (BLACKSHAW 1980). However, we have observed several examples elsewhere in the small bowel, stomach and large bowel of adults. This tumour is often advanced at presentation, with extensive infiltration through all layers of the bowel wall. However, unlike high grade polymorphic B cell lymphoma, Burkitt-type lymphoma is remarkably non-destructive. Fissuring ulceration and perforation are not features. Indeed the lymphoma, although deeply invading and widely permeating, shows little destruction of the muscularis propria (BLACKSHAW 1980). Another peculiarity of this tumour is that it seldom invades mesenteric lymph nodes, which may be seen uninvolved, although surrounded by infiltrating tumour cells. Even after radical surgery, recurrence is common and early widespread dissemination, especially within the peritoneal cavity, is another problem. Adjuvant chemotherapy should always be given.

The histological appearances of this tumour are characteristic. The tumour is composed of monotonous sheets of medium sized blast cells with little cytoplasm and a nucleus containing rather coarse chromatin with several inconspicuous nucleoli. The cells have a B phenotype. The very rapid cell turnover is reflected in the high mitotic index, wide areas of necrosis and the presence of apoptotic bodies. There may be plentiful reactive histiocytes containing these apoptotic bodies, and the liberal distribution of these cells gives the tumour its characteristic, although not universal, starry sky appearance.

9.6 Pure Centroblastic and Immunoblastic Lymphomas

We now regard centroblastic and B immunoblastic lymphomas as extremely rare gut primaries. We find it very difficult to pick out from our series, tumours which are composed of pure populations of either centroblasts or B immunoblasts. Most tumours containing large numbers of centroblasts and/or B immunoblasts we now classify as high grade polymorphic B cell lymphomas (see Sect. 9.1). However, should the reader prefer to regard such tumours as centroblastic or B immunoblastic lymphomas then the remarks above concerning behaviour, presentation, spread, treatment and prognosis of high grade polymorphic B cell lymphomas can also be applied to these lymphomas.

That T immunoblastic lymphomas occur in the gut is now indisputable: large cell pleomorphic T cell lymphomas are essentially T immunoblastic tumours. T immunoblastic lymphomas, however, apart from the setting of coeliac disease, are relatively rare gut primaries, but do occur (MOUBAYED et al. 1987; SHEPHERD et al. 1987).

9.7 T Cell Lymphomas

At the time of writing there has been no published systematic classification of primary T cell lymphomas of the gut. It is only recently that such a classificaton has been proposed for T cell lymphomas of nodes (SUCHI et al. 1987; STANSFELD et al. 1988). Descriptive terms have been applied to groups of gut T cell lymphomas, e.g. enteropathy-associated T cell lymphoma (O'FARRELLY et al. 1986) and malignant lymphoma with eosinophilia (SHEPHERD et al. 1987), and such terms are in current usage. Our proposed classification of gut T cell lymphomas (Table 2) attempts to incorporate such terms within a framework which is in line with current Kiel nomenclature, the published literature and our own experience.

It is generally agreed that enteropathy-associated T cell lymphomas exhibit a wide range of tumour cell appearance (ISAACSON and WRIGHT 1980), from small pleomorphic to large pleomorphic cells, though in most cases medium to large cells predominate. Also we have certainly seen tumours morphologically identical to enteropathy-associated T cell lymphomas, but outwith the context of coeliac disease (enteropathy). It therefore seems sensible to us to employ Kiel terms such as small/medium/large cell pleomorphic T cell and to indicate whether or not such tumours are associated with enteropathy. Our own experience of primary T cell lymphomas of gut comprises over 50 cases of pleomorphic T cell lymphoma, about half of which are enteropathy (coeliac disease) associated, and including 28 cases of malignant lymphoma with eosinophilia (SHEPHERD et al. 1987), eight of which are coeliac associated. We have also seen one small cell T cell tumour which showed very marked epitheliotropism, and one large cell anaplastic T cell lymphoma associated with Crohn's disease (SHEPHERD et al. 1989). The vast majority of our T cell lymphomas are in small bowel, but we have seen occasional examples in stomach, as have others (MOUBAYED et al. 1987), and colon. Pleomorphic T cell lymphoma and its subgroup malignant lymphoma with eosinophilia are considered in more detail below (Sects. 9.8 and 9.9).

9.8 Pleomorphic T Cell Lymphoma

We favour this term to "enteropathy-associated T cell lymphoma" (ISAACSON et al. 1985; LOUGHRAN et al. 1986; O'FARRELLY et al. 1986) as this tumour is not exclusively related to coeliac disease. Until 1985 it was widely known as malignant histiocytosis of the intestine (ISAACSON and WRIGHT 1978, 1980) in the mistaken belief that the tumour cells were true histiocytes, but there is now convincing evidence that it is a T cell tumour (ISAACSON et al. 1985; SALTER et al. 1986). the relationship between this tumour, coeliac disease and ulcerative jejunitis is discussed in Sect. 7.1. Recent studies have indicated that there are immunophenotypic similarities between normal T lymphocytes that are found in association

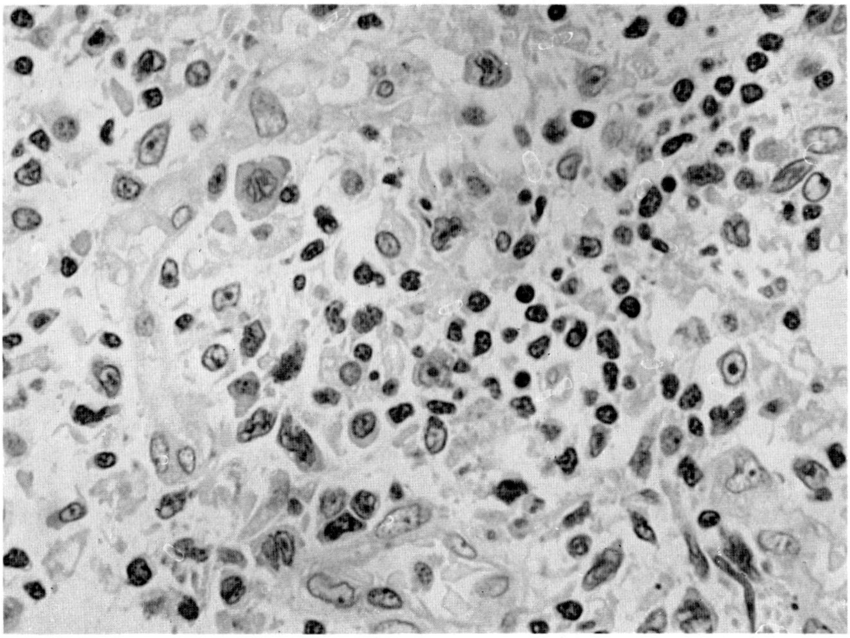

Fig. 12. A non-enteropathy-associated pleomorphic T cell lymphoma of jejunum. Large neoplastic pleomorphic T cells are scattered amongst small inflammatory lymphoid cells. The appearances are indistinguishable from enteropathy-associated pleomorphic T cell lymphoma. HE, × 625

with the surface epithelium and the neoplastic cells in enteropathy-associated pleomorphic T cell lymphomas (ISAACSON et al. 1987).

This tumour occurs particularly in the fifth to seventh decades with an equal incidence in males and females. Presenting features include return of steatorrhoea in a previous responder to a gluten-free diet, weight loss, abdominal pain and diarrhoea. Pyrexia, finger clubbing and an ichthyotic skin rash are sometimes seen (HODGES et al. 1979). Perforation of the tumour with peritonitis is common and this may recur following surgery. Some cases present with peripheral lymphadenopathy due to disseminated tumour.

Macroscopic appearances are variable. The tumour may occur in any part of the small intestine, but is most common in the jejunum. It is often multifocal, appearing as multiple ulcers or strictures or alternatively as larger plaques, nodules or areas of diffuse thickening. The mesentery is often tickened and mesenteric lymph nodes are often enlarged. Sometimes there is no obvious macroscopic lesion.

The histological appearances are also very variable. At one end of the spectrum one sees a predominantly mixed inflammatory infiltrate containing only occasional tumour cells of relatively bland appearance, but with large irregular indented nuclei (Fig. 12). At the other end of the spectrum one finds sheets of clearly malignant cells also with large somewhat less irregular nuclei and showing a high mitotic rate. The inflammatory infiltrate sometimes contains abundant eosinophils and the picture merges with malignant lymphoma with eosinophilia (see below). Pleomorphic T cell lymphoma, like many other primary gut lymphomas, may diffusely infiltrate blood vessel walls, and is also sometimes associated with a granulomatous response (ISAACSON and WRIGHT 1980). When lymph nodes are involved it is predominantly the T zones which are infiltrated and here it may be easier to recognise the neoplastic nature of the process as there may be fewer associated inflammatory cells than in the bowel wall.

In the majority of cases the tumour is disseminated when the diagnosis is made. Mesenteric lymph nodes are first involved, but spleen, liver and bone marrow are common sites and in these the subtle nature of the malignant infiltrate can easily be missed unless searched for very diligently. The prognosis is generally regarded as poor though exact survival figures are not available.

9.9 Malignant Lymphoma with Eosinophilia

In our series of primary gut lymphomas, which now stands at over 250 cases, we have observed 28 cases of a lymphoma with distinctive histological features, characterised by a massive tissue eosinophilia (SHEPHERD et al. 1987). The relatively high incidence in our series, we are sure, does not reflect the state of affairs in a standard population as many of these cases were secondary referrals due to local difficulty with the diagnosis. We were most often asked – is this reactive or neoplastic, or could it be Hodgkin's disease? Two of the tumours were present in the stomach (Fig. 13) and 26 in the small intestine. Eight of the latter were associated with coeliac disease.

On low power microscopy a characteristic zoning phenomenon was regularly seen. This comprised an innermost zone consisting of an ulcer base of fibrinous debris with extensive tissue necrosis and granulation tissue; beneath this was a cellular zone with the areas of intense tissue eosinophilia and scattered neoplastic lymphoid cells (Fig. 14); the outermost zone was densely fibrotic, of variable depth and in most cases replaced the muscularis propria. This zone contained numerous eosinophils and capillary blood vessels, but tumour cells were scanty or absent. Fissuring ulceration with perforation and fistula formation were common findings. High power examination showed the tumour cells to be large and pleomorphic with irregular nuclear morphology and prominent nucleoli (Fig. 14). Though eosinophils were the predominant associated inflammatory cells, plasma cells, epithelioid histiocytes and small lymphocytes were also present. Veins often showed invasion of walls and luminal narrowing. Both arteries and veins, particularly in the fibrotic zone, showed intimal fibrosis. Involved lymph nodes showed gross expansion of the paracortex

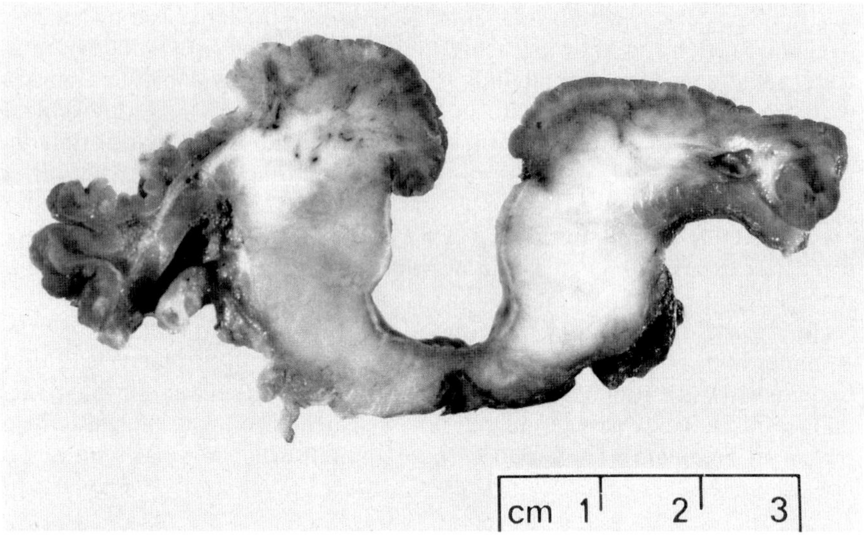

Fig. 13. Malignant lymphoma with eosinophilia of stomach, showing full thickness involvement and ulceration

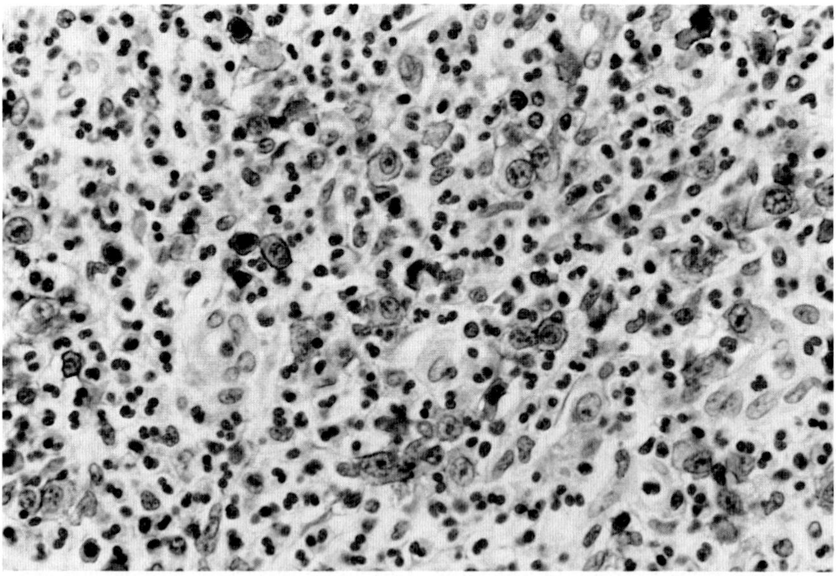

Fig. 14. Malignant lymphoma with eosinophilia of jejunum. Scattered, large pleomorphic T lymphocytes, confirmed by membrane staining with UCHL1, among abundant eosinophil polymorphs showing no cytoplasmic or membrane staining. UCHL1 immunoperoxidase, × 500

by tumour, often with relatively fewer eosinophils than in the primary tumour. Immunohistochemical studies (Fig. 14) showed that the lymphoma was probably of T cell origin (SHEPHERD et al. 1987).

Of 24 patients on whom we had full clinical follow-up information, 12 had died at a mean of 11 months from the time of diagnosis. Most of the survivors were recently diagnosed, but two had survived for 12 and 13 years respectively. Surgical resection was the mainstay of therapy. There was no evidence in our series that radiotherapy or chemotherapy was useful.

10 Immunohistochemistry and Gene Rearrangement Studies

These techniques have an important role in research into the biology of gut lymphomas. Their diagnostic role is more limited but, in certain circumstances, important. Most diagnostic problems concerning gut lymphomas do not become apparent until after the specimen is fixed and paraffin sections have been examined. We shall therefore concentrate on markers which may be employed with paraffin sections.

One recurring problem, particularly with high grade gut lymphomas, is their distinction from anaplastic carcinomas. This can now be achieved in most instances in paraffin sections by the use of antibodies to leucocyte common antigen (CD45), which react with most lymphomas, and antibodies to various cytokeratins (particularly CAM 5.2) which react with most carcinomas (GATTER et al. 1984; DEAN et al. 1987). Antibodies to epithelial membrane antigen are, in our view, generally less useful in making this particular distinction as they react with some lymphoid cells as well as most epithelial cells (DELSOL et al. 1984; HALL et al. 1988a).

There is now a range of monoclonal antibodies commercially available which will distinguish the B cell, T cell, or macrophage lineage of cells in paraffin sections (SHEPHERD et al. 1987, 1988; HALL et al. 1988a). We have found it necessary in our studies to employ panels of antibodies to be sure of the lineage of tumours (SHEPHERD et al. 1987, 1988). Great care must be exercised in interpreting the results of UCHL1 staining, where only distinct cell membrane positivity can be taken as evidence of T cell phenotype.

Another problem area in which immunohistochemistry can sometimes help is in the distinction between reactive and neoplastic lymphoid infiltrates. The demonstration of immunoglobulin light chain restriction is useful evidence in favour of a clonal population and thus is supportive of a diagnosis of lymphoma. Until recently only cytoplasmic immunoglobulin could be demonstrated in formalin-fixed paraffin-embedded tissues and surface immunoglobulin required cryostat sections for its demonstration. However, the use of the ABC (avidin biotin complex) system (HSU et al. 1981; NORTON and ISAACSON 1987; HALL, unpublished) and the IGS (immunogold silver) methods (HOLGATE et al. 1983; SMITH G et al. 1987) now allows surface immunoglobulin to be reliably demonstrated in conventionally processed material. Such methods are of great value in the assessment of light chain restriction. Similar methods for the demonstration of clonal T cell populations using immunohistochemistry can still only be performed on cryostat sections and are not yet widely applicable (CLARK et al. 1986).

Ideally, tissue from all suspected gut lymphomas should be snap-frozen and stained with the full range of immunohistochemical markers routinely employed for nodal lymphomas. It is only through the use of frozen tissue, at present, that one can distinguish between subsets of T lymphocytes, e.g. helper and suppressor, and even more precisely characterise such tumours. Such information is certainly of histogenetic interest though not currently of therapeutic importance. Frozen tissue is also required for the detection of CD5 immunoreactivity which is present in centrocytic lymphomas, but not in polymorphic B cell tumours, though other means of making this differential diagnosis are usually reliable.

Gene rearrangement studies are not routinely available in most hospitals. However, such techniques have already proved useful in settling arguments regarding the lineage of certain tumours. Demonstration of rearranged T cell receptor beta chain genes (ISAACSON et al. 1985) has helped to confirm that lymphomas complicating coeliac disease are predominantly of T cell type and not histiocytic. In IPSID, the demonstration of monoclonal heavy and light chain gene rearrangements at all stages of the disease has suggested that it is neoplastic even in its early stages despite responsiveness to antibiotics (SMITH WJ et al. 1987). Similar studies in patients with IPSID have so far failed to detect the same gene rearrangements in circulating cells in humans, suggesting that such malignant cells do not belong to a recirculating pool. Further studies of this type can be expected to advance our understanding of this enigmatic group of tumours.

11 Concluding Comment

The main fuction of gut-associated lymphoid tissue is to provide an adaptive protective mechanism to help defend the body from exogenous antigens. This complex function requires the co-ordination of various cellular elements including B and T lymphocytes, macrophages and the epithelial cells of the gut. The control mechanisms for this are largely unknown but almost certainly involve humoral factors acting in a paracrine and autocrine manner, and direct cell-cell interactions. Disruption of these mechanisms must be involved in, and is likely to be fundamental to, the development and behaviour of gut lymphomas. Although conventional histopathology is likely to remain the mainstay of diagnosis and patient management, it seems probable that further significant advances in the understanding, diagnosis and therapy of gastrointestinal lymphomas will require a greater knowledge of these control mechanisms and the molecules involved therein.

Acknowledgements. We wish to thank particularly Drs. Alfred Stansfeld and Basil Morson, our mentors in lymphoma and gut pathology, to whom many of the cases studied by us were originally referred. We also thank Dr. Neil Shepherd for his recent considerable work in documenting the Bart's/St Mark's series of gut lymphomas. Drs. Shepherd and Stansfeld also critically reviewed the text. We thank Miss Gillian Taylor and Mr. Peter Crocker respectively for excellent secretarial and photographic work.

Addendum

Since the completion of this chapter several important advances have been reported in our understanding of the molecular basis of the immune system of the gut. BUTCHER and colleagues have reported the preliminary characterisation of an evolutionarily highly conserved series of endothelial antigens (WU et al. 1988) that are involved in the homing of lymphocytes to gastrointestinal (STREETER et al. 1988a) and nodal (STREETER et al. 1988b) sites and the fact that these interactions can be blocked by specific antibodies. Such mechanisms are of obvious relevance to the characteristic localisation of gastrointestinal lymphoma. A second advance has been the recognition that T lymphocytes associated with epithelia, and in particular gastrointestinal epithelia, do not employ the $\alpha\beta$ heterodimer T cell receptor as seen in nodal T lymphocytes. Instead a second pair of T cell receptor genes are used, γ and δ (BONEVILLE et al. 1988; GOODMAN and LEFRANCOIS 1988), which may be phylogenetically older and serve a specific defence function at epithelial sites (JANEWAY 1988; JANEWAY et al. 1988). This does, however, lead to a paradox: why have some primary gut T cell lymphomas been shown to have rearranged β T cell receptor genes?

That T lymphocytes of the gut, and tumours derived from them, differ from nodal T cells is supported by the recent observations of SPENCER et al. (1988) and STEIN et al. (1988), who have reported independently that the antibody HML-1 recognises intra-epithelial gastrontestinal T lymphocytes and associated tumours. Although purported to be a marker of enteropathy-associated tumours (SPENCER et al. 1988), we consider this claim to be premature in view of the small number of enteropathy-associated cases ($n = 9$) so far reported, and the complete absence of non-enteropathy-associated gut lymphomas in the reported series. HML-1 may well prove to mark gut-associated T cell lymphomas regardless of an association with enteropathy, and the nature of the antigen recognised will certainly be of interest.

These recent data concerning molecular aspects of the immune system of the gut and its associated tumours strengthen the argument for a separate, site-specific, nomenclature. Since submission of this manuscript we have proposed such a classification which is similar to, and extends, that described in this chapter (HALL et al. 1988c). We hope that this interim classification is seen as a pragmatic approach to the subject, given our present imperfect understanding of the immune system of the gut. We are aware of the meeting of the European Association of Haematopathology (Geneva, April 1988) in which a consensus on a provisional classification of gut lymphomas was reached (as yet unpublished) and we understand from discussions with delegates that this view is not dissimilar from that proposed previously (HALL et al. 1988c) and in this chapter.

References

Adjukiewicz AB, Youngs GR, Bouchier IAD (1972) Nodular lymphoid hyperplasia with hypogammaglobulinaemia. Gut 13:589–595

Al-Bahrani Z, Bakir F (1971) Primary intestinal lymphoma: a challenging problem in abdominal pain. Ann R Coll Surg Engl 49:3–13

Allen AW, Donaldson G, Sniffen RC, Goodale F (1954) Primary malignant lymphoma of the gastrointestinal tract. Ann Surg 140:428–438

Al-Saleem T, Al-Bahrani Z (1973) Malignant lymphoma of the small intestine in Iraq. Cancer 31:291–294

Anscombe AM, Wright DH (1985) Primary malignant lymphoma of the thyroid – a tumour of mucosa associated tissue: review of seventy six cases. Histopathology 9:81–97

Armitage JO, Dick FR, Corder MP (1978) Diffuse histiocyte lymphoma complicating chronic lymphocytic leukaemia. Cancer 41:422–427

Asselah F, Slavin G, Sowter G, Asselah H (1983) Immunoproliferative small intestinal disease in Algerians. I. Light microscopic and immunochemical studies. Cancer 52:227–237

Azzopardi JG, Menzies T (1960) Primary malignant lymphoma of the gastrointestinal tract. Br J Surg 47:358–366

Berg JW (1969) Primary lymphomas of the gastrointestinal tract. Nat Cancer Inst Monogr 32:211–216

Bienenstock J, McDermott M, Befus D, O-Neill M (1978) A common mucosal immunologic system involving breast, bronchus and bowel. Adv Exp Med Biol 107:53–62

Blackledge G, Bush H, Dodge OG, Crowther D (1979) A study of gastrointestinal lymphoma. Clin Oncol 5:209–219

Blackshaw AJ (1980) Non-Hodgkin's lymphomas of the gut. In: Wright R (ed) Recent advances in gastrointestinal pathology. WB Saunders, London, pp 213–240

Bockman DE, Boydston WR, Beezhold DH (1983) The role of epithelial cells in gut associated immune reactivity. In: McGhee JR, Mestecky J (eds) The secretory immune system. The New York Academy of Sciences, New York pp 129–144

Boneville M, Janeway CA, Ito K, Haser W, Ishida I, Nakanishi N, Tonegawa S. (1988) Intestinal intraepithelial lymphocytes are a distinct set of $\gamma-\delta$ T cells. Nature 336:479–481

Brandt L, Hagander B, Norden A, Stentsam M (1978) Lymphoma of the small intestine in adult coeliac disease. Acta Med Scand 204:467–470

Brown TC, Peter MV, Bergsagel DE, Reid J (1975) A retrospective analysis of the clinical results in relation to the Rappaport histological classification. Br J Cancer. [Suppl II]:174–186

Brunt PW, Sircus W, MacLean N (1969) Neoplasia and the coeliac syndrome in adults. Lancet I:180–184

Burkes RL, Meyer PR, Gill PS, Parker JW, Rasheed S, Levine AM (1986) Rectal lymphoma in homosexual men. Arch Intern Med 146:913–915

Burman SO, van Wyk FAK (1956) Lymhomas of the small intestine and caecum. Ann Surg 143:349–359

Bush RS, Ash CL (1969) Primary lymphoma of the gastrointestinal tract. Radiology 92:1349–1354

Camilleri JP, Diebold J (1972) Sarcomes lymphorecticulaires de l'intestin grele. Ann Gastroenterol Hepatol 8:279–297

Clark DM, Boylston AW, Hall PA, Carrel S (1986) Antibodies to T-cell antigen receptor beta chain families detect monoclonal T-cell proliferations. Lancet II:835–837

Clarke RE, Simonds JP (1951) Primary lymphosarcoma of the appendix. Cancer 4:994–998

Coggon DNM, Rose DH, Ansell ID (1981) A large bowel lymphoma complicating renal transplantation. Br J Radiol 54:418–420

Connors J, Wise L (1974) Management of gastric lymphomas. Am J Surg 127:102–108

Coonley CL, Straus DJ, Filippa D, Watson R (1984) Hodgkin's disease presenting with rectal symptoms in a homosexual male. Cancer Invest 2(4):279–284

Cornes JS (1961) Multiple lymphmatous polyposis of the gastrointestinal tract. Cancer 14:249–257

Cornes JS, Wallace MH, Morson BC (1961) Benign lymphomas of the rectum and anal canal. J Pathol Bacteriol 82:371–382

Crabbe PA, Bazin H, Eyssen H, Huemans JF (1968) The normal microbial flora as a major stimulus for proliferation of plasma cells sythesising IgA in the gut. Int Arch Allergy Appl Immunol 34:362–375

Cruveilhier J (1835–1842) Anatomie Pathologique du Corps Humain. J.B. Bailliere, Paris, vol 2, Sect 34 pp 1–6

Davies SW, Scarrow GD, Macaulay MB (1970) Mutltiple lymphomatous polyposis of the gastrointestinal tract. Br J Surg 57:125–131

Dawson IMP, Cornes JS, Morson BC (1961) Primary malignant lymphoid tumours of the gastrointestinal tract. Ann Surg 191:593–598

Dean PJ, Moinuddin SM, Emmerson LD (1987) Application of anti-leukocyte common antigen and anti-cytokeratin antibodies to the biopsy diagnosis of gastric large cell lymphoma. Hum Pathol 18:918–923

Delsol G, Gatter KC, Stein H, Erber WN, Pulford KA, Zinne K, Mason DY (1984) Human lymphoid cells express epithelial membrane antigen. Implications for diagnosis of human neoplasms. Lancet II:1124–1128

Dixon MF, Wyatt JL, Burke DA, Rathbone BJ (1988) Lymphocytic gastritis – relationship to Campylobacter pylori infection. J Pathol 154:125–132

Dorreen MS, Gregory WM, Wrigley PFM, Stansfeld AG, Lister TA (1986) Second primary malignant neoplasms in patients treated for Hodgkin's disease at St Bartholomew's Hospital. Haematol Oncol 4:149–161

Drexler HG,Jones DB, Diehl V, Minowada J (1988) Is the Hodgkin's cell a T- or B-lymphocyte? Haematol Oncol (In press)

Eimoto T, Futami K, Naito H, Takeshita M, Kikuchi M (1985) Gastric pseudolymphoma with monotypic cytoplasmic immunoglobulin. Cancer 55:788–793

Elston CO, Heck JA, Strober W (1979) T-cell regulation of murine IgA synthesis. J Exp Med 149:636–643

Fairley NH, MacKie FP (1937) The clinical and biochemical syndrome in lymphadenoma and allied diseases involving the mesenteric glands. Br Med J I:375–380

Farris TD, Saltzstein SL (1964) Gastric lymphoid hyperplasia: a lesion confused with lymphosarcoma. Cancer 17:207–212

Ferguson A (1977) Progress report. Intraepithelial lymphocytes of the small intestine. Gut 18:921–937

Freeman C, Berg JW, Cutler SJ (1972) Occurrence and prognosis of extranodal lymphomas. Cancer 29:252–260

Friedman AI (1959) Primary lymphosarcoma of the stomach: a clinical study of 75 cases. Am J Med 26:783–796

Fromke VL, Weber LW (1974) Extensive leukaemic infiltration of the gastrointestinal tract in chronic lymphosarcoma cell leukaemia. Am J Med 56:879–882

Fu YS, Perzin KH (1972) Lymphosarcoma of the small intestine: a clinicopathologic study. Cancer 29:645–659

Fuller LM, Banker FL, Butler JJ, Gamble JF, Sullivan MP (1975) The natural history of non-Hodgkin's lymphomata stages I and II. Br J Cancer [Suppl II]:270–285

Galian A, Lecestre MJ, Scotto J, Bognel C, Matuchansky C, Rambaud JC (1977) Pathological study of alpha-chain disease with special emphasis on evolution. Cancer 39:2081–2101

Gall EA, Mallory TB (1942) Malignant lymphoma. A clinico-pathologic survey of 618 cases. Am J Pathol 18:381–429

Gatter KC, Alcock C, Heryet A et al. (1984) The differential diagnosis of routinely processed anaplastic tumours using monoclonal antibodies. Am J Clin Pathol 82:33–43

Givler RL (1968) Lymphocytic leukaemia with co-existent localised reticulum cell sarcoma. Cancer 21:1184–1192

Glick DD, Soule EH (1966) Primary malignant lymphoma of colon or appendix. Arch Surg 92:144–151

Goodman T, Lefrancois L (1988) Expression of the γ–δ T cell receptor on intestinal CD8+ intraepithelial lymphocytes. Nature 333:855–858

Goudie RB, MacFarlane PS, Lindsay MK (1974) Homing of lymphocytes to non-lymphoid tissues. Lancet I:292–293

Green JA, Dawson AA, Jones PF, Brunt PW (1979) The presentation of gastrointestinal lymphoma: study of a population. Br J Surg 66:798–801

Griscelli C, Vasalli P, McClusky RT (1969) The distribution of large dividing lymph node cells in syngeneic recipient rats after intravenous injection. J Exp Med 130:1427–1451

Grody WW, Magidson JG, Weiss LM, Hu E, Warnke RA, Lewin KJ (1985) Gastrointestinal lymphomas. Immunohistochemical studies on the cell of origin. Am J Surg Pathol 9:328–337

Haghighi P, Nabizadeh I, Asvadi S, Mohallatee EA (1971) Cancer in Southern Iran. Cancer 27:965–977

Halkin H, Meytes D, Militeanu J, Ramot B (1973) Multiple lymphomatous polyposis of the gastrointestinal tract. Isr J Med Sci 9:648–654

Hall JG, Parry DM, Smith ME (1972) The distribution and differentiation of lymph node immunoblasts after intravenous injection into syngeneic recipients. Cell Tissue Kinet 5:269–281

Hall JG, Hopkins J, Orlans E (1977) Migration pathways of lymphoid cells with reference to the gut, immunoglobulins and lymphomata. Biochem Soc Trans 5:1581–1583

Hall PA, d'Ardenne AJ, Stansfeld AG (1988a) Paraffin section immunohistochemistry I. Non-Hodgkin's lymphoma. Histopathology 13:149–160

Hall PA, d'Ardenne AJ, Stansfeld AG (1988b) Paraffin section immunohistochemistry II. Hodgkin's disease and large cell anaplastic (Ki1) lymphoma. Histopathology 13:161–169

Hall PA, Jass JR, Levison DA, Morson BC, Shepherd NA, Sobin LH, Stansfeld AG (1988c) Classification of primary gut lymphoma. Lancet II:958

Hall PA, Kingston J, Stansfeld AG (1988d) Extensive necrosis in malignant lymphoma with granulomatous reaction mimicking tuberculosis. Histopathology 13:339–346

Hayes HT, Burr HB (1952) Benign lymphomas of the rectum. Am J Surg 84:545–550

Henry K, Farrer-Brown G (1977) Primary lymphomas of the gastrointestinal tract. 1. Plasma cell tumours. Histopathology 1:53–76

Henry K, Bennett MH, Vaughan G (1987) Non-Hodgkin's lymphoma in treated Hodgkin's disease. The BNLI experience. J Clin Pathol 152:200 A

Hermans PE, Huizenga KA, Hoffman HN, Brown AL, Markowitz H (1966) Dysgammaglobulinaemia associated with nodular lymphoid hyperplasia of the small intestine. Am J Med 40:78–89

Herrmann R, Panahon AM, Barcos MP, Walsh D, Stutzman L (1980) Gastro-intestinal involvement in non-Hodgkin's lymphoma. Cancer 46:215–222

Hertzer NR, Hoerr SO (1976) An interpretive review of lymphoma of the stomach. Surg Gynecol Obstet 143:113–124

Hodges JR, Isaacson PG, Smith CI, Sworn MJ (1979) Malignant histiocytosis of the intestine. Dig Dis Sci 24:631–638

Hoerr SO, McCormack LJ, Hertzer NR (1973) Prognosis in gastric lymphoma. Arch Surg 107:155–158

Holgate CS, Jackson P, Lauder I, Cowen P, Bird CC (1983) Surface membrane staining of immunoglobulins in paraffin sections of non-Hodgkin's lymphoma using immunogold-silver staining techniques. J Clin Pathol 36:742–746

Holmes GKT, Stokes PL, Sorahan TM, Prior P, Waterhouse JAH, Cooke WT (1976) Coeliac disease, gluten-free diet and malignancy. Gut 17:612–619

Hsu SM, Raine L, Fanger H (1981) Use of avidin-biotin-peroxidase complex (ABC) in immunoperoxidase techniques: a comparison between ABC and unlabelled antibody (PAP) procedures. J Histochem Cytochem 29:577–580

Hughes RK (1955) Reticulum cell sarcoma: a case possibly originating in regional enteritis. Ann Surg 21:770–773

Husband AJ (1982) Kinetics of extravasation and redistribution of IgA-specific antibody containing cells in the intestine. J Immunol 128:1355–1359

Husband AJ, Gowans JL (1978) the origin and antigen dependent distribution of IgA-containing cells in the intestine. J Exp Med 148:1146–1160

Ioachim HL, Weinstein MA, Robbins RD, Sohn N, Lugo PN (1987) Primary anorectal lymphoma. A new manifestation of the acquired immune deficiency syndrome (AIDS). Cancer 60:1449–1453

Isaacson PG (1985) Middle Eastern intestinal lymphoma. Semin Diagn Pathol 2:210–223

Isaacson PG, Price SK (1985) Light chains in Mediterranean lymphoma. J Clin Pathol 38:601–607

Isaacson PG, Spencer J (1987) Malignant lymphoma of mucosa-associated lymphoid tissue. Histopathology 11:445–462

Isaacson PG, Wright DH (1978) Malignant histiocytosis of the intestine. Hum Pathol 9:661–677

Isaacson PG, Wright DH (1980) Malabsorption and intestinal lymphoma. In: Wright R (ed) Recent advances in gastrointestinal pathology. WB Saunders, London, pp 193–212

Isaacson PG, Wright DH (1987) Extranodal lymphoma. In: Anthony PP, MacSween RNM (eds) Recent advances in histopathology XIII. Churchill Livingstone, Edinburgh, pp 159–184

Isaacson PG, Wright DH, Judd MA, Mepham BL (1979) Primary gastrointestinal lymphomas: a classification of 66 cases. Cancer 43:1805–1819

Isaacson PG, MacLennan KA, Subbuswamy SG (1984) Multiple lymphomatous polyposis of the gastrointestinal tract. Histopathology 8:641–656

Isaacson PG, O-Connor NTJ, Spencer J et al. (1985) Malignant histiocytosis of the intestine: a T cell lymphoma. Lancet II:688–691

Isaacson PG, Spencer J, Finn T (1986) Primary B-cell gastric lymphoma. Hum Pathol 17:72–82

Isaacson PG, Cerf-Bensussan N, Jarry A, Brousse N, Krajewski S, Spencer J (1987) Enteropathy associated T-cell lymphoma (malignant histiocytosis of the intestine) is derived from intraepithelial T-cells. J Pathol 152:217 A

Jacobs DS (1963) Primary gastric malignant lymphoma and pseudolymphoma. Am J Clin Pathol 40:379–394

Janeway CA (1988) Frontiers of the immune system. Nature 333:804–806

Janeway CA, Jones B, Hayday A (1988) Specificity and function of T cells bearing $\gamma-\delta$ receptors. Immunol Today 9:73–76

Jensen F (1967) Primary gastric sarcoma. Acta Chir Scand 133:139–151

Joseph JI, Lattes R (1966) Gastric lymphosarcoma: clinicopathologic analysis of seventy-one cases and its relation to disseminated lymphosarcoma. Am J Clin Pathol 45:653–669

Kagnoff MF (1981) Immunology of the digestive system. In: Johnson LR (ed Physiology of the gastrointestinal tract. Raven, New York, pp 1337–1358

Kahn LB, Selzer G, Kaschula ROC (1972) Primary gastrointestinal lymphoma: a clinicopathologic study of fifty seven cases. Am J Dig Dis 17:219–232

Kay S (1964) Lymphoid tumours of the stomach. Surg Gynaecol Obstet 118:1059–1066

Khojasteh A, Haghshenass M, Haghighi P (1983) Immunoproliferative small intestinal disease. A "third world lesion". N Engl J Med 308:1401–1405

Kumararatne DS, Bazin H, MacLennan ICM (1981) Marginal zones: the major B-cell compartment of rat spleens. Eur J Immunol 11:858–864

Kwee WS, Wils JAM, van den Tweel JG (1985) Malignant lymphoma, immunoblastic with plasmacytic differentiation, complicating Crohn's disease. Histopathology 9:1115–1120

Lennert K in collaboration with Mohri N, Stein H, Kaiserling E, Muller-Hermelink HK (1978) Malignant lymphomas other than Hodgkin's disease. Springer, Berlin Heidelberg New York

Levine AM, Gill PS, Meyer PR et al. (1985) Retrovirus and malignant lymphoma in homosexual men. JAMA 254:1921–1925

Levison DA, Shepherd NA (1986) Pathology of gastric lymphomas and smooth muscle tumours. In: Preece PE, Cuschieri A, Wellwood JM (eds) Cancer of the stomach. Grune and Stratton, London, pp 47–72

Lewin KJ, Kahn LB, Novis BH (1976) Primary intestinal lymphoma of "Western" and "Mediterranean" type, alpha chain disease and massive plasma cell infiltration: a comparative study of 37 cases. Cancer 38:2511–2528

Lewin KJ, Ranchod M, Dorfman RF (1978) Lymphomas of the gastrointestinal tract. Cancer 42:693–707

Li IY (1948) Benign lymphoma of the rectum. Surgery 23:814–820

Lim FE, Hartman AS, Tan EGC, Cady B, Meissner WA (1977) Factors in the prognosis of gastric lymphoma. Cancer 39:1715–1720

Loehr WJ, Mujhahed Z, Zahn FD, Gray GF, Thorbjarnarson B (1969) Primary lymphoma of the gastrointestinal tract: a review of 100 cases. Ann Surg 170:232–238

Loughran TP, Kadin ME, Deeg HJ (1986) T-cell intestinal lymphoma associated with coeliac sprue. Ann Intern Med 104:44–47

MacLennan ICM, Gray D, Kumararatne DS, Bazin H (1982) The lymphocytes of splenic marginal zones: a distinct B-cell lineage. Immunol Today 3:305–307

Matuchansky C, Touchard G, Lemaire M et al. (1985) Malignant lymphoma of the small bowel associated with diffuse nodular lymphoid hyperplasia. N Engl J Med 313:166–171

Montgomery PC, Ayyildiz A, Lemaitre-Coelho IM, Vaerman JP, Rockey JH (1983) Induction and expression of antibodies in secretions: the ocular immune system. In: McGhee JR, Mestecky J (eds) The secretory immune system. New York Academy of Science, New York, pp 428–440

Moore I, Wright DH (1984) Primary gastric lymphoma – a tumour of mucosa-associated lymphoid tissue. A histological and immunohistochemical study of 36 cases. Histopathology 8:1025–1039

Morgan DR, Holgate CS, Dixon MF, Bird CC (1985) Primary small intestinal lymphoma: a study of 39 cases, J Pathol 147:211–221

Morson BC, Dawson IMP (1979) Gastro-intestinal pathology, 2nd edn. Blackwell Scientific, Oxford, p 412

Moubayed P, Kaiserling E, Stein H (1987) T-cell lymphomas of the stomach: morphological and immunological studies characterising two cases of T-cell lymphoma. Virchows Arch [A] 411:523–529

Myhre MJ, Isaacson PG (1987) Primary B-cell gastric lymphoma – a reassessment of its histogenesis. J Pathol 152:1–11

Naqvi MS, Burrows L, Kark AE (1969) Lymphoma of the gastrointestinal tract: prognostic guides based on 162 cases. Ann Surg 170:221–231

Nasr K, Haghighi P, Bakhshandeh K, Hagshenas M (1970) Primary lymphoma of the upper small intestine. Gut 11:673–678

Nicoloff DM, Haynes LB, Wangensteen OH (1963) Primary lymphosarcoma of the gastrointestinal tract. Surg Gynecol Obstet 117:433–437

Nikbin B, Banisadre M, Ala F, Mojtabai A (1979) HLA AW19 B12 in immunoproliferative small intestinal disease. Gut 20:226–228

Norton AG, Isaacson PG (1987) The immunocytochemical diagnosis of malignant lymphoma in routinely processed tissues (Letter). J Pathol 51:240–241

Novis BH (1979) Primary intestinal lymphoma in South Africa. Isr J Med Sci 15:386–289

O'Farrelly C, Feighery C, O'Briain DS, Stevens F, Connolly CE, McCarthy C, Weir DG (1986) Humoral response to wheat protein in patients with coeliac disease and enteropathy associated T-cell lymphoma. Br Med J 293:908–910

O'Leary AD, Sweeney EC (1986) Lymphoglandular complexes of the colon: structure and distribution. Histopathology 10:267–283

Owen RL (1977) Sequential uptake of horseradish peroxidase by lymphoid follicle epithelium of Peyer's patches in the normal unobstructed mouse intestine: an ultrastructural study. Gastroenterology 72:440–451

Owen RL, Jones AL (1974) Epithelial cell specialisation within human Peyer's patches: an ultrastructural study of intestinal lymphoid follicles. Gastroenterology 66:189–203

Pinkus GS, Wilson RF, Corson JM (1974) Reticulum cell sarcoma of the colon following renal transplantation. Cancer 34:2103–2108

Piris MA, Rivas C, Morente M, Oliva H, Rubio C (1986) Immature sinus histiocytosis, a monocytoid B-lymphoid reaction. J Pathol 148:159–167

Rambaud JC, Modigliani R, Nguyen Phuoc BK, Lejeune R (1980) Non-secretory alpha-chain disease in intestinal lymphoma. N Engl J Med 303:53

Ree HJ, Rege VB, Knisely RE, Thayer WR, D'Amico RP, Song JY, Crowley JP (1980) Malignant lymphoma of Waldeyer's ring following gastrointestinal lymphoma. Cancer 46:1528–1535

Renton P, Blackshaw AJ (1976) Colonic lymphoma complicating uclerative colitis. Br J Surg 63:542–545

Richards MA (1986) Lymphoma of the colon and rectum. Postgrad Med J 62:615–620

Riddell RH, Shove DC, Ritchie JK, Lennard-Jones JE, Morson BC (1978) Precancer in ulcerative colitis. In: Morson BC (ed) The pathogenesis of colorectal cancer. WB Saunders, London, Chap 9

Rilke F, Pilotte S, Clemente C (1978) Cytology of non-Hodgkin's lymphomas involving the stomach. Acta Cytol 22:71–79

Rudders RA, Ross ME, DeLellis RA (1978) Primary extranodal lymphoma: response to treatment and factors influencing prognosis. Cancer 42:406–416

Russo A, Grasso G, Sanfillipo G, Giannone G, Guerrera G (1978) Gastroscopy and directed biopsy in the diagnosis of gastric lymphomas. Report of 16 personal cases. Tumori 64:419–427

Salmela H (1968) Lymphosarcoma of the stomach: a clinical study of 39 cases. Acta Chir Scand 134:567–576

Salter DM, Krajewski AS, Dewar AE (1986) Immunophenotype analysis of malignant histiocytosis of the intestine. J Clin Pathol 39:9–15

Schmid U, Helbron D, Lennert K (1982) Development of malignant lymphoma in myoepithelial sialadenitis (Sjögren's syndrome). Virch Arch [A] 395:11–43

Schneck SA, Penn I (1971) De-novo brain tumours in renal transplant recipients. Lancet I:983–986

Selby W, Gallagher ND (1979) Malignancy in a 19 year experience of adult coeliac disease. Dig Dis Sci 24:684–688

Selzer G, Sacks M, Shermann G, Nagan L (1979a) Primary malignant lymphoma of the small intestine in Israel: changing incidence with time. Isr J Med Sci 15:390–396

Selzer G, Sherman G, Callihan TR, Schwartz Y (1979b) Primary small intestinal lymphomas and alpha-heavy-chain disease: a study of 43 cases from a pathology department in Israel. Isr J Med Sci 15:111–123

Shadid MJ, Alami SY, Nassar VH, Balikian JB, Salem AA (1975) Primary intestinal lymphoma with paraproteinaemia. Cancer 35:848–858

Shani M, Modan B, Goldman B, Brandstaeter S, Ramot B (1969) Primary gastrointestinal lymphoma. Isr J Med Sci 5:1173–1177

Sheahan DG, Martin F, Baginsky S, Mallory GK, Zamchek N (1971) Multiple lymphomatous polyposis of the gastrointestinal tract. Cancer 28:408–425

Sheibani K, Sohn CC, Burke JS, Winberg CD, Wu AM, Rappaport H (1986) Monocytoid B-cell lymphoma. A novel B-cell neoplasm. Am J Pathol 124:310–318

Shepherd NA, Blackshaw AJ, Hall PA et al. (1987) Malignant lymphoma with eosinophilia of the gastrointestinal tract. Histopathology 11:115–130
Shepherd NA, Hall PA, Coates PJ, Levison (1988) Primary malignant lymphoma of the colon and rectum. A histopathological and immunohistochemical analysis of 45 cases with clinicopathological correlations. Histopathology 12:235–252
Shepherd NA, Hall PA, Williams GT, Codling BW, Jones EL, Levison DA, Morson BC (1989). Primary malignant lymphoma of the large intestine complicating chronic inflammatory bowel disease. Histopathology (in press)
Smith G, Crocker J, Nar P, Chesner I, Leyland MJ (1987) Immunogold-silver technique applied to showing malignant B-cell infiltration of gastrointestinal tract in patients with chronic lymphocytic leukaemia and non-Hodgkin's lymphoma. J Clin Pathol 40:756–759
Smith WJ, Price SK, Isaacson PG (1987) Immunglobulin gene rearrangement in immunoproliferative small intestinal disease (IPSID). J Clin Pathol 40:1291–1297
Spencer J, Hall JG (1984) Studies on the lymphocytes of sheep. IV. Migration patterns of lung-associated lymphocytes efferent from the caudal mediastinal lymph node. Immunology 52:1–5
Spencer J, Finn T, Isaacson PG (1985a) Gut associated lymphoid tissue: a morphological and immunocytochemical study of the human appendix. Gut 26:672–679
Spencer J, Finn T, Pulford KAF, Mason DY, Isaacson PG (1985b) The human gut contains a novel population of B lymphocytes which resemble marginal zone cells. Clin Exp Immunol 62:607–612
Spencer J, Finn T, Isaacson PG (1986a) Human Peyer's patches; an immunohistochemical study. Gut 27:405–410
Spencer J, MacDonald TT, Finn T, Isaacson PG (1986b) The development of gut associated lymphoid tissue in the terminal ileum of foetal human intestine. Clin Exp Immunol 64:536–543
Spencer J, Cerf-Bensussan N, Jarry A et al. (1988) Enteropathy associated T cell lymphoma (malignant histiocytosis of the intestine) is recognised by a monoclonal antibody (HML–1) that defines a membrane molecule on mucosal lymphocytes. Am J Pathol 132:1–5
Stansfeld AG, Diebold J, Kapanci Y et al. (1988) Updated Kiel classification for lymphomas. Lancet I:292–293, 603
Stein H, Dienemann D, Sperling M, Zeitz M, Rieken E–O (1988) Identification of a T cell derived lymphoma derived from intestinal mucosa associated T cells. Lancet II:1053–1054
Stobbe JA, Dockerty MB, Bernatz PE (1966) Primary gastric lymphoma and its grades of malignancy. Am J Surg 112:10–19
Streeter PR, Berg EL, Rouse BTN, Bargatze RF, Butcher EC (1988a) A tissue specific endothelial cell molecule involved in lymphocyte homing. Nature 331:41–46
Streeter RP, Rouse BTN, Butcher EC (1988b) Immunohistologic and functional characterisation of a vascular addressin involved in lymphocyte homing into peripheral lymph nodes. J Cell Biol 107:1853–1862
Strindel H (1935) Bartel's "Tonsille des Mastdarmes" und ihre Stellung in der Pathologie des Lymphatischen Apparates des Mastdarmes. Zentralbl Chir 62:2594
Suchi T, Lennert K, Tu L–Y, Kikuchi M, Sato E, Stansfeld AG, Feller AC (1987) Histopathology and immunohistochemistry of peripheral T-cell lymphomas: a proposal for their classification. J Clin Pathol 40:995–1015
Sugarbaker ED, Craver LF (1940) Lymphosarcoma. A study of 196 cases with autopsy. JAMA 115:17–23, 112–117
Swinson CM, Coles EC, Slavin G, Booth CC (1983) Coeliac disease and malignancy. Lancet I:111–115
Thorbjarnarson B, Beale JM, Pearce JM (1956) Primary malignant lymphoid tumours of the stomach. Cancer 9:712–717
Vaerman JP, Andre C, Bazin H, Heremans JF (1973) Mesenteric lymph as a major source of serum IgA in guinea pigs and rats. Eur J Immunol 3:580–584

Van den Heule B, Van Kerkem C, Heimann R (1979) Benign and malignant lymphoid lesions of the stomach. A histological reappraisal in the light of the Kiel classification for non-Hodgkin's lymphomas. Histopathology 3:309–320

Welborn JK, Ponk JL, Rebuck JW (1965) Lymphoma of the stomach: a diagnostic and therapeutic problem. Arch Surg 90:480–487

Wu NW, Jalkanen S, Streeter PR, Butcher EC (1988) Evolutionary conservation of tissue-specific lymphocyte-endothelial cell recognition mechanisms involved in lymphocyte homing. J Cell Biol 107:1845–1851

Wychulis AR, Beahrs OH, Woolner LB (1966) Malignant lymphoma of the colon. Arch Surg 93:215–225

Zeigler JL, Becksted JA, Volberding PA et al. (1984) Non-Hodgkin lymphoma in 90 homosexual men. Relation to generalised lymphadenopathy and the acquired immunodeficiency syndrome. N Engl J Med 311:565–570

The Place of Quantitation in Diagnostic Gastrointestinal Pathology

J. M. SLOAN, D. C. ALLEN, P. W. HAMILTON, and P. C. H. WATT

1 Introduction

Diagnosis based on histopathological or cytopathological assessment frequently shows considerable interobserver variation. More efficient exchange of information over recent decades has improved diagnostic standards but the subjective nature of the interpretation involved means that the standardisation available in other branches of laboratory medicine cannot easily be achieved. For example despite detailed and widely publicised attempts to achieve more uniform assessment of dysplasia in gastric (MORSON et al. 1980; MING et al. 1984) and in colonic mucosa (RIDDELL et al. 1983) there is still widespread variation even among histopathologists experienced in this field.

The application of quantitative methods as an adjunct to routine interpretation of histological sections can provide more objective and reproducible assessment. Such application remains time consuming in spite of the introduction of computer-assisted methods and is unlikely to become part of every-day histological methodology in the foreseeable future. Nonetheless simple morphometric methods have proved useful in the diagnosis of jejunal villous atrophy in coeliac disease (DUNNILL and WHITEHEAD 1972) and in histological diagnosis of reflux oesophagitis (ISMAIL-BEIGI et al. 1970) over a number of years.

Application of morphometry may help direct the attention of the pathologist to particular cytological or architectural features within tissue sections which are especially relevant in the circumstances under consideration. The highlighting of such features together with identification of other features which are of little diagnostic importance may improve the accuracy of subjective assessment.

The purpose of this chapter is to outline current methods of quantitative analysis and review the application of such methods to gastrointestinal pathology.

2 Quantitative Methods

2.1 Morphometry

Histological examination of tissue is carried out on thin sections. This essentially produces a two-dimensional image of the tissue, but contains much information about the processes involved in the three-dimensional tissue structure. Pathologists are trained to recognise patterns from these two-dimensional images which relate to the pathology of the tissue as a whole. Image analysis is only one of several potential sources of error in reaching a diagnosis but is fundamental to the process (LANGLEY et al. 1983). Visual images, however, are not easy to analyse objectively, and are open to subjective interpretation. Morphometry permits derivation of quantitative geometric information from two-dimensional images. The relevance of this information to the histopathology of the tissue under review may then be determined. Quantitation of the histological image is objective, reproducible and produces numerical data about the size, shape, volume and number of histological elements or compartments which make up the tissue. These data can then be analysed statistically.

Morphometry can be divided into two forms of measurement. First 'planimetry', which takes into account measurement of two-dimensional geometric parameters (e.g. nuclear area, perimeter, diameter, nuclear-cytoplasmic ratio, number of mitoses per unit area, linear measurements of distance). These are direct measurements derived visually from the histological image. Second, there is 'stereology', which involves the mathematical derivation of three-dimensional parameters from the two-dimensional information available in the histological image (UNDERWOOD 1970; WEIBEL 1969). Stereological parameters generally include volume density measurements of various tissue compartments (e.g. lamina propria, epthelium). Planimetry and stereology, whilst producing very different information, are closely related and supplement each other in the quantitative assessment of histological tissue (BAAK and OORT 1983).

Morphometric measurements are carried out using three main technical methods. These may be termed (a) manual linear measurement or point-counting methods, (b) semi-automatic image analysis, and (c) fully automatic image analysis, and are of increasing technical complexity. Detailed accounts of these have been published previously outlining the mathematical background, potential applications, limitations and pitfalls, and the serious student should refer to these standards works (WEIBEL 1979; BRADBURY 1979; AHERNE and DUNNILL 1982; BAAK and OORT 1983). Only a brief discussion on each will be given here.

2.1.1 Manual Methods

In their simplest form manual methods involve direct linear measurement on a histological section using a micrometer attached to the microscope or on an enlarged projected image of the tissue section. Much of the original work related to villous atrophy in coeliac disease was based on such technique used alone (THURLBECK et al. 1960; SHINER and DONIACH 1960), or in combination with point counting (RUBIN et al. 1960). Point-counting involves derivation of quantitative measurements from a two-dimensional image by superimposing over the image a system of lines or points. The number of times the boundary of the feature under investigation intersects the lines, or the number of points which fall within the boundary, can be used to estimate the surface area or volume of the histological feature. Various mathematical formulae are used to derive morphometric variables in this way (AHERNE and DUNNILL 1982; WEIBEL

1979). This approach to morphometry was essentially devised for analysis of ultrastructural images but has also been used at light microscope level. It is an inexpensive method but can be very time consuming, especially when a large number of cases have to be measured.

Manual methods have previously been used successfully to quantitate the features of gastrointestinal mucosa, including surface/volume ratio (DUNNILL and WHITEHEAD 1972), and the number of cells in the lamina propria of duodenal biopsies (WHITEHEAD et al. 1975). A recent detailed study on gastric dysplasia (TOSI et al. 1987) shows that manual point-counting techniques are very useful for estimating the volume density of various architectural components and the surface density and shape of mucosal glands, even in comparison with computer-aided methods.

2.1.2 Semi-automatic Image Analysis

Image analyis is a term which, strictly speaking, may encompass any assessment of an image, including the examination of a histological slide by a pathologist, and the manual methods previously mentioned. Generally, however, the term is associated with computer-linked quantitation of an image, which is faster and less labour intensive than manual methods.

Semi-automatic image analysis (SAIA) is so called because although a computer is employed to calculate various geometric parameters, an operator is required to trace the individual elements to be measured. This is generally carried out using a graphic tablet and electromagnetic stylus or a 'light pen'. Images placed on the tablet (in the form of a projected image or photomicrograph) or transferred to a television monitor with graphic tablet overlay can be traced with the stylus. This tracing action is recorded by the tablet, which inputs into the computer the x- and y-coordinates of each point the stylus moves over. Instruments are available with specifically programmed software which allows geometric parameters to be calculated from these coordinates.

In this way nuclear or cellular outlines can be traced from a highly magnified histological image, and several variables calculated simultaneously for each nucleus or cell (Table 1, part I). In addition the area of various architectural components (Table 1, part II) can be easily measured, i.e. mucosal area, epithelial area etc. (SLAVIN et al. 1980; CORAZZA et al. 1985; ALLEN et al. 1988a). In addition to measurements related to area and shape, SAIA systems usually allow the operator to make linear measurements of length or distance (Table 1, part III). This can be used to measure accurately parameters such as mucosal thickness, crypt length and derived features such as length of epithelium per millimetre of muscularis mucosa (JENKINS et al. 1985; ALLEN et al. 1988a). In previous work (HAMILTON et al. 1987a) the authors used linear measurement to give an estimation of nuclear stratification by measuring the distance between the top of the nucleus and the cell apex (N–C AP Dist.) and the basement

Table 1. Possible variables that may be measured using a semi-automatic image analyser (Kontron: MOP Videoplan)

	Variable	Description	Application	
I	Area Perimeter Longest Axis Shortest Axis Dia. Circle Form Factor PE Form Factor AR Vol. Ellipse Vol. Sphere	Measurements related to enclosed structures, i.e. spheres, ellipses etc.	Cells Nuclei Nucleoli	
II	Area	Pure measurement of area with no associated parameters	Mucosal area Epithelial area Vascular area Nuclear–cytoplasmic ratio	
III	Length Direct distance Angle	Linear measurements	Nucleus–cell apex distance Basement membrane-nucleus apex dist	Nuclear Stratification
			Mucosal length Crypt Length Nuclear Polarity	
IV	Density	Number of elements occurring in a unit area	Inflammatory cell Density Cellularity Number of mitoses	

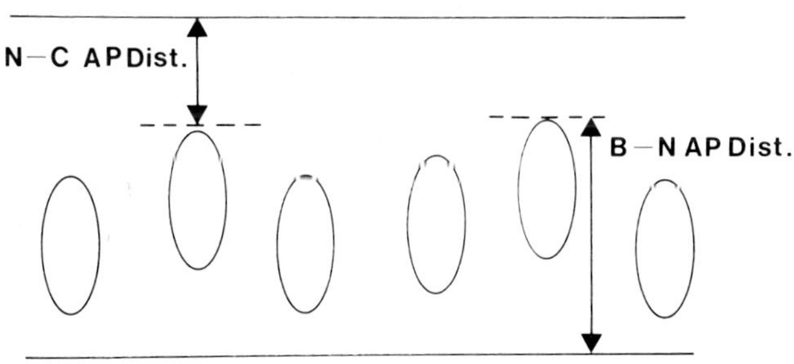

Fig. 1. Illustration of basement membrane to nuclear apex (*B–N AP Dist.*) and nuclear apex to cell apex distances (*N–C AP Dist.*) measured for each nucleus (HAMILTON et al. 1987)

membrane to nucleus apex distance (B–N AP Dist.) (Fig. 1). In the same study, they sought to estimate nuclear polarity by measuring the angle between the longitudinal symmetry line of the nucleus and the basement membrane and calculating its deviation from 90° (Table 1, part III) (Fig. 2). SAIA systems can be used to estimate the density of a particular cell within a particular field (Table 1, part IV). This entails measuring the area of a microscopic field and counting the number of times the feature

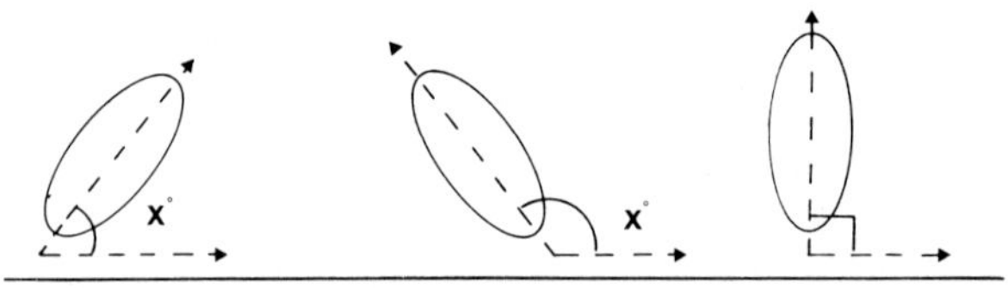

Fig. 2. Assessment of nuclear polarity was made by measuring angle X° and calculating the difference between X° and 90° for each nucleus (HAMILTON et al. 1987)

under investigation (inflammatory cell, mitoses etc.) occurs within that field (JENKINS et al. 1985; WATT et al. 1987). This can then be expressed as number of elements per unit area or unit length.

Thus SAIA systems are versatile due to the fact that the operator can choose the feature to be measured and the morphometric parameters necessary to describe the feature. The process is, however, fairly time consuming and can be tedious for the operator. In a study of malignant mucosal changes in ulcerative colitis (HAMILTON et al. 1987 a; ALLEN et al. 1987, 1988 a) morphometric parameters on 50 nuclei were measured in addition to assessment of nuclear-cytoplasmic ratio, nuclear stratification and nuclear polarity as well as six architectural measurements. Given familiarity with the image analyser, and this is readily achieved, the time taken to quantitate a single histological section varied between 1 and 2 hours. The use of discriminant analysis to select the most important parameters for separation of study groups can reduce the number of parameters which it is necessary to measure and consequently the time required.

In our experience, SAIA is essential to the morphometric study of gastrointestinal mucosa. Because of the anisotropic nature of gastrointestinal mucosa it is necessary to discriminate between the various architectural compartments and the different cell types within those compartments. SAIA systems retain the operator's ability to do this. He is responsible for recognising and defining the features or areas to be measured whilst the computer calculates the morphometric variables. The operator is free to measure areas of interest and to avoid areas where artefacts exist.

Semi-automatic image analysis has been widely applied in gastrointestinal studies. It has been used to assess the nuclear and architectural morphometry of gastric (JARVIS and WHITEHEAD 1985; TOSI et al. 1987), jejunal (SLAVIN et al. 1980; CORAZZA et al. 1985), duodenal (JENKINS et al. 1985) and colorectal (BROWN et al. 1985; HAMILTON et al.1987 a; ALLEN et al. 1987; ROSEKRANS et al. 1980 b) mucosa.

2.1.3 Automatic Image Analysis

Automatic image analysers basically consist of a television camera attached to a computer-linked analysing system and are the most sophisticated of the three methods described. The two-dimensional histological image is scanned by the T.V. system, which can detect the optical density or grey level (brightness or darkness) of the various parts of the image (OJA and COLLAN 1983). In this way dark and light areas can be separated, as can the varying intermediate grey areas. The computer can then create an enhanced digitised image of its own from the 'grey' values it receives and calculate morphometric parameters from the components it has detected from the image. Using this technique, nuclei (dark) can be separated from cytoplasm (light) and in this way, a field of 50 nuclei can be measured very rapidly in comparison with SAIA systems. Using grey levels to analyse an image applies to black and white images only as colour images need intensity levels for green, red and blue parts of the image (OJA and COLLAN 1983).

Although these systems are termed fully automatic, only rarely can they be used without intervention by the operator in the measuring process. Problems in automatic image analysis tend to increase with the complexity of the image. Folds in the tissue section may be dark enough to be mistaken for nuclei, or two overlapping nuclei may be counted together as one cumulative area (BAAK and OORT 1983). Most systems do allow the operator to 'edit' the image in order to alleviate these problems but this may not be sufficient in some circumstances. For example in an area of epithelium showing high grade dysplasia, in which the nuclei are overlapping and stratified, an automatic system would have difficulty in distinguishing between each nucleus due to lack of grey level discrimination, even with intervention 'editing' techniques. A semi-automatic system, however, has the advantage that the operator can identify the nuclei and measure only those with a clearly defined border.

Automatic image analysis has been found to be useful in assessing nuclear morphometry of gastric cytological smears (WEINREB et al. 1984) and other isotropic tissues, and can rapidly quantitate nuclear features in such cases. Gastrointestinal mucosa as seen in a histological section, however, presents an image which is anisotropic and much more complex. This complexity increases the problems associated with automatic image analysis and for this reason with the technology at present available its application to gastrointestinal pathology is limited.

2.2 DNA Content

In pathological change, not only do alterations occur in the geometry of histological features, but measurable changes in the quantities of cellular constituents can also be recognised. The measurement of nuclear DNA content (ploidy) has emerged as a powerful tool for the examination of abnormalities found in malignant and premalignant tissue (BARLOGIE et al. 1980).

Normal cells have a range of DNA content which corresponds to the different stages of the cell cycle. It ranges from the diploid DNA comple-

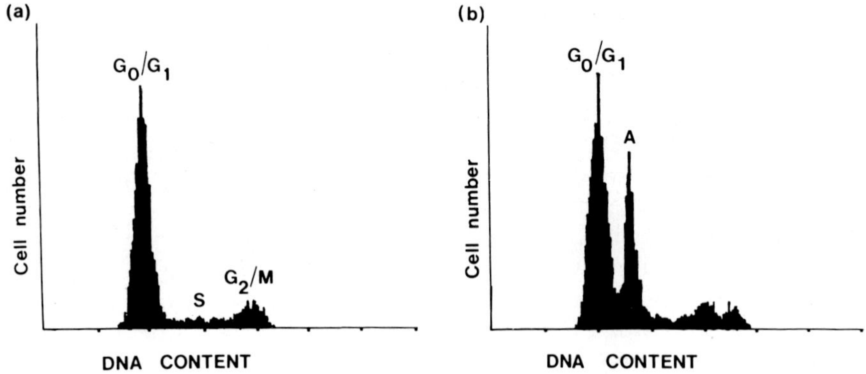

Fig. 3a, b. Diagrammatic representation of **a** normal DNA distribution with a diploid (G_0/G_1) DNA stem line, synthetic phase (*S*) and G_2/M peak and **b** aneuploid distribution showing an abnormal DNA stem line (*A*) which is distinguished from the normal G_0/G_1 peak

ment (G_0/G_1) through a DNA synthetic phase (S-phase) to double the diploid chromosomal number (G_2) before the cell undergoes mitosis (M). The diploid DNA content (2C), therefore, doubles its value (4C) with a transitional increase in DNA content between the two (KIEFER and SANDRITTER 1976). In addition, some normal tissues, such as liver, possess increasing multiples (tetraploid, octaploid etc.) of the diploid DNA complement. DNA aneuploidy is defined as the presence of an abnormal DNA stem line which is distinguishable from the diploid stem line (QUIRKE and DYSON 1986) (see Fig. 3). In principle, two methods are used for the quantitative measurement of DNA content.

2.2.1 Photocytometry

The simplest approach to estimating the amount of nuclear DNA is to stain the DNA (Feulgen stain) and measure the intensity of transmitted light through the stained nucleus. This is termed absorption cytophotometry and can be carried out on a histological section or cytological smear. It is based on the principle that the density of the stain is proportional to the DNA content, i.e. the more darkly stained a nucleus is, the greater the amount of DNA present. The transmitted light (unabsorbed by the stain) is detected by a photometer, and its intensity converted into units of optical density.

The DNA within a nucleus, however, is not always evenly distributed throughout the nucleus (e.g. nucleoli, heterochromatin). This causes a 'distributional error' when using absorption techniques, which may be corrected by taking several measurements within each nucleus for analysis (BAAK and OORT 1983) or by using an integrated scanning system.

An alternative and more precise approach to quantifying DNA content is to stain specifically the DNA using a fluorescent dye. When the stain is excited by a light source, the resulting fluorescence can be measured using a microfluorometer and quantified. (For a full discussion on fluorescence cytophotometry, see BOHM and SPRENGER 1968.)

In both types of measurement, the DNA content of each nucleus measured is usually plotted in the form of a DNA histogram which illustrates where the main populations of cells lie in relation to their DNA content, and from which information can be obtained regarding the stem line DNA content and the various stages of the cell cycle.

As DNA content is measured in arbitrary units, it is necessary to obtain a diploid reference value with which to compare the population of cells under investigation. This reference value is taken from DNA measurements of cells known to have a diploid DNA content, e.g. lymphocytes, granulocytes. Ideally these reference nuclei should be measured from the same slide as the cells under investigation (BOHM and SANDRITTER 1975).

Photocytometric techniques (principally those of fluorescence cytometry) have been used to investigate the significance of DNA content in oesophageal carcinoma (SUGIMACHI et al. 1983), gastric adenocarcinoma (INUI and OOTA 1965; SPRENGER et al. 1974; BOHM and SANDRITTER 1975) and the growth patterns of early gastric cancer (INOKUCHI et al. 1983). Similarly, photocytometry has been used to examine the ploidy of colorectal carcinomas (LEUCHTENBERGER et al. 1954; STICH et al. 1960; BOHM and SANDRITTER 1975; FORSSLUND et al. 1984; ENBLAD et al. 1985) as well as benign adenomatous polyps (STICH et al. 1960) and dysplasia in ulcerative colitis (CUVELIER et al. 1987).

2.2.2 Flow Cytometry

Technically, flow cytometry is a much more advanced method for measuring DNA content. Whilst photocytometric techniques are carried out on histological sections or smears, flow cytometry requires the tissue to be disaggregated and the cells dispersed in a monosuspension and stained using a DNA-specific fluorescent dye, e.g. propidium iodide. Initially, this was only possible on fresh tissue, but recently introduced methods allow formalin-fixed, paraffin-embedded tissue to be deparaffinised, disaggregated and converted into a nuclear suspension (HEDLEY et al. 1983, 1985; SCHUTTE et al. 1985; COON et al. 1986). Using hydrodynamic methods, the cells are brought into a very narrow stream which intercepts a beam of light (either from a mercury arc lamp or more usually a laser). As each individual cell passes down the stream, it is interrogated by the light source, which the stain absorbs and re-emits at a longer wavelength. This emitted fluorescence is then directed to specific detectors and quantitated. For a detailed account of the principles of flow cytometry, see LOVETT et al. (1984) and QUIRKE and DYSON (1986).

The advantage of such a technique is the extreme speed of the process. Between 1000 and 5000 cells/second can be analysed for their DNA content. As with photocytometric estimations of DNA content, the data are presented as a DNA distribution (Fig. 3) but because of the large number of cells involved the degree of statistical significance is much greater (LOVETT et al. 1984).

Because flow cytometry can now be carried out on paraffin-embedded tissue, archival material can be retrieved for analysis. This has prompted many comprehensive retrospective studies investigating the significance of ploidy in relation to prognosis, principally in colorectal carcinoma (WOLLEY et al. 1982; ARMITAGE et al. 1985; MELAMED et al. 1986; QUIRKE et al. 1987b). The significance of DNA content in gastric cancer and its prognosis has recently been examined (BENNETS et al. 1979; MACARTNEY et al. 1986; WYATT et al. 1987). Colonic polypi (VAN DEN INGH et al. 1985; BANNER et al. 1987) and dysplasia in ulcerative colitis (MELVILLE et al. 1987) have also been investigated, and found to contain aneuploid cells.

A major disadvantage of flow cytometry is that the morphology of the tissue is lost in the resultant suspension. As a result there may be uncertainty about the population of cells being analysed, and for this reason the worker must ensure that the block of tissue to be disaggregated contains a predominance of the cell he is interested in. If there is widespread abnormality within a tissue block it is likely that disaggregation will result in a suspension containing a predominance of abnormal cells. However, small lesions or focal areas of abnormality may be masked by the predominance of surrounding normal cells. MACARTNEY et al. (1986) have drawn attention to difficulties which arise in interpretation of flow cytometry results and in identifying aneuploidy. The influence of fixation is considerable, good fixation resulting in a much lower coefficient of variation. In addition histological factors such as pattern of growth correlate with S-phase fractions in gastric cancer, so for comparative studies several aspects have to be clearly defined.

3 Statistical Analysis of Morphometric Data

Quantitative studies produce numerical data derived from the histological features of the tissue in question. Statistical procedures must be employed in the analysis of the data in order to understand the significance of the measured variables.

Statistical comparisons involving one variable are relatively simple and can be carried out on most basic statistical computer packages or as described in any standard statistical textbook. Morphometric studies, however, generally involve the measurement of several variables (as many as 15 in some studies) for each patient, patients often being divided into a number of clinical groups. These data are therefore multivariate, and as the variables are likely to be correlated in some way, they ought to be studied simultaneously and not as individuals. Multivariate statistical techniques can achieve this and thereby elucidate relationships between variables and summarise the data. Such techniques usually require the use of a computer and suitable software packages. Generally, three multivariate techniques have been found valuable in analysing data derived from morphometric studies.

3.1 Principal Components Analysis

Principal components analysis is a useful technique in the initial evaluation of morphometric data as it attempts to reduce the multidimensional nature of the data into fewer dimensions. By examining variables simultaneously, it expresses the major sources of variation within the multivariate dataset as 'principal components'. The first component comprises the weighted combination of the variables which account for the maximum amount of variation in the data. The second component accounts for the maximal remaining variance after the first principal component has been extracted, and so on. In this way the overall dataset can be simplified into a few components responsible for decreasing amounts of variation. It may be possible to give each component a descriptive name depending on which variables are weighted heavily in the component and this may reveal an underlying structure to the data (ALLEN et al. 1987).

3.2 Discriminant Analysis

Morphometric measurements are often made in order to determine their importance in distinguishing two or more predefined groups. A single measured variable may give some discrimination between groups but usually a combination of two or more variables increases discrimination, giving a better separation. Discriminant analysis defines the weighted combination of variables which are best at discriminating the predefined groups. This combination of variables is termed a discriminant function. These variables can be identified and others discarded. In addition, an allocation or classification rule can be derived from this combination of variables. The discriminatory effectiveness of this rule can be examined by calculating the percentage of cases correctly classified by the rule into the predefined histological groups.

If a classification rule is evaluated on the data from which it was derived, falsely optimistic results may be obtained. For this reason, discriminant analysis generally requires two sets of cases: a 'training' set from which the classification rule is derived, and a 'test' set of different cases on which the performance of the classification rule can be examined. If the discriminatory performance of the classification rule does not deteriorate when tested on a new set of cases, it may then be used to allocate a 'new' case into one of the predefined groups. This may be of value when investigating the use of morphometry in differential histological diagnosis.

If a test set of cases is not available, for instance due to lack of histological material, an alternative form of discriminant analysis can be applied to the training set. This technique is termed "jack-knifing" and involves each case being eliminated in turn from the analysis and classified according to a rule derived from the remaining cases. As each case is not involved in its own classification, this reduces the bias which is encoutered in using the training set alone to evaluate the classification rule.

Discriminant analysis applied to morphometric data in the endometrium has been described by BEZEMER et al. (1977). In the gastrointestinal tract discriminant analysis of morphometric data has been used to help discriminate between various grades of dysplasia, in the stomach (TOSI et al. 1987) and in the colorectum (ALLEN et al. 1987).

3.3 Cluster Analysis

A prerequisite of discriminant analysis is the need for predefined groups on which to carry out the discrimination. These groups are usually defined using histological criteria which may be subjective and lacking in reproducibility. The basis of such a study (i.e. the grouping) is, therefore, not totally reliable and this introduces an underlying weakness into an otherwise objective study. For this reason, some workers have used cluster analysis to group histological changes statistically without using predefined groups.

Cluster analysis partitions a set of cases into groups (i.e. clusters) on the basis of the distance between cases in multidimensional space (cases which are close to each other will tend to fall in the same cluster). Various mathematical algorithms and measures of distance can be used to define clusters and in some methods the number of clusters to be identified can be specified. Thus the grouping of cases is carried out quantitatively, removing subjectivity from the analysis.

The resulting clusters of cases can then be analysed in a normal statistical fashion. The mathematically defined clusters can be compared with the histologically defined groups in order to examine the similarity between the effectiveness of the two methods of grouping cases. TOSI et al. (1987) used such an approach to examine the morphometric characteristics of increasing grades of gastric dysplasia. JENKINS et al. (1985) used cluster analysis to define quantitatively grades in duodenitis and proceeded to use discriminant analysis to examine discrimination between clusters.

This is a highly simplified overview of complex statistical methods. It is unlikely that many pathologists possess the necessary knowledge of how best to analyse a particular dataset. For this reason it is wise to seek advice from a competent statistician at the outset of a morphometric study.

4 Application of Quantitative Methods in Gastrointestinal Pathology

4.1 Oesophagus

The clinical assessment of oesophagitis is notoriously difficult as symptoms may be atypical and the endoscopic appearance normal. In view of these problems, attempts have been made to establish histological criteria for non-ulcerative oesophagitis. The presence of subepithelial lymphocytes does not indicate oesophagitis, and neutrophil infiltration, while being relatively specific, is an insensitive marker. In 1970 ISMAIL-BEIGI et al. proposed the hypothesis that reflux causes accelerated exfoliation of epithelial cells with consequent basal zone hyperplasia and lengthening of stromal papillae. They showed that these features could be measured and established positive criteria for oesophagitis, namely basal zone thickening greater than 15% and papillary length greater than 66% of total epithelial thickness. These were based on a study of 33 subjects with and 21 without subjective and objective evidence of oesophageal reflux. Subsequently BEHAR and SHEAHAN (1975) applied less stringent criteria, i.e. basal zone height greater than 15% and papillary length greater than 50%, but these are less specific.

These quantitative criteria for oesophagitis have not been universally accepted. SEEFELD et al. (1977) in a morphometric study found that reflux patients did not have basal zone hyperplasia and that elongation of stromal papillae had only a poor association with reflux. WEINSTEIN et al. (1975) found hyperplastic changes in over half the biopsies taken within 2.5 cm proximal to the gastro-oesophageal junction in asymptomatic subjects. These changes were not infrequent in more proximal biopsies. COLLINS et al. (1985) in a study of 56 patients concluded that the diagnostic use of the Ismail-Beigi criteria, while specific, was only moderately sensitive. In biopsies taken 5.0 cm proximal to the gastro-oesophageal junction 64% of patients with clinical and endoscopic evidence of oesophagitis fulfilled the criteria.

The accurate measurement of papillary length and basal zone height requires relatively large well orientated biopsies preferably taken by a suction technique. Grasp biopsies which can be taken during a routine endoscopy are often poorly orientated and frequently do not lend themselves to the relevant measurements. In order to get over this JARVIS et al. (1985) suggested that certain morphometric measurements made in poorly orientated oesophageal biopsies would give an indication of increased epithelial cell turnover and therefore provide an objective assessment of oesophagitis. They reasoned that increased mitotic division in the basal layer would result in more nuclei per unit length, elongated nuclei due to physical crowding, and smaller, more variable nuclear size due to a higher proportion of dividing cells. Other changes were postulated in the intermediate layer. The authors were able to detect statistically significant changes in the measurements they made in a group of patients before and after drug therapy for oesophagitis. HAMILTON et al. (1987b), however, used similar morphometric measurements and showed poor correlation with reflux measured by 24-h oesophageal pH monitoring although they were able to demonstrate differences between those with and those without endoscopic oesophagitis.

As yet no distinct improvement on the simple morphometric criteria of ISMAIL-BEIGI et al. (1970) has emerged. These criteria are easily and rapidly applied, provided a well orientated section is available, but the histological assessment of reflux oesophagitis remains relatively insensitive.

In an investigation into the pathogenesis of bleeding from oesophageal varices, simple morphometric methods were applied to the histological examination of oesophageal transection rings from patients with varices. Results indicated that oesophagitis is not an important factor and that bleeding occurs from rupture of small superficial blood-filled channels within the squamous epithelium which connect with underlying larger vessels (SPENCE et al. 1983, 1984).

MUKADA et al. (1978) examined DNA content in oesophageal dysplasia and carcinoma using cytophotometry. DNA values were significantly increased in severe dysplasia and carcinoma in situ but this was not always the case in invasive carcinoma.

4.2 Stomach and Duodenum

4.2.1 Gastritis and Duodenitis

Inflammatory changes in the stomach have traditionally been studied qualitatively, widely used classifications being those of WHITEHEAD (1985) and OWEN (1984). Although these classifications are useful in routine surgical diagnosis their descriptive nature makes them difficult to use in investigative circumstances where statistical analyses are necessary. Interobserver variation in the interpretation and grading of gastritis probably contributes to the confusion in the literature on the relationship between histological gastritis, endoscopic findings and symptomatology. In addition a wide range of inflammatory cell infiltration can be found in healthy volunteers (KREUNING et al. 1978).

An alternative approach is to ignore subjective grading of gastritis and to quantitate actual numbers of inflammatory cells. Thus PARL et al. (1979), using a quantitative technique, showed that alcoholic patients have a higher incidence of antral gastritis than non-alcoholics. In a detailed study of non-ulcer dyspepsia patients by TOUKAN et al. (1985), counts were made of inflammatory cells in gastric body, antrum and duodenal biopsies. This showed that patients with non-ulcer dyspepsia have significantly more neutrophils in both stomach and duodenal mucosa than controls. Duodenal mononuclear cells and eosinophils were also increased in the dyspeptic patients, albeit to a lesser extent than neutrophils. This did not apply to the stomach. Thus it appears from this study that active gastroduodenal inflammation as characterised by neutrophils is a feature of non-ulcer dyspepsia. These authors maintain that much of the disagreement in the literature on this subject is due to lack of controls and objective data in other work.

A similar study was carried out by WATT et al. (1987), who measured mononuclear cells and neutrophils in the epithelium and lamina propria of both stomach and duodenum. Patient groups included those with duodenal ulcer, duodenitis, non-ulcer dyspepsia and controls. In essence this work showed that duodenal ulcer patients had significant degrees of gastritis in the antrum and fundus whereas duodenitis and non-ulcer dyspepsia patients had lesser degrees not significantly different from controls. Further work showed that all three symptomatic groups had increased numbers of neutrophils in duodenal biopsies in either the lamina propria or epithelium, this being in broad agreement with TOUKAN et al.'s (1985) findings with respect to non-ulcer dyspepsia. It is tempting to suggest that duodenal ulcer, duodenitis and at least some cases of non-ulcer dyspepsia represent a spectrum of inflammatory gastroduodenal disease the activity of which is related to the numbers of mucosal inflammatory cells. Confirmation of this speculation must, however, await further pathophysiological investigations.

It appears, therefore, that quantitation of gastric inflammatory cells produces objective data which can be used to make statistical comparisons between patient groups. The major drawback is that for routine use or in the study of a large number of patients it is time consuming. HAMILTON et al. (1987c), however, showed that a more rapid semi-quantitative technique can be used. They compared the grading of biopsies by cell counting techniques with grading by a pathologist who assessed each biopsy with reference to a set of standard photomicrographs taken to represent obvious examples of each grade. This showed good correlation for assessment of gastric biopsies but not for duodenal biopsies.

A number of studies have concentrated on the quantitative aspects of duodenitis. WHITEHEAD et al. (1975) studied 747 duodenal biopsies and graded each one subjectively from 0 to 3. Subsequent morphometric and stereological measurements of representative biopsies from each group showed statistically significant differences between them, thus justifying the subjective classification. JENKINS et al. (1985) used a different approach in that they made morphometric and stereological measurements on duodenal biopsies and then applied cluster analysis to the data. Thus instead of comparing subjectively defined groups they used cluster analysis to generate groups based on the statistical association of histological changes. Detailed measurements of mucosal architectural features and various cell counts (e.g. polymorphs, eosinophils) were made in each field.

From these measurements derived values were obtained as indications of villous atrophy (ratio of total length of surface epithelium to length of muscularis mucosa) and of mucosal oedema (area of lamina propria per unit length of muscularis mucosa). The most successful clustering was into three groups. Group I was considered to comprise normal biopsies and included cases which would fall into the mild duodenitis classification of WHITEHEAD et al. (1975). Group II biopsies were regarded as mild duodenitis and showed a plasma cell response, oedema with intra-epithelial polymorphs and gastric metaplasia. Group III (severe duodenitis) biopsies were characterised by an appreciable polymorph response with villous atrophy but a decreased plasma cell response. The authors believe that quantitative statistical techniques have shown that mild duodenitis has in the past been overdiagnosed on the basis that such cases fall into the same group as 'normals'. The justification for this is not absolute since these authors did not use asymptomatic controls. However, the study does demonstrate that duodenitis can be divided into quantitative groups which roughly parallel the descriptive grading of WHITEHEAD et al. (1975).

4.2.2 Gastric Dysplasia and Carcinoma

Follow-up studies on patients with gastric dysplasia show that the lesion may regress, may not change or most importantly may progress to carcinoma (OEHLERT et al. 1979). This indicates the importance of accurate histopathological assessment of possible premalignant gastric biopsies. This area of gastric pathology has, however, been dogged by two problems: firstly the distinction between epithelial regenerative change and dysplasia and secondly the intra- and interobserver variation in the grading of dysplastic lesions. Both these problems are predictable since histological assessment of gastric dysplasia relies heavily on subjective criteria. Gastric dysplasia therefore appears to be a fruitful area in which to apply the various subjective techniques for quantitation.

JARVIS and WHITEHEAD (1985) studied gastric dysplasia using computer-aided morphometry. A large number of segments of epithelium were graded as regenerative, mild, moderate or severe dysplasia or cancer. Each segment was then subject to a series of detailed measurements aimed at quantitating the major cytological features of dysplasia such as nuclear-cytoplasmic ratio, nuclear size and variability, crowding of nuclei, nuclear elongation and epithelial thickness. Discriminant analysis was carried out which reduced the original variables to a set of three discriminant functions. The first function described over 90% of the variance in the data; the others contributed little. Of the first and most important function, nuclear area contributed the major part, followed by the standard deviation (i.e. the variability) of nuclear area. These criteria were related to nuclear size and thus the first discriminant function was termed 'nuclear size' factor.

Further analysis of the data produced a set of classification coefficients which were used to calculate classification scores for membership of a particular case to the defined groups. The original cases were classified and predicted and actual groups compared. Overall only 46.9% of the cases were correctly classified but most errors occurred in the regenerative category. This study is helpful in that it shows the relative weight of the cytological criteria used by an experienced pathologist in his assessment and focuses attention on them. Hoewever, only cytological features were measured; architectural features were not considered. Furthermore as the authors state, the cases were initially classified using routine subjective criteria which may not have been correct.

These two problems were addressed in a later study by TOSI et al. (1987). These authors studied 54 consecutive antral biopsies in which agreement on the grade of dysplasia had been reached between four independent pathologists. In addition to cytological measurements architectural parameters were measured using point-counting and semi-automatic image analysis techniques. Discriminant analysis indicated that the volume density of glands (a measure of gland crowding and quantity of epithelium) and the nuclear distance (distance between the centre of gravity of the nucleus and the epithelial basement membrane, i.e. an indication of stratification) were the features of greatest importance in the first discriminant function, thus underlining the importance of architectural features.

The authors recognised the need for a reliable training set in discriminant analysis and the fact that this is not possible in gastric dysplasia due to its subjective nature. Therefore within the statistical analysis they employed cluster analysis, a statistical technique in which predefined groups are not required (see Sect. 3). Using eight stereological and morphometric parameters an analysis was carried out aimed at producing three clusters. The comparison of the three grades of dysplasia made by the pathologist (mild, moderate and severe) with the three clusters showed a total disagreement of 35.2% although no cases of mild dysplasia were classified into cluster 3 and no cases of severe dysplasia into cluster 1. These authors therefore produced a quantitatiave method of classifying dysplasia which did not rely on predefined subjective groupings. As they point out, only follow-up prospective studies will indicate whether subjective or quantitative grading is the superior predictor of prognosis.

Morphometry has been used by a number of workers to assist the interpretation of gastric cytological smears. DANNO (1975) showed the importance of nuclear-cytoplasmic ratio in distinguishing benign from malignant gastric epithelial cells. BOON et al. (1981) carried out a detailed investigation of the use of morphometry on the cytodiagnosis of gastric smears. Measurements included nuclear perimeter, nuclear area, cell perimeter, cell area, nuclear-cytoplasmic ratio and their standard deviations. Discriminant analysis showed that a classification rule could be calculated using mean nuclear-cytoplasmic ratio and standard deviation of nuclear area. This rule gave 100% correct classification of 33 test cases of known histology. In addition a further 39 cases were examined in which the initial cytodiagnosis was said to be difficult. This gave encouraging results with no false positives and only two cases wrongly categorised as benign. These authors advocated the use of morphometry routinely in difficult cases in which 25 or more cells could be measured in order to refine cytodiagnosis. WEINREB et al. (1984) used a more sophisticated quantitative technique to distinguish normal from malignant gastric cells. In addition to morphometric assessment they measured light absorbance of each cell. This produced a computer-generated three-dimensional image in which the cell shape was represented by x- and y-axes while the light absorbance (grey value) was represented by the z-axis. The grey values thus gave a quantitative measurement of hyperchromasia and irregularity of chromatin pattern. Statistical analysis gave 100% discrimination between benign and malignant cells, with the best discriminant factor being maximal grey area value in the core (representing nuclear staining intensity) followed by several features related to cell size. Thus the major cellular features assessed subjectively by the cytologist were quantitated. Quantitation successfully distinguished between benign and malignant cells.

Studies on DNA content of gastric carcinoma have produced variable results. PETROVA et al. (1980) examined the ploidy of a series of gastric cancers. Surprisingly they found that more differentiated adenocarcinomas showed aneuploidy whilst undifferentiated carcinomas showed diploid distributions which did not differ much from those seen in normal cells. A similar trend to this was shown in a study by MACARTNEY et al. (1986), who also found no relationship between tumour stage and ploidy abnormality. This work supports an earlier study by INUI and OOTA (1965).

These results contrast with those of INOKUCHI et al. (1983), who found that ploidy abnormalities were greater in advanced gastric carcinoma compared with early lesions. WYATT et al. (1987) found that, of a number of prognostic indicators assessed, stage-related factors (e.g. intramural spread, number of lymph nodes involved) related to prognosis but among grade-related factors only DNA aneuploidy was prognostic.

MACARTNEY et al. (1986) point out that flow cytometry results are influenced by other factors such as quality of fixation and histological growth patterns and must thus be interpreted with caution.

Studies on DNA content of chronic atrophic gastritis have also produced variable results. Using cytophotometry, WEISS et al. (1980) found that 7% of cases of atrophic gastritis studied showed increased proliferative activity and carcinoma-like DNA distribution patterns. No comment was made as to the presence of dysplasia within these cases. Using flow cytometry, DEINLEIN et al. (1983) confirmed increased cell proliferative activity but no DNA aneuploidy in atrophic gastritis while TEODORI et al. (1984) reported DNA aneuploidy in almost 50% of cases examined. The findings of MACARTNEY and CAMPLEJOHN (1986) did not support this. They found evidence of DNA aneuploidy only in severe dysplasia or carcinoma. Chronic atrophic gastritis with intestinal metaplasia and mild or moderate dysplasia showed diploid DNA tracings.

4.3 Coeliac Disease

Application of quantitative methods has contributed both to diagnostic accuracy and to better understanding of teh pathogenesis of coeliac disease. Using a method based on the point-counting technique devised by CHALKLEY (1943), RUBIN et al. (1960), noted that in jejunal biopsies in untreated coeliac disease epithelial surface area is significantly reduced and accompanied by blunting or loss of villi. Other workers using linear methods quantitated mucosal changes in coeliac disease. They recorded reduction in villous height, increased mitotic activity within crypts, increased mucosal thickness, reduction in the height of epithelial cells lining the villi and a reduction in the villous height to crypt depth ratio (SHINER and DONIACH 1960; THURLBECK et al. 1960). The importance of obtaining well orientated sections cut at right angles to the mucosal surface was repeatedly emphasised (THURLBECK et al. 1960; RUBIN et al. 1960). Despite the limitations of the methods used (DUNNILL and WHITEHEAD 1972), these observations have provided the basis for the histological diagnosis of coeliac disease, provided allowance is made for geographical variations. The value of reduced villous height to crypt depth ratio and mucosal surface to volume ratio as a marker of untreated coeliac disease has been repeatedly confirmed in adults (DUNNILL and WHITEHEAD 1972; SLAVIN et al. 1980; CORAZZA et al. 1985), and in children (ROSEKRANS et al. 1981 a).

DUNNILL and WHITEHEAD (1972) introduced a stereological method for quantitating small intestinal biopsies which obviated certain difficulties associated with linear measurement. This uses a template devised by WEIBEL (1963) to assess mucosal surface to volume ratio using the method devised by CHALKLEY et al. (1949). Assessment is rapid and can be applied to routinely processed paraffin sections. The value of a significant reduction in surface to volume ratio as a marker of untreated coeliac disease was reinforced. This stereological method is cheap and highly efficient in distinguishing between biopsies from controls and patients with coeliac disease. Its value has been confirmed when used to assess less marked morphological changes in giardiasis (WRIGHT and TOMKINS 1978).

SLAVIN et al. (1980) described a semi-automatic computer-aided method of image analysis for quantitating jejunal biopsies. Using a 'light pen' to outline specific components of the histological section the volume occupied by each component is calculated by computer and in addition direct linear measurements can be carried out. Thus ratios such as mucosal height to crypt depth and epithelial volume to mucosal volume are easily calculated. Results confirm a significant reduction in both of these ratios in untreated coeliac disease. The volume of the lamina propria of the mucosa is also increased, a feature which has been noted by other workers (GUIX et al. 1979; DHESI et al. 1984).

This semi-automatic method has the advantage of using direct measurement of areas within the histological field rather than stereologically derived estimates. It requires more expensive equipment than methods based on the use of a graticule and appears to take approximately the same amount of time as manual methods. In a recent comparative study of morphometric methodology, CORRAZZA et al. (1985) showed that computer-aided methods are no more efficient than cheaper stereological methods in distinguishing patients with coeliac disease from controls. Nonetheless the potential applications for such computer-based but observer-controlled equipment seem considerable. Similar methodology has been used to quantify morphological changes in jejunal mucosa in giardiasis (ROSEKRANS et al. 1981 a) and in food allergy (ROSEKRANS et al. 1980 a).

In addition to studies based on mucosal architecture quantitation of individual cell types within jejunal mucosa in coeliac disease has yielded much information. This work was stimulated by a report by FERGUSON and MURRAY (1971) of increased numbers of intra-epithelial lymphocytes (IELs) in relation to the number of villous epithelial cells in coeliac disease. This increase reverted toward normal following treatment with gluten-free diet and appeared to be a useful marker of active coeliac disease in that such an increase in IEL numbers was not seen in other intestinal diseases. This finding has been challenged by others (GUIX et al. 1979; MARSH 1980; CORAZZA et al. 1984) who pointed out that when IELs are counted per unit length of muscularis mucosa, which is unaltered in coeliac disease, the numbers of these cells are not increased in comparison with controls, thus raising a question mark over the role of IELs in epithelial damage (MARSH 1980). Decreased numbers of IELs in untreated coeliac disease have been reported when the cells are counted overlying a fixed area of muscularis mucosa (MARSH 1980; CORAZZA et al. 1984). This discrepancy arising between IEL counts in relation to epithelial cells or in relation to unit length of muscularis mucosa was confirmed when both methods of quantitation were applied in the same study (ROSEKRANS et al. 1981 a; CORAZZA et al. 1984).

Careful observation by MARSH (1980) revealed increased flux of lymphocytes across the basal lamina of the epithelium in jejunal mucosa in untreated coeliac disease. In addition there was increased blast transformation and mitotic activity among IELs. These findings were interpreted as evidence of increased activation of the cells together with increased loss of lymphocytes into the gut lumen in association with desquamation of enterocytes. All of these abnormalities reverted toward normal following treatment.

Intra-epithelial lymphocytes in the jejunum have been identified as consisting predominantly of suppressor/cytotoxic T cells (SELBY et al. 1981 a, b). This is not altered in coeliac disease but further evidence of increased migration and stimulation of these cells in coeliac disease has been provided by the identification of Leu-1 and T2 antigens on an increased proportion of the cells (SELBY et al. 1983; MALIZIA et al. 1985). More T helper cells in the lamina propria were also stimulated, suggesting an alternation of immune tolerance to dietary gluten in coeliac disease (MALIZIA et al. 1985).

While there is argument regarding absolute numbers of IELs in jejunal mucosa in coeliac disease, there appears to be general agreement that the density of the cells is increased. The role of these cells is uncertain. Quantitation of IELs by LEIGH et al. (1985) over several days following low dose gluten challenge in treated coeliac disease patients showed that there is a significant increase in numbers, reaching a peak after 12 h and reverting towards normal after 60 h. This was not accompanied by any immediate mucosal damage. The authors thus questioned the significance of increased lymphoid infiltration in relation to mucosal damage. Nonetheless there is evidence of altered humoral and cell-mediated immunity in coeliac disease. The latter is reflected by reports of activation among IELs already mentioned and suppported by further evidence of altered cell marker patterns indicating an active cytotoxic role among IELs rather than simple passive crowding (JENKINS et al. 1986).

Marked increase in proliferative activity among crypt enterocytes in coeliac disease has been well documented (WATSON and WRIGHT 1974) but mitotic activity amongst IELs is also increased. Quantitation of this increase by counting mitotic figures within 3000 IELs per specimen has been carried out (MARSH 1982). The results indicated a particularly high mitotic rate in coeliac disease or related conditions, separating this group from controls and other patients with gastrointestinal disease. The author recommends this as a reliable diagnostic feature in gluten-related disease, distinguishing it from unrelated causes of mucosal flattening and cutting out the need to perform further biopsies (MARSH 1985). Caution regarding the value of this feature as a diagnostic indicator for coeliac disease or related conditions has been expressed. FERGUSON and ZIEGLER (1986) found that IEL mitoses increase in proportion to the numbers of IELs present and that high mitotic counts are not specific for coeliac disease. The counting technique in their study has been criticised (WHITEHEAD 1986; MARSH 1986) and the value of IEL mitoses as a diagnostic feature of coeliac disease defended (MARSH 1986). However, it is likely that the procedure will be reserved for research purposes or occasional problematical cases.

4.4 Colorectal Disease

Colorectal biopsies or operative specimens constitute a significant proportion of the diagnostic work-load of the general histopathologist. Application of quantitative methods to this material may improve the accuracy of diagnosis and assessment of disease severity in addition to providing insight into the pathogenesis of lesions produced. Furthermore construction of quantitative scoring systems can provide an index of prognosis in established disease. This section discusses the use of quantitation in various colorectal disorders to elucidate their pathogenesis and diagnosis.

4.4.1 Diverticular Disease and Abnormalities of Colorectal Muscle

A fall in the consumption of dietary fibre in Western society has resulted in a high incidence of diverticular disease (PAINTER and BURKITT 1975). It is thought that mucosal extrusion occurs as a consequence of raised intraluminal pressure (PAINTER 1964) associated with an abnormality of the muscularis propria in the sigmoid colon (MORSON and DAWSON 1979). The width of both muscle layers is greatly increased but quantitation showed no evidence of hyperplasia or hypertrophy of muscle cells in either the circular muscle coat or the taenia coli (WHITEWAY and MORSON 1985). However, a marked increase in elastin content of the taeniae was noted. From these findings the authors postulate that there is contracture of the taenia due to increased elastin content with resultant concertina-like folding of the circular muscle coat and bowel shortening. This results in short, segments of high intraluminal pressure between opposed circular muscle folds and subsequent formation of diverticular pouches.

Simple morphometric techniques on ganglion and nerve fibre counts have contributed to the understanding and diagnosis of Hirschsprung's disease and its related variants, such as aganglionosis and neuronal colonic dysplasia (MEIER-RUGE 1974).

4.4.2 Chronic Inflammatory Bowel Disease

The cause of ulcerative colitis and Crohn's disease remains unknown but recently some insight into their pathogenesis has been gained from studies enumerating cell populations and their functions (for overview see MACDERMOTT 1986). Mucosal biopsy plasma cell counting is a reliable, reproducible investigation (SELDENRIJK et al. 1986) and when linked to immunoglobulin staining shows immunocyte numbers in ulcerative colitis to be increased by a factor of 4, predominantly due to a 30-fold increase in IgG-containing cells (BRANDTZAEG et al. 1974). KEREN and co-workers (1984) obtained similar results and others have confirmed elevated plasma cell counts to varying extents in the different immunoglobulin classes (ROSEKRANS et al. 1980b). The total mucosal plasma cell counts correlate with the level of disease activity (SCOTT et al. 1983) and are predominantly IgG cells (STRICKLAND et al. 1975). It is postulated that antigen exposure leads to a local mucosal IgA and IgG immunoglobulin response and that these antibodies in turn may co-contribute to disease pathogenesis by immune cross-reactivity or complex formation (MACDERMOTT 1986). There is variation in the reporting of the relative distribution of the Ig classes in

Crohn's disease and ulcerative colitis and as to whether these profiles aid in their discrimination (VAN SPREEUWEL et al. 1986).

Mucosal quantitation has characterised the inflammation in non-specific proctitis (HYWEL-JONES et al. 1973; JENKINS et al. 1988). The number and type of immunoglobulin-containing cells (VAN SPREEUWEL et al. 1985), total mucosal cellularity and the distribution of inflammatory cells within the lamina propria (JENKINS et al. 1988) help to differentiate normal mucosa, acute infectious colitis and chronic inflammatory bowel disease. Bacterial colitis shows a preferential increase in IgA-producing plasma cells (SCOTT et al. 1983; VAN SPREEUWEL et al. 1985). Crohn's disease and ulcerative colitis show increased cellularity, with disproportionately heavy inflammation in the deepest one-third of the mucosa (JENKINS et al. 1988) consisting of IgA immunocytes (VAN SPREEUWEL et al. 1985). Eosinophil numbers have been postulated to be an index of activity (SARIN et al. 1987) and prognosis in proctocolitis (HEATLEY and JAMES 1979) and mast cell counts have been established in normal mucosa (SANDERSON 1985) as a baseline for further investigation in disease (SARIN et al. 1987).

Using graticule measurements clinical improvement in ulcerative colitis correlates with normalisation of architectural variables such as mucous membrane thickness, crypt depth and epithelial height (NOGALLER et al. 1983). Normal mucosa, ulcerative colitis in remission and chronic active disease score differently on assessment of the features glandular lumen diameter, gland density and the linear space of lamina propria between consecutive glands (RUBIO et al. 1982a, 1984). Inflamed mucosa has enlarged, sparse glands set in abundant lamina propria (RUBIO et al. 1982b). Image analysis has shown the ratios of surface to mucosal epithelial lengths and surface to crypt epithelial heights, in combination with lamina propria cellularity, to be highly predictive for chronic inflammatory bowel disease (JENKINS et al. 1988). Surface villous regeneration, which is one of the most reproducible biopsy criteria for assessing ulcerative colitis (GIARD et al. 1985; SURAWICZ and BELIC 1984; DUNDAS et al. 1987), has been confirmed with an increase in mucosal depth (THOMPSON et al. 1985), due predominantly to inflammatory expansion of the lamina propria (ROSEKRANS et al. 1980b; ALLEN et al. 1988a), and also in the surface to mucosal epithelial lengths ratio (JENKINS et al. 1988).

The difficulty in distinguishing some cases of ulcerative colitis from Crohn's colitis is reflected in morphometric studies. THOMPSON et al. (1985) found that no variables reliably separated the two. The most successful feature was the ratio of surface epithelial height to crypt epithelial height, which is significantly reduced in ulcerative colitis, probably reflecting increased surface damage in this condition.

The role of quantitation in the diagnosis of premalignancy in chronic inflammatory bowel disease is discussed below.

4.4.3 Collagenous Colitis

The term 'collagenous colitis' describes an unusual clinical syndrome of chronic watery diarrhoea associated with thickening of the mucosal subepithelial collagen table (LINDSTROM 1976, see pp. 219–227). The normal collagen layer is elaborated by the pericryptal fibroblast sheath and measures up to 7 μm (GARDINER et al. 1974). In collagenous colitis the thickness of the layer can increase to 50 μm and appears as an eosinophilic subepithelial hyaline band (NIELSEN et al. 1980). The exact relationship of the presence of a thickened collagen layer and chronic diarrhoea remains controversial (WILLIAMS and RHODES 1987).

4.4.4 Transitional Colonic Mucosa

Transitional colonic mucosa contains hyperplastic, branched glandular crypts composed of dilated goblet cells secreting sialomucins instead of the usual sulphomucins (FILIPE 1969). Controversy exists as to its biological significance (WILLIAMS 1985). It has been interpreted as an early premalignant change due to its frequent occurrence in the mucosa adjacent to colorectal carcinoma (FILIPE 1984). On the other hand it may occur secondary to mucosal inflammation, ischaemia or prolapse, and present in conjunction with dysplastic or malignant tissues as a consequence of maturation from them (ALLEN et al. 1988b). Quantitation shows increased mucosal height in transitional mucosa (range 0.8–2 mm, normal range 0.4–0.5 mm) (HAMILTON et al. 1988; SAFFOS and RHATIGAN 1977; LEV et al. 1985). Densitometry confirms goblet cell 0-acyl sialomucin levels intermediate between those of normal mucosa and carcinoma (DAWSON et al. 1978). Analysis of multiple nuclear and cellular variables failed to show any differences from control mucosa or the trend encountered in other premalignant colonic conditions (see below). The suggestion that transitional mucosa represents early neoplastic change is not therefore supported by morphometry (HAMILTON et al. 1988).

4.4.5 Epithelial Dysplasia

Epithelial dysplasia is a precancerous lesion of the mucosa with a variable potential for progression to adenocarcinoma. It is present in sporadic colorectal adenomatous polyps, familial polyposis coli and a proportion of patients with long-standing ulcerative colitis. The recognition of dysplasia and assessment of its grade are subject to inter- and intra-observer variation (BROWN et al. 1985; RIDDELL et al. 1983). It is assessed by architectural and cytological changes and both of these variables, along with estimation of nuclear DNA content, are amenable to quantitation.

Table 2. The percentages of aneuploidy found on flow cytometry of colorectal adenomas < 2 cm and > 2 cm in diameter

	Polyp Diameter		
	< 1 cm	1–2 cm	> 2 cm
QUIRKE et al. 1985 b	1.5%		42%
VAN DEN INGH et al. 1985	0%	30%	50%

4.4.5.1 Adenomatous Polyps

The histogenesis of tubular adenoma formation is postulated as glandular growth due to the infolding of proliferating surface epithelium between normal, pre-existing glands. The proliferative region in normal mucosa is confined to the lower one-third of the gland but in villous adenomas there is an increase in the proliferative region with extension of epithelial and mesenchymal proliferation up to the crypt neck, resulting in upward papillary projections (MASKENS 1979). Stereological (ELIAS et al. 1981) and scanning electron microscope studies of adenomas (PHELPS et al. 1979) confirm this, showing increased epithelial surface area thrown into villi consisting of branched folia and intervening crypts. Low resolution image analysis can separate normal mucosa, adenomas and adenocarcinoma using the following variables: the minimum diameter of glands, minimum distance between and number of neighbouring glands, and area and circumference of glands (KAYSER et al. 1985). Ultrastructural analysis of nuclear size achieves similar results (SATO et al. 1981). Significant cytological features showing a morphometric trend between the grades of dysplasia in adenomas are: nuclear-cytoplasmic ratio, nuclear size variation and stratification (BROWN et al. 1985; SASSI et al. 1986

The concept of a dysplasia-carcinoma sequence is now well established (KONISHI and MORSON 1982), with evidence arising from several studies. These show a greater likelihood of malignant change where adenomas are multiple (BUSSEY 1978; EIDE 1986), are greater than 2 cm in diameter (50% malignancy rate), and show a villous architeture and severe dysplasia (DAY and MORSON 1978; KONISHI and MORSON 1982). Flow cytometry and densitometry ploidy patterns support this dysplasia-carcinoma sequence. Adenomas predominantly possesss a diploid DNA profile. The detection of aneuploidy varies but several studies have found it be more frequent if the adenoma is greater than 2 cm in diameter (Table 2) and in those with severe epithelial dysplasia (Table 3). It is also more prevalent when a villous pattern (QUIRKE et al. 1985 b, VAN DEN INGH et al. 1985; BANNER et al. 1987) and enlarged nuclear size are present (JARVIS et al. 1987). In contrast to these results, two studies using tissue densitometry failed to detect aneuploidy in colorectal adenomas (Table 3). The reported higher

Table 3. The percentages of aneuploidy related to the grade of dysplasia in colorectal adenomas

	Dysplasia Mild	Moderate	Severe
Flow cytometry			
GOH and JASS 1986	4%	18%	36%
QUIRKE et al. 1985 b	0%	5.5%	12%
VAN DEN INGH et al. 1985	21%	29%	43%
Tissue densitometry			
WHITEHEAD et al. 1985	All in diploid range (n = 19)		
JARVIS et al. 1987	All in diploid range (n = 10)		

rate of aneuploidy in adenocarcinoma suggests that the dysplasia-cancer sequence behaves in a stepwise fashion, with ploidy abnormalities either initiating the process of invasion occurring as a consequence of it (GOH and JASS 1986; WHITEHEAD et al. 1985).

Quantitation studies on adenomas can therefore lead to more consistent grading and identification of those most likely to contain carcinoma. This has obvious implications for the pathologist examining an individual lesion and for the clinician in patient follow-up.

4.4.5.2 Familial Polyposis Coli

Flow cytometry of adenomas in familial polyposis coli indicates an aneuploidy rate of 10% but bearing no relationship to polyp size, histological pattern or grade of dysplasia. There was an increased proliferative index in polyps greater than 5 mm in diameter. Ploidy patterns were not found to be a good predictor of the presence of carcinoma (QUIRKE et al. 1987 a).

4.4.5.3 Ulcerative Colitis with Dysplasia and Carcinoma

Patients with long-standing ulcerative colitis have an increased risk of mucosal dysplasia and carcinoma (RIDDELL 1976; LENNARD-JONES et al. 1983). The designation of dysplasia in inflammatory bowel disease is sub ject to observer variation and its distinction from regenerative change is difficult. This distinction is important in patient follow-up and treatment (RIDDELL et al. 1983). Image analysis of multiple nuclear and cellular geometric variables gives an insight into the morphological differences between histological groups and allows the construction of classification rules in an attempt to achieve more accurate and reproducible categorisation of individual lesions. Analysis of normal mucosa, regenerative mucosa, dysplasia and carcinoma in ulcerative colitis identifies three principal components responsible for variation in the dataset (ALLEN et al. 1987). These are: (a) nuclear size, nuclear-cytoplasmic ratio and nuclear stratification; (b) the variation of nuclear size; and (c) nuclear shape and polarity. This is

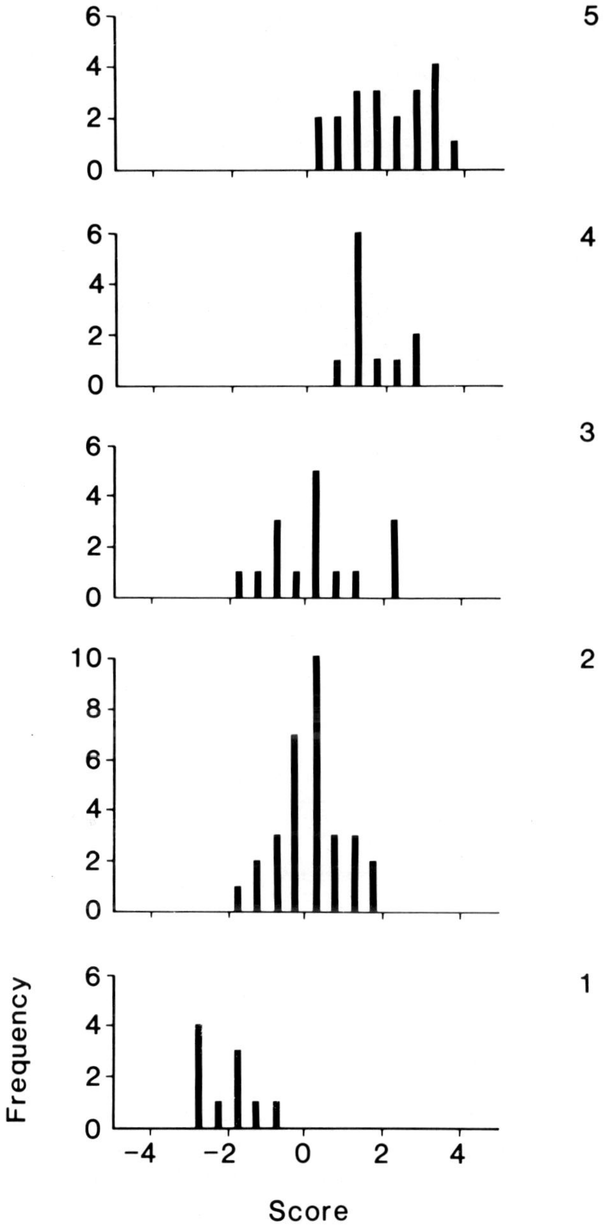

Fig. 4. Discriminant scores for colonic mucosal lesions plotted by histological groups. Tumour (*5*) and high grade dysplasia (*4*) are grouped together and separate from normal mucosa (*1*). Regeneration (*2*) and low grade dysplasia (*3*) lie intermediate between the other groups. There is complete discrimination between normal and carcinoma. (ALLEN et al. 1987)

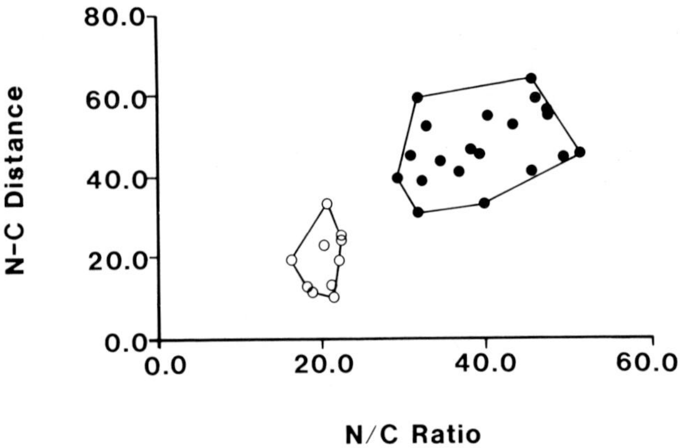

Fig. 5. Scatter plot of mean nuclear–cytoplasmic ratio against coefficient of variation of nucleus to cell apex distance. There is complete separation of normals (*left* ○) and carcinoma (*right* ●). (HAMILTON et al. 1987)

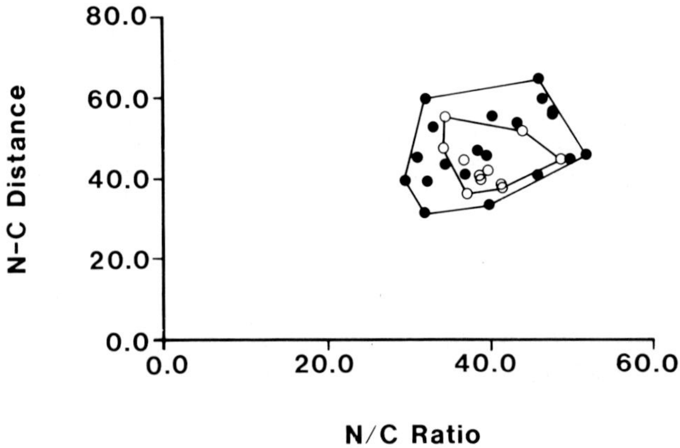

Fig. 6. Scatter plot showing grouping of high grade dysplasia (○) with adenocarcinoma (●) (ALLEN et al. 1987)

of value to the pathologist in that it emphasises the subjective features that are useful in diagnosis. Discriminant analysis of the dataset selects those variables that make significant contributions in distinguishing the predefined histological groups. The chosen variables are used to construct an allocation rule or scoring system and each lesion is scored accordingly. In this way HAMILTON and co-workers (1987 a) have separated normal mucosa and adenocarcinoma. The results may be represented as frequency histograms of the lesion scores (Fig. 4) or scatter plots of the two discriminating variables (Fig. 5). The system may be verified with further test set data. Using this classification rule, based on the variables nuclear-cytoplasmic ratio and the coefficient of variation of nucleus to cell apex

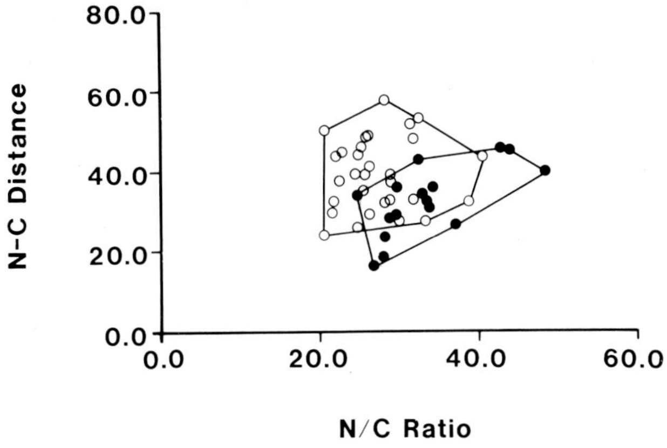

Fig. 7. Scatter plot showing overlap of regeneration (○) and low grade dysplasia (●) (ALLEN et al. 1987)

distance, the diagnostic categories of regeneration and low and high grade dysplasia were assessed (ALLEN et al. 1987). This led to grouping of high grade dysplasia with adenocarcinoma and the intermediate placement of regeneration and low grade dysplasia (Fig. 4). The close correlation between high grade dysplasia and adenocarcinoma (Fig. 6) suggests that quantitation may be used to confirm this diagnosis, which is an indication for colectomy. Furthermore the overlap between regeneration and low grade dysplasia emphasises the trend of morphological changes between these categories. When sections in the overlap areas of the scatter plots of these two groups (Fig. 7) were reviewed histologically it was seen that factors such as active inflammation at an ulcer edge, polyp margin or crypt base dilute the significance of any epithelial changes. This feedback on subjective assessment allows refinement of lesion allocation to the various diagnostic groups and this has implications for patient colonoscopic surveillance (ALLEN et al. 1987).

In a parallel study low power image analysis of architectural variables was carried out on ulcerative colitis (ALLEN et al. 1988a). This showed the dataset variation to be due to the area of mucosa and the relative proportions of lamina propria and epithelium per unit length of muscularis mucosae, along with the mucosal and epithelial heights. Regeneration results in a thicker mucosa due to inflammatory expansion of the lamina propria. Dysplasia shows a biphasic enlargement of the epithelial and lamina propria compartments due to an increase in epithelial proliferation along with an associated mesenchymal response, which is in part contributed to by an inflammatory component. A classification rule based on the discriminating variables, epithelial height and lamina propria area completely separated normal mucosa and high grade dysplasia. Low grade dysplasia was allocated to the same grouping as the high grade category and 60% of regeneration cases to the normal group (Fig. 8). Scatter plots

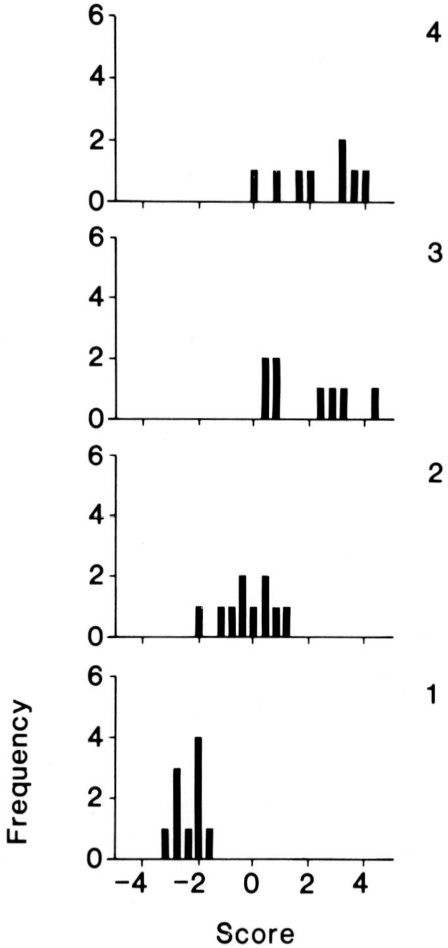

Fig. 8. Discriminant scores for the lesions plotted by histological groups and derived from the variables epithelial height and lamina propria area. Normals (*1*) are separated from high grade dysplasia (*4*) with a threshold value of zero. Low grade dysplasia (*3*) is allocated to the high grade category and 60% of regenerative lesions (*2*) to the normal group (ALLEN et al. 1988 a)

successfully distinguised regenerative epithelium from dysplasia (Fig. 9). Future work will be aimed at combining architectural and cytological features in a quantitative index as a basis for classification of biopsy material and it is hoped that this will provide further refinement and form the basis of an adjunct to the pathologist's subjective opinion.

Cytophotometry studies have noted increasing DNA content with worsening grades of dysplasia, the 62.5% aneuploidy rate in high grade dysplasia being recommended as a potential prognostic marker for the presence of invasion (CUVELIER et al. 1987). Flow cytometry has shown aneuploidy in colitic dysplasia and been advocated as augmenting colonoscopic surveillance (HAMMARBERG et al. 1984; MCKINLEY et al. 1985) but its exact role is not yet defined. FOZARD and co-workers (1986) found a dysplasia-associated aneuploidy rate of approximately 20% correlating with the disease duration but unrelated to dysplasia grade and no more

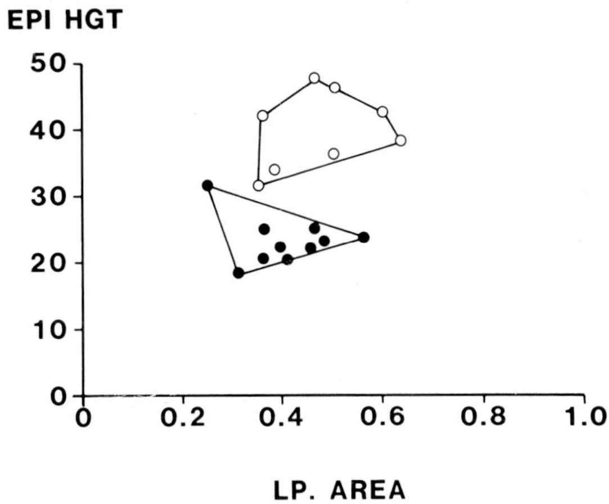

Fig. 9. Scatter plot of epithelial height (*EPI HGT*) and lamina propria (*LP AREA*) separating regeneration (●) from high grade dysplasia (○) (ALLEN et al. 1988a)

prevalent than in regenerative controls. MELVILLE et al. (1987) detected aneuploidy in 30% of dysplastic lesions correlating with dysplasia grade, while regenerative cases were diploid. Both of these studies, together with LOFBERG et al. (1987), described cases with abnormal ploidy patterns in mucosa well away from areas of dysplasia and suggested its use for detecting potentially malignant changes in the absence of histological changes.

4.4.6 *Colorectal Adenocarcinoma*

Quantitation by both light and electron microscopy separates normal mucosa from adenocarcinoma. Significant discriminating variables are nuclear volume and nuclear-cytoplasmic ratio (NAKAMURA et al. 1974) and a combination of the latter with the coefficient of variation of nucleus to cell apex distance (HAMILTON et al. 1987a). In the latter study discrimination was achieved with high reproducibility by an observer with minimal histological knowledge who was unaware of the diagnosis. SATO and coworkers (1981) have shown a trend of nuclear and nucleolar enlargement correlating with malignant transformation from normal mucosa through dysplasia to carcinoma. They suggested a possible role for the quantitative diagnosis of epithelial lesions by measuring the area of 50 nuclei and their nucleoli. LOWE et al. (1986) noted an aneuploidy rate of 51% in a group of Dukes' stage B carcinomas. Morphometric differences from the diploid tumours were in the mean nuclear profile area (62.9 μm^2 vs 48.2 μm^2: $P < 0.001$) and the percentage of large nuclei in a given carcinoma (6.2% vs 1%: $P < 0.001$). Their findings allowed the construction of a simple algorithm to determine nuclear size by a single linear graticule measurement taken over six fields. This gave a 74% accurate prediction of ploidy status and it was recommended for use in routine histological assessment.

DNA photometry has noted the frequent occurrence of non-diploid cell populations in adenocarcinomas (STICH et al. 1960). Tumours containing a higher proportion of cells exceeding the upper diploid limit were associated with worse survival and greater likelihood of local recurrence. They also correlated with tumour stage and grade (FORSSLUND et al. 1984). Several flow cytometry studies indicate the poorer prognosis of aneuploid tumours (WOLLEY et al. 1982; ARMITAGE et al. 1985; SCOTT et al. 1987; QUIRKE et al. 1987 b). QUIRKE and co-workers (1985 a) have also demonstrated ploidy heterogeneity within a given tumour but with no difference between the superficial and deep aspects of a given lesion or its secondary deposits. They have found that ploidy relates to staging, that 54% of colorectal carcinomas are aneuploid, and that a combination of the ploidy profile and index of cell proliferation are good prognostic markers. High cell turnover was associated with an infiltrative growth pattern and worse prognosis (QUIRKE et al. 1987 b).

In contrast MELAMED et al. (1986) demonstrated no correlation between tumour ploidy and staging or survival and GOH et al. (1987) found the influence of ploidy on survival to be small.

Recently a new system of prognostic categorisation for colorectal carcinoma has been introduced (JASS et al. 1987). This is based on a scoring system derived from several variables, including depth of tumour invasion, infiltrating or expanding tumour edge, number of affected lymph nodes and degree of peritumoural lymphocytic infiltration. The system has improved prediction of prognosis and appears to be a refinement of the longstanding and widely used Dukes' classification (JASS and MORSON 1987).

4.4.7 Leiomyomatous Tumours

Irrespective of their site within the gastrointestinal tract, suggested predictors of behaviour are tumour size (> 7.5 cm). Other prognostic factors include mitotic count (> 5 per 10 high power fields) and their ploidy profile (COOPER et al. 1987).

5 Conclusion

Quantitation has increased our understanding of the pathogenesis and biological behaviour of gastrointestinal disease. To be of value to the practicising pathologist methods of quantitation must be easily applied, be inexpensive in terms of both equipment and time and impart additional useful information.

The above conditions can be met to some extent by semi-quantitative methods based on experience and careful observation of features easily visible and partly quantifiable in routine pathological specimens without special equipment. DUKES' staging of colorectal carcinoma (1932) is an example which is of proven value as a prognostic indicator. The recent refinement and extension of this system (JASS et al. 1987) may well enhance its value further.

The use of more detailed and sophisticated quantitative methods is still largely confined to research studies and while these methods have undoubtedly improved the diagnostic acumen of those acquainted with them, they have not yet created a widespread impact. Semi-automatic image analysis is relatively cheap but can be time consuming. At present its main role appears to lie in directing the pathologist towards the most useful histological features on which to base his diagnosis. A logical extension of this is the use of computer-aided assessment to reach a diagnosis and the capability of the methodology in this respect has been demonstrated in borderline ovarian carcinoma (BAAK et al. 1981). In gastrointestinal pathology there is considerable evidence that the technique is useful in identifying critical features in perennially difficult problems such as distinguishing regenerative from dysplastic epithelium, grading dysplasia, improving prognostic indicators in malignancy and in problematical cases of jejunal villous atrophy.

Flow cytometry is rapid, easily used and requires only small amounts of tissue. No doubt in time problems such as cell specificity and debris masking cell populations will be solved and it may have a defined role as prognostic marker in established tumours and perhaps even in detection of premalignant states. However, the equipment remains expensive and thus by necessity is centralised, demands on such equipment may multiply and some doubts exist about interpretation of results and the relationship between ploidy and prognosis.

The approach of LOWE et al. (1986) in using flow cytometry and image analysis as research tools to devise an algorithm capable of predicting tumour ploidy and applicable to simple measurement using a microscope eyepiece graticule is to be commended. It seems unlilkely that sophisticated equipment or the time to carry out the necessary research will become universally available. If simple methods emerge from the research which can be widely applied to improving and standardising diagnosis this will make a significant contribution to diagnostic pathology.

Acknowledgements. The authors gratefully acknowledge the assistance of Miss Kate McAteer and Mrs. Bridie Kelly in the preparation and typing of this manuscript.

References

Aherne WA, Dunnill MS (1982) Morphometry. Arnold, London

Allen DC, Hamilton PW, Watt PCH, Biggart JD (1987) Morphometrical analysis in ulcerative colitis with dysplasia and carcinoma. Histopathology 11:913–926

Allen DC, Hamilton PW, Watt PCH, Biggart JD (1988a) Architectural morphometry in ulcerative colitis with dysplasia. Histopathology 12:611–621

Allen DC, Connolly NS, Biggart JD (1988b) High iron diamine – alcian blue mucin profiles in benign, premalignant and malignant colorectal disease. Histopathology 13:399–412

Armitage NC, Robins RA, Evans DF, Turner DR, Baldwin RW, Hardcastle JD (1985) The influence of tumour cell DNA abnormalities on survival in colorectal cancer. Br J Surg 72:828–830

Baak JPA, Oort J (1983) A manual of morphometry in diagnostic pathology. Springer, Berlin Heidelberg New York

Baak JPA, Agrafojo Blanco A, Kurver PHJ et al. (1981) Quantitation of borderline and malignant mucinous ovarian tumours. Histopathology 5:353–360

Banner BF, Chacho MS, Roseman DL, Coon JS (1987) Multiparameter flow cytometric analysis of colon polyps. Am J Clin Pathol 87:313–318

Barlogie B, Drewinko B, Schumann J et al. (1980) Cellular DNA content as a marker of neoplasia in man. Am J Med 69:195–203

Behar J, Sheahan DG (1975) Histological abnormalities in reflux oesophagitis. Arch Pathol 99:387–391

Bennets R, Stroehlein J, Barlogie B (1979) Ploidy determination by DNA flow cytometry of malignant and benign gastric tissue obtained by endoscopic biopsy. Gastroenterology 76:1099

Bezemer PD, Baak JPA, de With C (1977) Discriminant analysis, exemplified with quantitative features of endometrium. Eur J Obstet Gynecol Reprod Biol 7(3):209–214

Bohm N, Sandritter W (1975) DNA in human tumours: a cytophotometric study. Curr Top Pathol 60:151–181

Bohm N, Sprenger E (1968) Fluorescence cytophotometry: a valuable method for the quantitative determination of nuclear fuelgen-DNA. Histochemie 16:100–118

Boon ME, Kurver PJH, Baak JPA, Thompson HT (1981) The application of morphometry in gastric cytological diagnosis. Virchows Arch [A]393:159–164

Bradbury S (1979) Microscopical image analysis: problems and approaches. J Microscopy 115:137–150

Brandtzaeg P, Baklien K, Fausa O, Hoel PS (1974) Immunohistochemical characterization of local immunoglobulin formation in ulcerative colitis. Gastroenterology 66:1123–1136

Brown LJR, Smeeton NC, Dixon MF (1985) Assessment of dysplasia in colorectal adenomas: an observer variation and morphometric study. J Clin Pathol 38:174–179

Bussey HJR (1978) Multiple adenomas and carcinomas. In: Bennington JL (ed) Major problems in pathology, vol 10. The pathogenesis of colorectal cancer. WB Saunders, Philadelphia, pp 72–80

Chalkley HW (1943) Methods for the quantitative morphologic analysis of tissues. J Natl Cancer Inst 4:47–53

Chalkley HW, Cornfield J, Park H (1949) A method for estimating volume-surface ratios. Science 110:295–297

Collins BJ, Elliott H, Sloan JM, McFarland RJ, Love AHG (1985) Oesophageal histology in reflux oesophagitis. J Clin Pathol 38:1265–1272

Coon JS, Landay AL, Weinstein RS (1986) Flow cytometric analysis of paraffin-embedded tumours: implications for diagnostic pathology. Hum Pathol 17:435–437

Cooper PN, Quirke P, Hardy GJ, Bird CC, Dixon MF (1987) Prediction of the behaviour of smooth muscle tumours of the gastrointestinal tract. J Pathol 152:217A

Corrazza GR, Frazzoni M, Gasbarrini G (1984) Jejunal intraepithelial lymphocytes in coeliac disease: are they increased or decreased? Gut 25:158–162

Corazza GR, Frazzoni M, Dixon MF, Gasbarrini G (1985) Quantitative assessment of the mucosal architecture of jejunal biopsy specimens: a comparison between linear measurement, stereology and computer aided microscopy. J Clin Pathol 38:765–770

Cuvelier CA, Morson BC, Roels HJ (1987) The DNA content in cancer and dysplasia in chronic ulcerative colitis. Histopathology 11:927–939

Danno M (1975) Statistical criteria for the cytology of gastric cancer. A proposal of distance index. Acta Cytol 20:446–468

Dawson PA, Patel J, Filipe MI (1978) Variations in sialomucins in the mucosa of the large intestine in malignancy: a quantimet and statistical analysis. Histochem J 10:559–572

Day DW, Morson BC (1978) The adenoma-carcinoma sequence. In: Bennington JL (ed) Major problems in pathology, vol 10. The pathogenesis of colorectal cancer. WB Saunders, Philadelphia, pp 58–71

Deinlein E, Schmidt H, Riemann J-F, Gra El-Pietrusky R, Hornstein OP (1983) DNA flow cytometric measurements in inflammatory and malignant human gastric lesions. Virchows Archiv [A]402:185–193

Dhesi I, Marsh MN, Kelly C, Crowe P (1984) Morphometric analysis of small intestinal mucosa. Virchows Arch [A]403:173–180

Dukes CE (1932) The classification of cancer of the rectum. J Pathol Bact 35:323–332

Dundas SAC, Kay R, Beck S, Cotton DWK, Coup aJ, Slater DN, Underwood JCE (1987) Can histopathologists reliably assess dysplasia in inflammatory bowel disease? J Clin Pathol 40:1282–1286

Dunnill MS, Whitehead R (1972) A method for the quantitation of small intestinal biopsy specimens. J Clin Pathol 25:243–246

Eide TJ (1986) Prevalence and morpological features of adenomas of the large intestine in individuals with and without colorectal carcinoma. Histopathology 10:111–118

Elias H, Hyde DM, Mullens RS, Lambert FC (1981) Colonic adenomas: stereology and growth mechanisms. Dis Colon Rectum 24:331–342

Enblad P, Glimelius B, Bengtssen A, Ponten J, Pahlmen L (1985) DNA content in carcinoma of the rectum and rectosigmoid. Acta Pathol Microbiol Immunol Scand [A]93:277–284

Ferguson A, Murray D (1971) Quantitation of intraepithelial lymphocytes in human jejunum. Gut 12:989–994

Ferguson A, Ziegler K (1986) Intraepithelial lymphocyte mitoses in a jejunal biopsy correlates with intraepithelial lymphocyte count irrespective of diagnosis. Gut 27:675–679

Filipe MI (1969) Value of histochemical reactions for mucosubstances in the diagnosis of certain pathological conditions of the colon and rectum. Gut 10:577–586

Filipe MI (1984) Mucins of normal, premalignant and malignant colonic mucosa. In: Wolman SR, Mastromarina AJ (eds) Progress in cancer research and therapy, vol 29. Raven, New York, pp 237–251

Forsslund G, Cedermark B, Ohman U, Erhardt K, Zetterberg A, Auer G (1984) The significance of DNA distribution pattern in rectal carcinoma. A preliminary study. Dis Colon Rectum 27:579–584

Fozard JBJ, Quirke P, Dixon MF, Giles GR, Bird CC (1986) DNA aneuploidy in ulcerative colitis. Gut 27:1414–1418

Gardiner GW, Goldberg R, Currie D, Murray D (1984) Colonic carcinoma associated with an abnormal collagen table. Cancer 54:2973–2977

Giard RWM, Hermans J, Ruiter DJ, Hoedemaeker PHJ (1985) Variations in histopathological evaluation of non-neoplastic mucosal abnormalities: assessment and clinical significance. Histopathology 9:535–541

Goh HS, Jass JR (1986) DNA content and the adenoma-carcinoma sequence in the colorectum. J Clin Pathol 39:387–392

Goh HS, Jass JR, Atkin WS, Cuzick J, Northover JMA (1987) Value of flow cytometric determination of ploidy as a guide to prognosis in operable rectal cancer. Int J Colorect Dis 2:17–21

Guix M, Skinner JM, Whitehead RW (1979) Measuring intraepithelial lymphocytes, surface area and volume of lamina propria in the jejunal mucosa of coeliac patients. Gut 20:275–278

Hamilton PW, Allen DC, Watt PCH, Patterson CC, Biggart JD (1987a) Classification of normal colorectal mucosa and adenocarcinoma by morphometry. Histopathology 11:901–911

Hamilton PW, Collins JSA, Watt PCH, Sloan JM, Love AHG (1987b) Morphometric assessment of oesophagitis in pinch biopsies and correlation with ambulatory pH data. J Pathol 151:78A

Hamilton PW, Watt PCH, Collins JSA, Sloan JM, Love AHG (1987c) Objective grading of gastritis and duodenitis: a comparison of two methods. J Pathol 152–228A

Hamilton PW, Watt PCH, Allen DC (1988) A morphometrical assessment of transitional mucosa in the colon. Histopathology 13:519–530

Hammarberg C, Slezak P, Tribukait B (1984) Early detection of malignancy in ulcerative colitis. A flow-cytometric DNA study. Cancer 53:291–295

Heatley RV, James PD (1979) Eosinophils in the rectal mucosa. A simple method of predicting the outcome of ulcerative proctocolitis? Gut 20:787–791

Hedley DW, Friedlander ML, Taylor IW, Rugg CA, Musgrove EA (1983) Method for analysis of cellular DNA content of paraffin-embedded pathological material using flow cytometry. J Histochem Cytochem 31:1333–1335

Hedley DW, Friedlander ML, Taylor IW (1985) Application of DNA flow cytometry to paraffin-embedded archival material for the study of aneuploidy and its clinical significance. Cytometry 6:327–333

Hywel-Jones J, Lennard-Jones JE, Morson BC (1973) Numerical taxonomy and discriminant analysis applied to non-specific colitis. Q J Med 42:715–732

Inokuchi K, Kodama Y, Sasaki O, Kamegawa T, Okamura T (1983) Differentiation of growth patterns of early gastric carcinoma determined by cytophotometric DNA analysis. Cancer 51:1138–1141

Inui N, Oata K (1965) DNA content of human tumour cell nucleus: a study on gastric carcinoma with special reference to its histological features. GANN 56:567–574

Ismail-Beigi F, Horton PF, Pope CE (1970) Histological consequences of gastroesophageal reflux in man. Gastroenterology 58:163–174

Jarvis LR, Whitehead R (1985) Morphometric analysis of gastric dysplasia. J Pathol 47:133–138

Jarvis LR, Dent J, Whitehead R (1985) Morphometric assessment of reflux oesophagitis in fibreoptic biopsy specimens. J Clin Pathol 38:44–48

Jarvis LR, Graff PS, Whitehead R (1987) Correlation of nuclear ploidy with histology in adenomatous polyps of colon. J Clin Pathol 40:26–33

Jass JR, Morson BC (1987) Reporting colorectal carcinoma. J Clin Pathol 40:1016–1023

Jass JR, Love SB, Northover JMA (1987) A new prognostic classification of rectal cancer. Lancet I:1303–1306

Jenkins D, Goodall A, Gillet FR, Scott BB (1985) Defining duodenitis: quantitative histological study of mucosal responses and their correlations. J Clin Pathol 38:1119–1126

Jenkins D, Goodall A, Scott BB (1986) T lymphocyte populations in normal and coeliac small intestinal mucosa defined by monoclonal antibodies. Gut 27:1330–1331

Jenkins D, Goodall A, Drew K, Scott BB (1988) What is colitis? Statistical approach to distinguishing clinically important inflammatory change in rectal biopsy specimens. J Clin Pathol 41:72–79

Kayser KK, Modlinger F, Postl K (1985) Quantitative low-resolution analysis of colon mucosa. Anal Qant Cytol Histol 7:205–212

Keren DF, Appelman HD, Dobbins WO et al. (1984) Correlation of histopathologic evidence of disease activity with the presence of immunoglobulin-containing cells in the colons of patients with inflammatory bowel disease. Hum Pathol 15:757–763

Kiefer G, Sandritter W (1976) DNA and the cell cycle. Beitr Pathol 158:332–362

Konishi F, Morson BC (1982) Pathology of colorectal adenomas: a colonoscopic survey. J Clin Pathol 35:830–841

Kreuning J, Bosman FT, Kuiper G, Wal AM, Lindeman J (1978) Gastric and duodenal mucosa in "healthy" individuals. An endoscopic and histopathological study of 50 volunteers. J Clin Pathol 31:69–77

Langley FA, Baak JPA, Oort J (1983) Diagnosis making: error sources. In: Baak JPA, Oort J (eds) A manual of morphometry in diagnostic pathology. Springer, Berlin Heidelberg New York, pp 6–14

Leigh RJ, Marsh MN, Crowe P, Kelly C, Garner V, Gordon D (1985) Studies of intestinal lymphoid tissue IX. Dose dependent gluten induced lymphoid infiltration of coeliac jejunal epithelium. Scand J Gastroenterol 20:715–719

Lennard-Jones JE, Morson BC, Ritchie JK, Williams CB (1983) Cancer suveillance in ulcerative colitis. Experience over 15 years. Lancet II:149–152

Leuchtenberger C, Leuchtenberger R, Davis A (1954) A microspectrophotometric study of the deoxyribonucleic acid (DNA) content in cells of normal and malignant human tissues. Am J Pathol 30:65–85

Lev R, Lance P, Camara P (1985) Histochemical and morphologic studies of mucosa bordering rectosigmoid carcinomas: comparisons with normal, diseased and malignant colonic epithelium. Hum Pathol 16:151–161

Lindstrom CG (1976) "Collagenous colitis" with watery diarrhoea: a new entity? Pathologia Europaea 11:87–89

Lofberg R, Tribukait B, Ost A, Brostrom O, Reichard H (1987) Flow cytometric DNA analysis in longstanding ulcerative colitis: a method of prediction of dysplasia and carcinoma development? Gut 28: 1100–1106

Lovett EJ, Schnitzer B, Keren DF, Flint A, Hudson JL, McClatchey KD (1984) Application of flow cytometry to diagnostic pathology. Lab Invest 50:115–153

Lowe J, Kent J, Armitage NC, Ballantyne KC, Hardcastle JD (1986) Nuclear morphometry and nuclear DNA content in rectal carcinoma. In: Fourth International Symposium on Morphometry in Morphological Diagnosis. The Royal Society of Medicine, London, p 19

Macartney JC, Camplejohn RS (1986) DNA flow cytometry of histological material from dysplastic lesions of human gastric mucosa. J Pathol 150:113–118

Macartney JC, Camplejohn RS, Powell G (1986) DNA flow cytometry of histological material from human gastric cancer. J Pathol 148:273–277

MacDermott RP (1986) Symposium on cell-mediated immunity in human disease. Part II. Cell-mediated immunity in gastrointestinal disease. Hum Pathol 17:219–233

Malizia G, Trejdosiewicz LK, Wood GM, Howdle PD, Janossy G, Losowsky MS (1985) The microenvironment of coeliac disease: T cell phenotypes and expression of the T_2 'T blast' antigen by small bowel lymphocytes. Clin Exp Immunol 60:437–446

Marsh MN (1980) Studies of intestinal lymphoid tissue III. Quantitative analysis of intraepithelial lymphocytes in the small intestine of human control subjects and of patients with coeliac spruce. Gastroenterology 79:481–492

Marsh MN (1982) Studies of intestinal lymphoid tissue IV – the predictive value of raised mitotic indices among jejunal epithelial lymphocytes in the diagnosis of gluten sensitive enteropahty. J Clin Pathol 35:517–525

Marsh MN (1985) Functional and structural aspects of the epithelial lymphocyte with implications for coeliac disease and tropical sprue. Scand J Gastroenterol [Suppl]114:55–75

Marsh MN (1986) Measurement of intra-epithelial lymphocytes. Gut 27:1516–1517

Maskens AP (1979) Histogenesis of adenomatous polyps in the human large intestine. Gastroenterology 77:1245–1251

McKinley M, Budman D, Caccese W, Weissman G, Scheidt N, Kahn E, Bronco R (1985) Evaluation of colonic neoplasia by flow cytometry of endoscopic biopsies. Am J Gastroenterol 80:47–49

Meier-Ruge W (1974) Hirschsprung's disease: its aetiology, pathogenesis and differential diagnosis. In: Grundmann E, Kirsten WH (eds) Curr Top Pathol 59:131–179

Melamed M, Enker WE, Banner P, Janov AJ, Kessler G, Darzynkiewicz Z (1986) Flow cytometry of colorectal carcinoma aith three year follow-up. Dis Colon Rectum 29:184–186

Melville DM, Jass JR, Shepherd NA (1987) DNA aneuploidy as a marker of neoplastic change in ulcerative colitis. J Pathol 152:215A

Ming S-C, Bajtai A, Correa P et al. (1984) Gastric dysplasia. Significance and pathologic criteria. Cancer 54:1794–1801

Morson BC, Dawson IMP (1979) Gastro-intestinal pathology, 2nd edn Blackwell Scientific, London

Morson BC, Sobin LH, Grundmann E, Johansen A, Nagayo T, Serch-Hanssen A (1980) Precancerous conditions and epithelial dysplasia in the stomach. J Clin Pathol 33:711–721

Mukada T, Sasano N, Sato E (1978) Evaluation of esophageal dysplasia by cytofluorometric analysis. Cancer 41:1399–1404

Nakamura K, Nakayo T, Sato E, Sasano N (1974) Ultramorphometry of the nucleus of human rectal cancer compared with normal mucosal gland. Tohoku J Exp Med 112:177–188

Nielsen VT, Vetner M, Harslof E (1980) Collagenous colitis. Histopathology 4:83–86

Nogaller AM, Nikonenko TN, Avirina TK (1983) Clinico-morphological and morphometric characteristics of chronic colitis. Klin Med (Mosk) 61:82–88

Oehlert W, Keller P, Henke M, Strauch M (1979) Gastric mucosal dysplasia: what is its clinical significance? Front Gastrointest Res 4:173–182

Oja E, Collan Y (1983) Basic principles of image analysis by computer. Acta Stereol 2:250–261

Owen DA (1984) Gastritis and duodenitis. In: Appleman HD (ed) Pathology of the oesophagus, stomach and duodenum. Churchill Livingstone, Edinburgh, pp 37–43

Painter NS (1964) The aetiology of diverticulosis of the colon with special reference to the action of certain drugs on the behaviour of the colon. Ann R Coll Surg Engl 34:98–119

Painter NS, Burkitt DP (1975) Diverticular disease of the colon is a 20th century problem. Clin Gastroenterol 4:3–21

Parl FF, Lev R, Thomas E, Pitchumuni CS (1979) Histologic and morphometric study of chronic gastritis in alcoholic patients. Hum Pathol 10:45–56

Petrova AS, Subrichina GN, Tschistjakova OV, Lukina TA, Weiss H, Wildner G (1980) Flow cytofluorometry, cytomorphology and histology in gastric carcinoma. Oncology 37:318–324

Phelps PC, Toker C, Trump BF (1979) Surface ultrastructure of normal, adenomatous and malignant epithelium from human colon. Scan Electron Microsc 3:169–176

Quirke P, Dyson JED (1986) Flow cytometry: methodology and applications in pathology. J Pathol 149: 79–87

Quirke P, Dyson JED, Dixon MF, Bird CC, Joslin CAF (1985 a) Heterogeneity of colorectal adenocarcinomas evaluated by flow cytometry and histopathology. Br J Cancer 51:99–106

Quirke P, Fozard JBJ, Dixon MF, Dyson JED, Giles GR, Bird CC (1985 b) DNA aneuploidy in colorectal adenomatous polyps with and without synchronous carcinoma. J Pathol 146:267A

Quirke P, Dixon MF, Fozard JBJ, Day D, Talbot IC, Bird CC (1987 a) DNA aneuploidy in familial polyposis coli: a flow cytometric study. J Pathol 151:76A

Quirke P, Dixon MF, Clayden AD, Durdey P, Dyson JED, Williams NS, Bird CC (1987 b) Prognostic significance of DNA aneuploidy and cell proliferation in rectal adenocarcinomas. J Pathol 151:285–291

Riddell RH (1976) The precarcinomatous phase of ulcerative colitis. In: Morson BC (ed) Current topics in pathology. Pathology of the gastrointestinal tract. Springer Berlin Heidelberg, New York, pp 179–219

Riddell RH, Goldman H, Ransohoff DF et al. (1983) Dysplasia in inflammatory bowel diseases: standardized classification with provisional clinical applications. Hum Pathol 14:931–968

Rosekrans PCM, Meijer CJLM, Cornelisse CJ, van der Wal AM, Lindemann J (1980 a) Use of morpohometry and immunohistochemistry of small intestinal biopsy specimens in the diagnosis of food allergy. J Clin Pathol 33:125–130

Rosekrans PCM, Meijer CJLM, van der Wal AM, Cornelisse CJ, Lindeman J (1980 b) Immunoglobulin containing cells in inflammatory bowel disease of the colon: a morphometric and immunohistochemical study. Gut 21:941–947

Rosekrans PCM, Meijer CJLM, Polanco I, Mearin ML, van der Wal AM, Lindeman J (1981 a) Long term morphological and immunohistochemical observations on biopsy specimens of small intestine from children with gluten sensitive enteropathy. J Clin Pathol 34: 138–144

Rosekrans PCM, Lindeman J, Meijer CJLM (1981 b) Quantitative immunological and immunohistochemical findings in jejunal biopsy specimens in giardiasis. Virchows Arch [A]393:145–151

Rubin CE, Brandbort LL, Phelps DC, Taylor HC (1960) Studies of celiac disease. I. Gastroenterology 38:28–49

Rubio CA, Johansson C, Kock Y (1982 a) A quantitative method of estimating inflammation in the rectal mucosa. II. Normal limits in symptomatic patients. Scand J Gastroenterol 17:1077–1081

Rubio CA, Johansson C, Kock Y (1982 b) A quantitative method of estimating inflammation in the rectal mucosa. III Chronic ulcerative colitis. Scand J Gastroenterol 17:1083–1087

Rubio CA, Johansson C, Uribe A, Kock Y (1984) A quantitative method of estimating inflammation in the rectal mucosa. IV. Ulcerative colitis in remission. Scand J Gastroenterol 19:525–530

Saffos RO, Rhatigan RM (1977) Benign (non-polypoid) mucosal changes adjacent to carcinoma of the colon. Hum Pathol 8:441–449

Sanderson IR, Slavin G, Walker-Smith JA (1985) Density of mucosal mast cells in the lamina propria of the colon and terminal ileum of children. J Clin Pathol 38:771–773

Sarin SK, Malhotra V, Gupta SS, Karol A, Gaur SK, Anand BS (1987) Significance of eosinophil and mast cell counts in rectal mucosa in ulcerative colitis. A prospective controlled study. Dig Dis Sci 32:363–367

Sassi I, Faravelli A, Freschi M, Ferrari AM, Cantaboni A (1986) Planimetric grading of dysplasia in colorectal adenomas: a step forward? In: Fourth International Symposium on Morphometry in Morphological Diagnosis. The Royal Society of Medicine, London, p 78

Sato E, Goto N, Nakamura T (1981) Nuclear ultrastructure in carcinoma, adenoma, Peutz-Jeghers polyp and dysplasia of the large bowel: a morphometric analysis. Gann 72:245–253

Schutte B, Reynders MMJ, Bosman FT, Blijham GH (1985) Flow cytometric determination of DNA ploidy level in nuclei isolated free from paraffin-embedded tissue. Cytometry 6:26–30

Scott BB, Goodall A, Stephenson P, Jenkins D (1983) Rectal mucosal plasma cells in inflammatory bowel disease. Gut 24:519–524

Scott NA, Rainwater LM, Vieand HS, Weiland LH, Pemberton JH, Beart RW, Lieber NM (1987) The relative prognostic value of flow cytometric DNA analysis and conventional clinicopathologic criteria in patients with operable rectal carcinoma. Dis Colon Rectum 30:513–520

Seefeld U, Kreys GJ, Siebermann RE, Blum AL (1977) Esophageal histology in gastroesophageal reflux. Morphometric findings on suction biopsies. Dig Dis Sci 22:956–964

Selby WS, Janossy G, Jewell DP (1981 a) Immunohistological characterisation of intraepithelial lymphocytes of the human gastrointestinal tract. Gut 22:169–176

Selby WS, Janossy G, Goldstein G, Jewell DP (1981 b) T lymphocyte subsets in the human intestinal mucosa: the distribution and relationship to MHC-derived antigens. Clin Exp Immunol 44:453–458

Selby WS, Janossy G, Bofill M, Jewell DP (1983) Lymphocyte subpopulations in the human small intestine. The findings in normal mucosa and in the mucosa of patients with adult coeliac disease. Clin Exp Immunol 52:219–228

Seldenrijk CA, Hendriks G, Baak JPA, Van Spreejuwel JP, Smeulders AWM, Meuwissen SGM, Meijer CJLM (1986) Plasma cell counting in colonic biopsies. In: Fourth International Symposium on Morphometry in Morphological Diagnosis. The Royal Society of Medicine, London, p 79

Shiner M, Doniach I (1960) Histopathologic studies in steatorrhoea. Gastroenterology 38:419–440

Slavin G, Sowter C, Robertson K, McDermott S, Paton K (1980) Measurement in jejunal biopsies by computer aided microscopy. J Clin Pathol 33:254–261

Spence RAJ, Sloan JM, Johnston GW, Greenfield A (1983) Oesophageal mucosal changes in patients with varices. Gut 24:1024–1029

Spence RAJ, Sloan JM, Johnston GW (1984) Histologic factors of the oesophageal transection ring as clues to the pathogenesis of bleeding varices. Surg Gynecol Obstet 159:253–259

Sprenger E, Witte S, Schaden M (1974) The differential diagnostic role of nuclear DNA content in gastric cytology. In: Sprenger E, Witte S, Schaden M (eds) Early gastric cancer. Springer, Berlin Heidelberg New York, pp 154–158

Stich HF, Florian SF, Emson HE (1960) The DNA content of tumour cells. I. Polyps and adenocarcinomas of the large intestine of man. J Natl Cancer Inst 24:471–482

Strickland RG, Husby G, Black WC, Williams RC Jr (1975) Peripheral blood and intestinal lymphocyte sub-populations in Crohn's disease. Gut 16:847–853

Sugimachi K, Inokuchi K, Matsuura H, Okamura T, Sasaki O (1983) Cytophotometric DNA analysis of early esophageal carcinoma. Jpn J Surg 13:37–41

Surawicz CM, Belic L (1984) Rectal biopsy helps to distinguish acute self-limited colitis from idiophatic inflammatory bowel disease. Gastroenterology 86:104–113

Teodori L, Capurso L, Cordelli E et al. (1984) Cytometrically determined relative DNA content as an indicator of neoplasia in gastric lesions. Cytometry 5:63–70

Thompson EM, Price AB, Altman DG, Sowter C, Slavin G (1985) Quantitation in inflammatory bowel disease using computerised interactive image analysis. J Clin Pathol 38:631–638

Thurlbeck WM, Benson JA, Dudley HR (1960) The histopathological changes of sprue and their significance. Am J Clin Pathol 34:108–117

Tosi P, Luzi P, Baak JPA, Miracco C, Vindigni C, Lio r, Barbini P (1987) Gastric dysplasia: a stereological and morphometrical assessment. J Pathol 152:83–94

Toukan AU, Kamal MF, Amr SS, Arnaout MA, Abu-Romiyeh AS (1985) Gastro-duodenal inflammation in patients with non-ulcer dyspepsia. A controlled endoscopic and morphometric study. Dig Dis Sci 30:313–320

Underwood EE (1970) Quantitative Steriology. Addison Wesley, Reading Mass

Van den Ingh HF, Griffioen G, Cornelisse CJ (1985) Folw cytometric detection of aneuploidy in colorectal adenomas. Cancer Res 45:3392–3397

Van Spreeuwel JP, Lindeman J, Meijer CJLM (1985) A quantitative study of immunoglobulin containing cells in the differential diagnosis of acute colitis. J Clin Pathol 38:774–777

Van Spreeuwel JP, Meijer CJLM, Rosekrans PCM, Lindeman J (1986) Immunoglobulin containing cells in gastrointestinal pathology – diagnostic applications. Pathol Annu 21:295–310

Watson AJ, Wright NA (1974) Morphology and cell kinetics of the jejunal mucosa in untreated patients with coeliac disease. Clin Gastrenterol 3:11–31

Watt PCH, Collins JSA, Hamilton PW, Sloan JM, Love AHG (1987) A quantitative assessment of mucosal inflammation in patients with non-ulcer dyspepsia, duodenitis and duodenal ulcer. J Pathol 152:228 A–229 A

Weibel ER (1963) Principles and methods for morphometric study of the lung and other organs. Lab Invest 12:131–155

Weibel ER (1969) Stereological principles for morphometry in electron microscopic cytology. Int Rev Cytol 26:235–302

Weibel ER (1979) Stereological methods, vol I. Practical methods for biological morphometry. Academic, London

Weinreb M, Zajicek G, Levij IS (1984) Discrimination betweeen normal and malignant gastric epithelial cells by computer image analysis. Anal Quant Cytol 6:206–210

Weinstein WM, Bogoch ER, Bowes KL (1975) The normal human oesophageal mucosa: a histological reappraisal. Gastroenterology 68:40–44

Weiss H, Gutz H-J, Wildner GP, Ebeling K, Schmidt W (1980) Characterisation of chronic atrophic gastritis by means of pulse cytophotometry. Acta Pathol Microbiol Scand [B] [Suppl] 274:412–416

Whitehead F, Jarvis LR, Skinner JM, Whitehead R (1985) Ploidy studies in adenomatous polyps of the colon J Clin Pathol 38:1261–1264

Whitehead R (1985) Mucosal biopsy of the gastrointestinal tract. WB Saunders, London

Whitehead R (1986) Measurement of intraepithelial lymphocytes. Gut 27:1399

Whitehead R, Roca M, Meikle DD, Skinner J, Truelove SC (1975) The histological classification of duodenitis in fibre-optic biopsy specimens. Digestion 13:129–136

Whiteway J, Morson BC (1985) Elastosis in diverticular disease of the sigmoid colon. Gut 26:258–266

Williams GT (1985) Commentary. Transitional mucosa of the large intestine. Histopathology 9:1237–1243

Williams GT, Rhodes J (1987) Collagenous colitis: disease or diversion? Br Med J 294:855–856

Wolley RC, Schreiber K, Koss LG, Karas M, Sherman A (1982) DNA distribution in human colon carcinomas and its relationship to clinical behaviour. J Natl Cancer Inst 69:15–22

Wright SG, Tomkins AM (1978) Quantitative histology in giardiasis. J Clin Pathol 31:712–716

Wyatt JI, Quirke P, Ward D, Johnson DJ, Dixon MF, Bird CC (1987) Comparison of histopathological and flow cytometric parameters in the prediction of prognosis in gastric cancer. J Pathol 152:233 A

Topics in Colorectal Biopsy Diagnosis

A Collagenous Colitis

W. V. BOGOMOLETZ

Collagenous colitis (CC) is characterised by a band-like collagenous deposit under the surface epithelium of the colorectal mucosa. Chronic watery diarrhoea is the main clinical symptom. LINDSTROM (1976) recorded the first description of this previously unrecognised entity and coined the term 'collagenous colitis'. Since 1980, over 100 cases of CC have been reported in the literature, mostly as individual case reports. Two large series of 17 and 21 cases respectively have been published recently (WANG et al. 1987; WIDGREN et al. 1988). There have also been a few reviews and editorials on CC (BOGOMOLETZ 1983; ANONYMOUS 1986; WILLIAMS and RHODES 1987; RAMS et al. 1987). In addition to published cases, a substantial number of unpublished cases of CC have been observed and diagnosed by pathologists throughout the world. This review on the different clinicopathological aspects of CC is based on our own experience of about 30 cases referred for consultation and data from the literature.

1 Clinical Aspects

Collagenous colitis occurs predominantly in women (about 90% of published cases). Cumulated data from 61 case reports of CC show a wide age range, from 19 to 86 years old, with a mean of 53.4. Most patients with CC present with chronic watery diarrhoea, described as continuous or intermittent and lasting for weeks, months or years despite treatment. Bacteriological investigations of stools have been consistently negative for ova and pathogens, both on microscopy and on culture. Mucus and blood are seldom present in the watery stools of CC. Most patients have undergone a wide range of biochemical and haematological investigations which have generally been negative or shown only minor and transient abnormalities.

In addition to chronic watery diarrhoea, many patients also complain of colicky abdominal pain. Nausea and vomiting have not been recorded features. Despite the intractable chronic watery diarrhoea, patients with CC have generally shown a remarkably preserved general health, with few recorded instances of weight loss or dehydration.

In general, patients with CC do not have malabsorption, functioning endocrine tumours, arthropathy or systemic connective tissue disease and there is no association with laxative abuse or previous abdominal irradiation. Diagnostic features of chronic ulcerative colitis, Crohn's disease, infectious (acute self-limited) colitis or ischaemic colitis are not present.

Conventional and double contrast radiology of the upper and lower gastrointestinal tract are normal, although rarely minor radiological abnormalities of the colonic mucosa have been noted but not illustrated.

The endoscopic appearances of the colorectal mucosa in CC have usually been reported as normal or showing mild and non-specific changes, such as oedema, congestion or flattening of mucosal folds. Fissuring and ulceration have not been described.

The clinical course of patients with CC varies. Despite some form of treatment, most patients continue to suffer from persistent chronic watery diarrhoea. Alternating remissions and relapses have been described in some treated and untreated cases (EAVES et al. 1983; FOERSTER and FAUSA 1985; DEBONGNIE et al. 1984; TEGLBJAERG et al. 1984; KINGHAM et al. 1986; PALMER et al. 1986). In a few cases reduction of the thickness of the collagenous deposit to normal has been recorded (EAVES et al. 1983; DEBONGNIE et al. 1984).

Colonic perfusion studies have been carried out in only a few patients with CC and have shown a net sodium chloride and water loss into the colonic lumen (RASK-MADSEN et al. 1983; GIARDELLO et al. 1985; LOO et al. 1985). One perfusion study demonstrated passive sodium secretion and active chloride secretion, persisting despite fasting (RASK-MADSEN et al. 1983). Another study reported abnormalities of bile salt absorption in two patients (GIARDELLO et al. 1985).

2 Histological Features

On routine light microscopy of haematoxylin-eosin stained sections, CC is characterised by a conspicuous eosinophilic, band-like thickening of the subepithelial basement membrane (Fig. 1). This collagenous band is birefringent with polarised light. In contrast with CC, the subepithelial base-

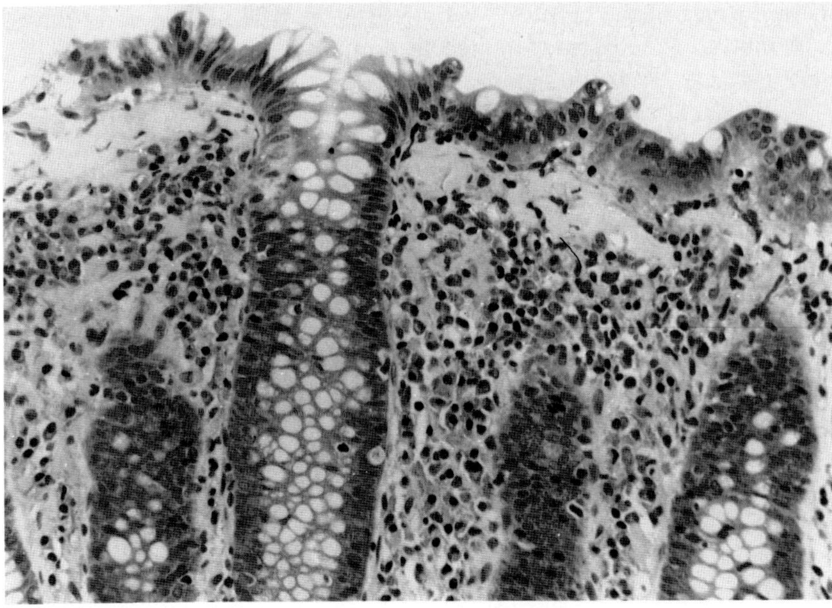

Fig. 1. Collagenous colitis showing the typical band-like thickening under the surface epithelium. Some chronic inflammatory cells and fibroblasts are entrapped within the collagenous deposit. HE, × 125

ment membrane of normal colorectal mucosa is inconspicuous or barely resolvable. The characteristic band-like thickening of CC is most pronounced under the surface epithelium between the crypts, the so-called intercryptic portion. However, in severe cases, the collagenous thickening can also extend around the upper third of the crypts. The homogeneous eosinophilic material reacts positively as collagen when stained with different trichrome methods for connective tissue demonstration (van Gieson and Masson techniques). On the other hand, staining for amyloid is consistently negative. Reticulin staining shows a dense network of reticulin fibrils. Some plasma cells, lymphocytes, histiocytes and fibroblasts are usually entrapped within the collagenous deposit.

Capillaries and fibroblasts of the uppermost lamina propria are often found closely applied to the undersurface of the collagenous band. The lamina propria usually contains an excess of lymphocytes and plasma cells but neutrophils are absent or scarce. Eosinophilia is not a feature of CC. An increased population of mast cells in the lamina propria, including some mast cells entrapped within the collagenous deposit, has been reported in four cases (FLEJOU et al. 1984). The surface epithelium often shows degenerative cell changes, including epithelial desquamation (JESSURUN et al. 1987), but these could represent traumatic artefacts. The overall height of the colorectal mucosa is normal or slightly reduced. The crypts are regular and show no significant impairment of mucus secretion. The uppermost part of the crypts or 'mouth area' may be narrowed. The muscularis mucosae and submucosa appear normal.

3 Measurement of the Collagen Band Thickness

The thickness of the characteristic collagenous band of CC has been reported as varying widely between 7 μm and 70 μm. Several independent factors may contribute to this discrepancy. The apparent thickness of any form of basement membrane deposit may alter depending on the mode of tissue fixation and processing. Authors reporting cases of CC have often used different tissue fixatives, ranging from formaldehyde-containing fixatives to picric acid fixatives such as Bouin's fluid. The accuracy of measurements of any thickened basement membrane also depends on the method used for carrying out these measurements. Some published reports lack methodological detail while others specify the use of a calibrated eye-piece graticule, considered to be a reliable histometric procedure.

A given basement membrane considered as 'abnormally thickened' should always be compared with measurements from a control population. In reported cases of CC, this comparison has only been performed in a few instances. Even then, the nature of the control groups has varied considerably: biopsies of normal colorectal mucosa, biopsies of patients suffering from a wide range of large bowel inflammatory conditions, or surgical specimens of colorectal carcinoma. The thickness of the basement membrane in 'normal' rectal biopsies has been variously reported to be 4.6–6.9 μm (BOGOMOLETZ et al. 1980), 3.8 μm (DEBONGNIE et al. 1984) and 1.25–6.26 μm (MOGENSEN et al. 1984). Another report has quoted a normal thickness of up to 3 μm, this figure being derived from autopsy colon specimens (GLEDHILL and COLE 1984).

Collagenous thickening in CC may represent an uneven process along the length of the large bowel mucosa. Hence, in a given patient, multiple mucosal biopsies taken at different levels may show different degrees of thickening. The collagenous band in CC is probably thickest in the proximal colon, and tends to be less prominent in the rectum (MASON and JEWELL 1985; HAMILTON et al. 1986).

4 Electron Microscopy

The ultrastructural features of the colorectal mucosa in CC have been well described and illustrated in several reports (BOGOMOLETZ et al. 1980; TEGLBJAERG and THAYSEN 1982; FOERSTER and FAUSTA 1985; HWANG et al. 1986). The collagenous deposit is located immediately underneath the basal lamina (which appears uninvolved) and consists of morphologi-

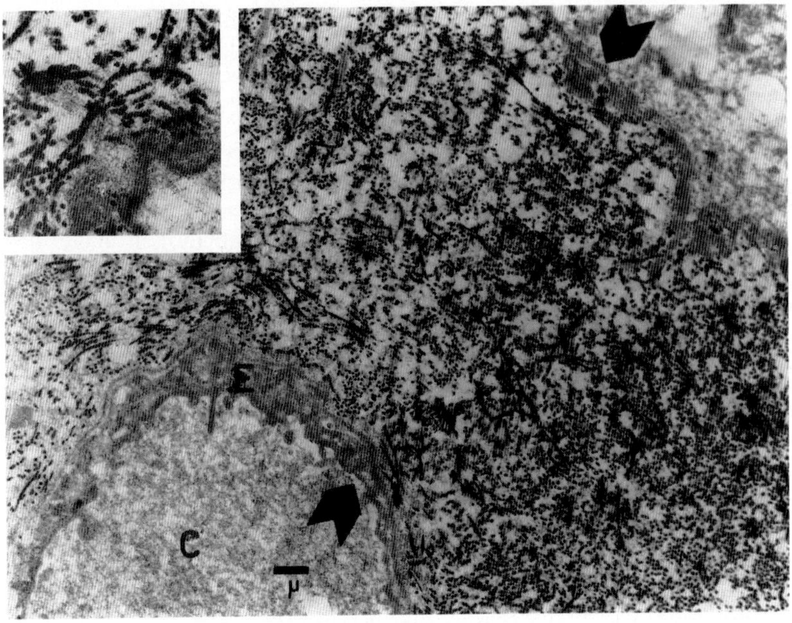

Fig. 2. Electron micrograph of collagenous colitis. The band-like thickening (*arrowed*) consists of collagen fibres of typical appearance and axial periodicity (detail in *inset*). *C*, capillary lumen; *E*, endothelial cell. (BOGOMOLETZ et al. 1980) Silver methenamine, × 5000

cally normal collagen fibres with typical axial periodicity (Fig. 2). Some chronic inflammatory cells, histiocytes, fibroblasts and mast cells are embedded within these collagen fibres. The so-called colonic pericryptal fibroblast sheath becomes separated from the crypt epithelium, its constituent fibroblasts showing evidence of cellular activation. The normal fenestrated capillaries of the uppermost lamina propria are closely apposed to the undersurface of the collagenous deposit.

Recent electron microscopic studies have identified characteristic features of myoid cells in the 'fibroblasts' making up the pericryptal sheath and occasionally entrapped within the collagenous deposit of CC (HWANG et al. 1986; WIDGREN et al. 1988). The myofibroblastic nature of these cells has also been confirmed by immunohistochemistry (WIDGREN et al. 1988).

5 Immunohistochemical Approach

Collagen typing has been carried out immunohistochemically in several cases of CC (BIREMBAUT et al. 1982; FLEJOU et al. 1984; MASON and JEWELL 1985). The collagenous deposit shows strong positivity with immune serum against collagen type III. On the other hand, the uninvolved basal lamina overlying the collagenous deposit shows marked positivity for collagen IV, as well as for laminin and fibronectin. These findings, therefore, confirm ultrastructural observations that the collagenous deposit in CC is quite distinct from the epithelial basal lamina. Moreover, immunotyping raises the possibility that the collagenous deposit in CC could result from an abnormal protein synthesis by the disturbed pericryptal fibroblast sheath. A recent report has suggested that the collagenous deposit also contains collagen VI, which is rich in disulfide bonds (LOO et al. 1985). Immunoglobulin, complement, albumin or fibrinogen have not been identified within the collagenous deposit and circulating immune complexes have not been described in patients with CC.

6 Therapeutic Problems

Most patients with CC have shown a disappointing response to conventional antidiarrhoeal drugs (opiates, loperamide, cholestyramine, codeine phosphate etc.), which have proven ineffective in the long-term control of the chronic watery diarrhoea. Some relief of symptoms has been reported in a few individual cases with mepacrine, metronidazole, prednisolone, betamethasone and sulphasalazine. However, these drugs have not alleviated symptoms when tried in other patients with CC. Considerable difficulty, therefore, persists in the treatment and long-term control of most patients with CC.

7 Coexisting Diseases

Osteoarthritis or some other form of degenerative joint disease has been reported in 12 patients with CC (ERLENDSSON et al. 1983; HWANG et al. 1986; MAROY 1986; PALMER et al. 1986; JESSURUN et al. 1987; WANG et al. 1987). More intriguing has been the recent description of four patients with CC and malabsorption with histologically proven subtotal villous atrophy of the small bowel (HAMILTON et al. 1986; HWANG et al. 1986; BREEN et al. 1987). Small bowel biopsies of two of these patients also showed a patchy thickening of the basement membrane, in addition to the subtotal villous atrophy (HAMILTON et al. 1986). Subepithelial collagen deposition within the basement membrane of the small intestine in patients with malabsorption was first described under the term 'collagenous sprue' and regarded as a special form of adult coeliac disease. Subsequent studies have shown that collagenous sprue is not a specific entity (BOSSART et al. 1975). Prior to the reporting of these four unusual cases of CC with concomitant malabsorption, other reported patients with CC had not shown clinical, laboratory or biopsy evidence of coeliac disease. It is tempting to suggest a causal relationship between the changes seen in the small bowel and those in the colon. However, chance association is a more plausible explanation and until further data are obtained, CC should not be considered as synonymous with or related to coeliac disease. Some patients with CC have also shown thyroid function disturbance (PARIENTE et al. 1985; JESSURUN et al. 1987; WANG et al. 1987; WIDGREN et al. 1988).

8 Aetiology and Pathogenesis

The study of CC raises a number of questions. Is CC related to inflammatory bowel disease? Which mechanisms are responsible for producing both the collagenous deposit and the chronic watery diarrhoea? The characteristic collagenous thickening of CC has not been reported in the vast literature on inflammatory bowel disease, regardless of type (ulcerative colitis, Crohn's disease, ischaemic colitis, infectious colitis, amoebic colitis etc.), nor in connective tissue disorders involving the colon or in the so-called transitional mucosa adjacent to colorectal carcinoma (RIDDELL and LEVIN 1977). Moreover, as mentioned earlier, patients with CC have not shown convincing evidence of coexisting inflammatory bowel disease.

Could CC be preceded by some form of 'colitis'? So far, no convincing evidence has been published to support this hypothesis. Two recent reports of patients with CC (KINGHAM et al. 1986; JESSURUN et al. 1986) have suggested that so-called microscopic colitis could be a possible precursor. However, it should be pointed out that the histological appearances of CC and microscopic colitis are quite different, even though patients with both conditions present with chronic watery diarrhoea. The characteristic band-like thickening of CC has not been described in microscopic colitis. Conversely, the typical excess of neutrophils seen in microscopic colitis (KINGHAM et al. 1982; BO-LINN et al. 1985) is not a feature of CC.

PASCAL and co-workers (PASCAL et al. 1968; KAYE et al. 1968) have shown that the subepithelial basement membrane of the normal colorectal mucosa is closely associated with the pericryptal fibroblast sheath. Its constituent fibroblasts arise from around the lower part of the crypts and migrate towards the surface. Moreover, these fibroblasts are responsible for collagen production and deposition within the basement membrane. The band-like thickening of CC could therefore result from some disorder of collagen synthesis by the fibroblasts or the myofibroblasts of the pericryptal sheath. An inflammatory or toxic injury to these cells could be responsible for excess collagen synthesis and hence its accumulation underneath the basement membrane. The resulting collagenous deposit could interfere with the colonic resorption of water and electrolytes, thereby accounting for the watery diarrhoea.

On the other hand, could the collagenous thickening of CC represent a consequence rather than the cause of the watery diarrhoea? The latter hypothesis seems unlikely because the different types of inflammatory bowel disease usually associated with chronic diarrhoea do not show evidence of such collagenous thickening. It is interesting to note that collagenous thickening somewhat similar to that of CC has been described associated with the basement membrane of colorectal hyperplastic polyps (FLEJOU et al. 1984).

In summary, despite some reservations, CC has become accepted as a distinctive, albeit somewhat mysterious, disorder of colorectal mucosa. The aetiology, the pathogenesis, the true incidence and the clinical significance of CC need more clarification.

References

Anonymous (1986) Collagenous colitis. Lancet II:1136–1137

Birembaut P, Adnet JJ, Feydy P, Bogomoletz WV (1982) Colite collagène: approche immunomorphologique de la lésion. Gastroenterol Clin Biol 6:833

Bogomoletz WV (1983) Collagenous colitis: a clinicopahtological review. Surv Dig Dis 1:19–25

Bogomoletz WV, Adnet JJ, Birembaut P, Feydy P, Dupont P (1980) Collagenous colitis; and unrecognised entity. Gut 21:164–168

Bo-Linn GW, Vendrell DD, Lee E, Fordtran JS (1985) An evaluation of the significance of microscopic colitis in patients with chronic diarrhoea. J Clin Invest 75:1559–1569

Bossart R, Henry K, Booth CC, Doe WF (1975) Subepithelial collagen in intestinal malabsorption. Gut 16:18–22

Breen EG, Farren C, Connoly CE, McCarthy CF (1987) Collagenous colitis and coeliac disease. Gut 28:364

Debongnie JC, De Galocsy C, Caholessur MO, Haot J (1984) Collagenous colitis: a transient condition? Report of two cases. Dis Colon Rectum 27:672–676

Eaves ER, McIntyre RLE, Wallis PL, Korman MG (1983) Collagenous colitis: a recently recognised reversible clinicopathological entity. Aust NZ J Med 13:630–632

Erlendsson J, Fenger C, Meinicke J (1983) Arthritis and collagenous colitis. Report of a case with concomitant chronic polyarthritis and collagenous colitis. Scand J Rheumatol 12:93–95

Flejou JF, Grimaud JA, Molas G, Baviera E, Potet F (1984) Collagenous colitis. Ultrastructural study and collagen immunotyping of four cases. Arch Pathol Lab Med 108:977–982

Foerster A, Fausa O (1985) Collagenous colitis. Pathol Res Pract 180:99–104

Giardello FM, Bayless TM, Jessurun J, Hamilton SR (1985) Collagenous colitis: physiologic and pathologic studies. Gastroenterology 88:1392

Gledhill A, Cole FM (1984) Significance of basement membrane thickening in the human colon. Gut 25:1085–1088

Hamilton I, Sanders S, Hopwood D, Bouchier IAD (1986) Collagenous colitis associated with small intestinal villous atrophy. Gut 27:1394–1398

Hwang WS, Kelly JK, Shaffer EA, Hershfield NB (1986) Collagenous colitis: a disease of pericryptal fibroblast sheath? J Pathol 149:33–40

Jessurun J, Yardley JH, Lee EL, Vendrell DD, Schiller LR, Fordtran JS (1986) Microscopic and collagenous colitis: different names for the same condition? Gastroenterology 91:1583–1584

Jessurun J, Yardley JH, Giardello FM, Hamilton SR, Bayless TM (1987) Chronic colitis with thickening of the subepithelial collagen layer (collagenous colitis): histopathologic findings in 15 patients. Hum Pathol 18:839–848

Kaye GI, Lane N, Pascal RR (1968) Colonic pericryptal fibroblast sheath: replication, migration and cytodifferentiation of a mesenchymal cell system in adult tissue. II. Fine ultrastructural aspects in normal rabbit and human colon. Gastroenterology 54:852–865

Kingham JGC, Levison DA, Ball JA, Dawson AM (1982) Microscopic colitis – a cause of chronic watery diarrhoea. Br Med J 285:1601–1604

Kingham JGC, Levison DA, Morson BC, Dawson AM (1986) Collagenous colitis. Gut 27:570–577

Lindström CG (1976) "Collagenous colitis" with watery diarrhoea – a new entity? Pathol Eur 11:87–89

Loo FD, Wood CM, Soergel KH, Komorowski RA, Cheung H, Gay RE (1985) Abnormal collagen deposition and ion transport in collagenous colitis. Gastroenterology 88:1481

Maroy B (1986) Effet du Collagénan sur l'arthropathie associée à la colite collagène. Presse Med 15:1974

Mason CH, Jewell DP (1985) Collagenous colitis: a report of five cases. Gut 26:A1152

Mogensen AM, Olsen JH, Gudman-Hoyer E (1984) Collagenous colitis. Acta Med Scand 216:535–540

Palmer KR, Berry H, Wheeler PJ, Williams CB, Fairclough P, Morson BC, Silk DBA (1986) Collagenous colitis – a relapsing and remitting disease. Gut 27:578–580

Pariente EA, Chaumette MT, Maître F, Delchier JC, Soulé JC, Bader JP (1985) Colite collagène, déficit en IgA, maladie de Basedow et gastrite atrophique. Gastroenterol Clin Biol 9:738–741

Pascal RR, Kaye GI, Lane N (1968) Colonic pericryptal fibroblast sheath: replication, migration and cytodifferentiation of a mesenchymal cell system in adult tissue. I. Autoradiographic studies of normal rabbit colon. Gastroenterology 54:835–851

Rams H, Rogers AI, Ghandur-Mnaymneh L (1987) Collagenous colitis. Ann Intern Med 106:108–113

Rask-Madsen J, Grove O, Hansen MGJ, Buckhave K, Henrik-Nielsen R (1983) Colonic transport of water and electrolytes in a patient with secretory diarrhoea due to collagenous colitis. Dig Dis Sci 28:1141–1146

Riddell RH, Levin B (1977) Ultrastructure of the "transitional" mucosa adjacent to large bowel carcinoma. Cancer 40:2509–2522

Teglbjaerg PS, Thaysen EH (1982) Collagenous colitis: an ultrastructural study of a case. Gastroenterology 82:561–563

Teglbjaerg PS, Thaysen EH, Jensen HH (1984) Development of collagenous colitis in sequential biopsy specimens. Gastroenterology 84:703–709

Wang KK, Perrault J, Carpenter HA, Schroeders KW, Tremaine WJ (1987) Collagenous colitis: a clinicopathologic correlation. Mayo Clin Proc 62:665–671

Widgren S, Jlidi R, Cox JN (1988) Collagenous colitis: histologic, morphometric, immunohistochemical and ultrastructural studies. Report of 21 cases. Virchows Arch [A] 413:287–296

Williams GT, Rhodes J (1987) Collagenous colitis: disease or diversion. Br Med J 294:855–856

B Ischaemic Colitis

A. B. PRICE

1 Introduction

In a retrospective study of 81 patients presenting with colitis after the age of 50 years, ischaemic colitis was diagnosed in 75%, one-half of whom had an original discharge diagnosis of ulcerative colitis or Crohn's disease. The authors (BRANDT et al. 1981) claimed ischaemic colitis is the commonest cause of colitis in this age group. Whether or not this is the case, ischaemic bowel disease is an underdiagnosed entity. It is clearly important for the pathologist to recognise the basic patterns of ischaemic bowel disease and not to overdiagnose Crohn's disease and ulcerative colitis with their consequent major clinical and social implications. Recognition of ischaemic damage in a biopsy will direct the clinician's attention to investigate the vascular system, either the major vessels, or, in the correct setting, causes of systemic vasculitis. Drugs may be implicated in some cases (RIDDELL 1982), as may mechanical factors such as mucosal prolapse (DU BOULAY et al. 1983). Ischaemia has always been thought to play a role in severe bowel infections, in particular those due to *Clostridia* spp., via the vasoconstrictive effects of released bacterial toxins (MARSTON 1977). Ischaemia therefore envelops a wide spectrum of disease entities in which the basic event is an insufficient blood supply for the needs of the mucosa.

The precise biopsy picture of ischaemic colitis or proctitis depends on the rate of onset of the ischaemic insult and when in the natural history the biopsy is taken. This in turn depends on the aetiology of the ischaemia. In broad terms this may be an occlusive event or the consequence of a low flow state (non-occlusive). The final surgical report issued relies on knowing the clinical story, colonoscopic features and radiological picture. For example, ischaemia in the geriatric patient is likely to be due to degenerative vascular disease affecting the mesenteric vessels, whereas in the middle-aged patient with a long history of rheumatoid arthritis a vasculitis should be sought. An ischaemic picture in a young woman might prompt an inquiry about use of the contraceptive pill. The clinicopathological range is from infarction and gangrene to fleeting attacks of abdominal pain and bleeding per rectum in which full mucosal recovery can be swift. Between the two extremes is ischaemia of slower onset and a more chronic nature. It is in this group that biopsy generally has its main role.

2 Pathophysiology and Natural History

Prior to a description of the diagnostic biopsy features it is useful to appreciate the mechanism and evolution of the ischaemic lesion. The superior mesenteric artery supplies the proximal half of the large bowel whilst the inferior mesenteric and branches of the iliac arteries reach the distal half. The splenic flexure is believed to be most susceptible to ischaemic damage as it is the area of anastomosis between the superior and inferior vessels (ALSCHIBAJA and MORSON 1977). However, injection studies have failed to substantiate the concept of a watershed area at this site (BINNS and ISAACSON 1978). Furthermore in a study of 1000 cases of ischaemic colitis (REEDERS et al. 1984) the distribution of disease was right colon 8%, transverse colon 15%, splenic flexure 23%, descending colon 27%, sigmoid colon 23% and rectum 24%.

The causes of ischaemia can be grouped into major vessel arterial occlusion, small vessel disease, venous occlusion, mechanical and non-occlusive factors (Table 1). It is likely that more than one factor frequently operates and non-occlusive factors related to perfusion pressures can have a dominant role in over 30% of patients (RENTON 1972). The complex relation of pressure and lumenal dimension is apparent from the observation that ischaemic symptoms are unlikely until the patency of major vessels is

Table 1. The causes of large bowel ischaemia

Arterial occlusion	
Superior mesenteric artery (commonly thrombo-atheromatous disease)	
Inferior mesenteric artery (commonly surgical intervention)	
Small vessel disease	
Diabetes mellitus	
Amyloidosis	
Irradiation vasculopathy	
Arteritis (see Table 2)	
Renal transplantation/immunosuppression	
Venous occlusion	
Thrombosis:	Idiopathic
	Portal hypertension
	Acute pancreatitis
	Hypercoagulability states
Mechanical factors	
Direct extrinsic pressure – tumours, bands etc.	
Intrinsic factors – prolapse	
Non-occlusive factors	
Shock	
Dehydration	
Drugs	
Large bowel obstruction:	Tumours
	Hirschsprung's disease
	Volvulus
	Diverticular disease

reduced by 50%–80% (DICK et al. 1967; MAY et al. 1963), but even then the correlation of symptoms with degrees of stenosis is poor (CROFT et al. 1981). These generalisations obviously do not apply to focal ischaemic lesions caused by a local vasculitis.

If the vascular insult is sufficient to overcome the effectiveness of the collateral circulation then cell death occurs from the mucosal aspect outwards. The extent of the vascular deprivation, be it due to occlusion or non-occlusive factors, determines the degree of damage. Non-occlusive, or low flow states, usually produce more extensive damage (RENTON 1972) which takes the form of acute haemorrhagic infarction or one of the various forms of 'necrotising colitis' (ALSCHIBAJA and MORSON 1977; MARSTON 1986). Major surgery rather than biopsy is the usual outcome. With lesser degrees of vascular deprivation a phase of repair occurs following the initial mucosal damage. Granulation tissue is produced, then fibrosis and re-epithelialization (WHITEHEAD 1976). The final phase will be a stricture if damage was severe, or complete recovery if damage was limited. The pattern of pathology has close parallels to that of ischaemic damage in the heart. Interpretation of the pathology of ischaemic colitis depends on when in this progression the biopsy is taken.

3 Endoscopic Features

The appearence of the colonic mucosa and the distribution of the changes are essential information, especially if the biopsy features prove to be inconclusive. Like the pathology, the endoscopic features also reflect the rate of onset of ischaemia. In acute episodes the clinician will normally see focally swollen bluish-purple mucosa that is oedematous and which bleeds on contact (DAWSON and SCHAEFER 1971; SCOWCROFT et al. 1981). Focal ulceration is common and whilst this predominates on the left side the aetiology of the ischaemia determines the precise site. In chronic ischaemia, if a stricture has formed, a distinction from Crohn's disease is more difficult. Chronic ischaemia in the rectum is rare but when present white mucosal scars can be detected during sigmoidoscopy (DEVROEDE et al. 1982).

4 Biopsy Appearences

4.1 Gangrenous Ischaemia

Biopsy is seldom performed in this dangerous phase of ischaemic colitis. On the rare occasions it has been carried out the mucosa and muscularis mucosae appear necrotic and suffused with blood. The ghost outline of the crypt positions may remain (WHITEHEAD 1976). Any submucosa present will contain free blood. The picture of infarcted mucosa is rarely a diagnostic problem.

4.2 Non-gangrenous Ischaemia

4.2.1 Acute Phase

The characteristic feature is the damage developing in the superficial half of the mucosa (WHITEHEAD 1976). Early on there is oedema, haemorrhage and degeneration of the lumenal half of the crypts (Fig. 1). The surface epithelium is progressively lost and the upper half of the crypts show varying degrees of degeneration. Where crypt cells survive, especially in the lower half of the mucosa, there is loss of mucin, the cells are flattened, they are basophilic and have hyperchromatic nuclei. There is an accompanying, mild to moderate, inflammatory cell infiltrate in the lamina propria of mixed pattern. Neutrophil leucocytes can be seen infiltrating in between the upper crypt cells but only in small numbers. The lamina propria is frequently haemorrhagic and, in addition, can possess an opaque

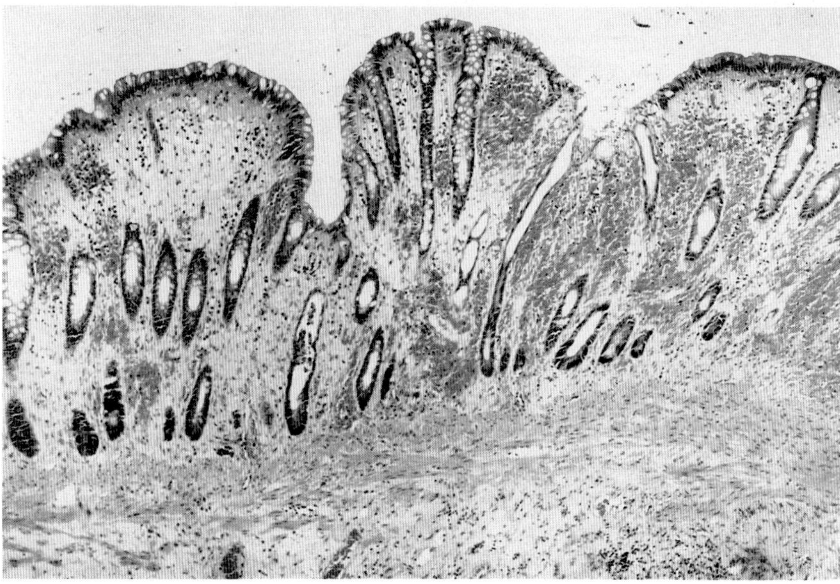

Fig. 1. In this early phase of acute ischaemia there is mucosal oedema, haemorrhage and characteristic crypt degeneration mostly in the superficial half of the mucosa. HE, × 102.5

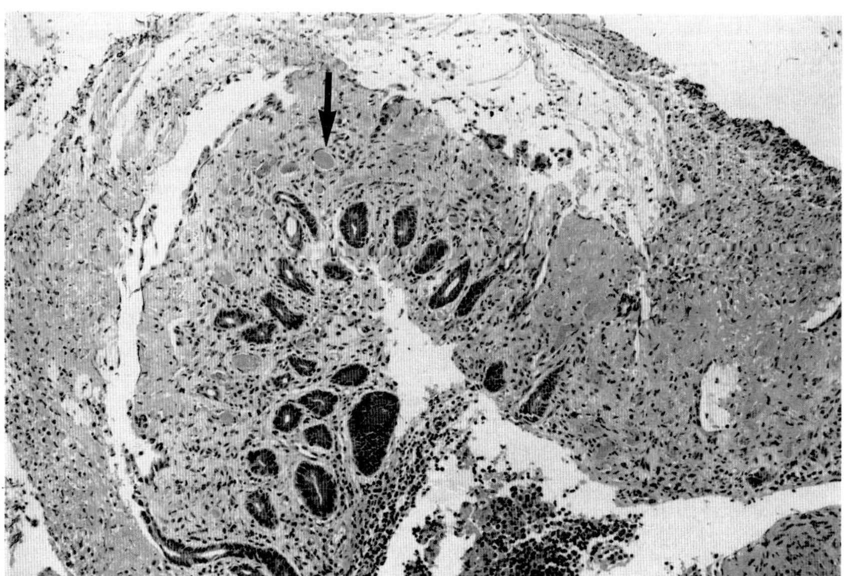

Fig. 2. More advanced acute ischaemia than in Fig. 1. The superficial half of the crypts are lost or degenerate. Deeper down they are hyperchromatic. the lamina propria has an opaque eosinophilia with fibrin plugs noted in small vessels (*arrowed*). Inflammation is present but minor. HE, × 157.5

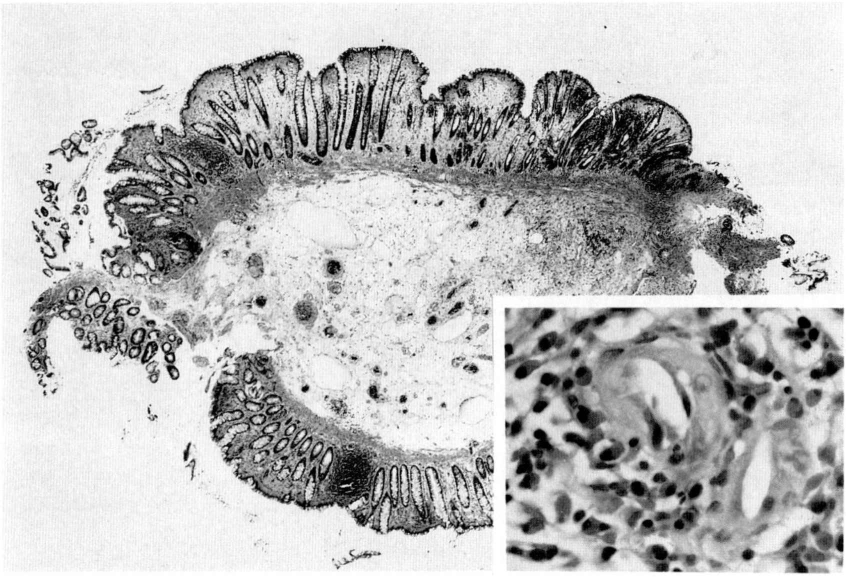

Fig. 3. A biopsy showing early ischaemic damage due to a cholesterol embolus (*inset*). HE, × 26, × 650

eosinophilic quality that can be mistaken for a collagen band (Figs. 2, 10a, b). This appears to be a combination of oedema and fibrinous material. Capillaries may contain fibrin plugs. Clearly the more severe the damage the more complete the crypt destruction, with a picture of full thickness mucosal necrosis being the end-point. Such a picture is not specific to ischaemia but it is helpful to search for the ghost outlines of crypts, the eosinophilia of the lamina propria and the limited inflammatory component as useful residual clues of the aetiology.

Any submucosa present in the biopsy is usually oedematous. This is the basis of the radiologists' 'thumb-print' sign. A careful inspection of vessels should always be made to try and identify an aetiological factor. Thus a vasculitis may be apparent, a thrombus or even a cholesterol embolus from a more central atheromatous plaque (Fig. 3) (DARSEE 1979). Any thrombus present must be evaluated in relation to an intact surface for beneath severely damaged and ulcerated mucosa it is likely to be secondary. Disseminated intravascular coagulation is an important cause of ischaemic disease in which thrombi in small vessels are the key feature (MARGARETTAN and MCKAY 1971; WHITEHEAD 1971).

4.2.2 Reparative Phase

It is convenient to consider this a separate phase but in practice the acute and healing stages occur alongside each other. The microscopic picture is

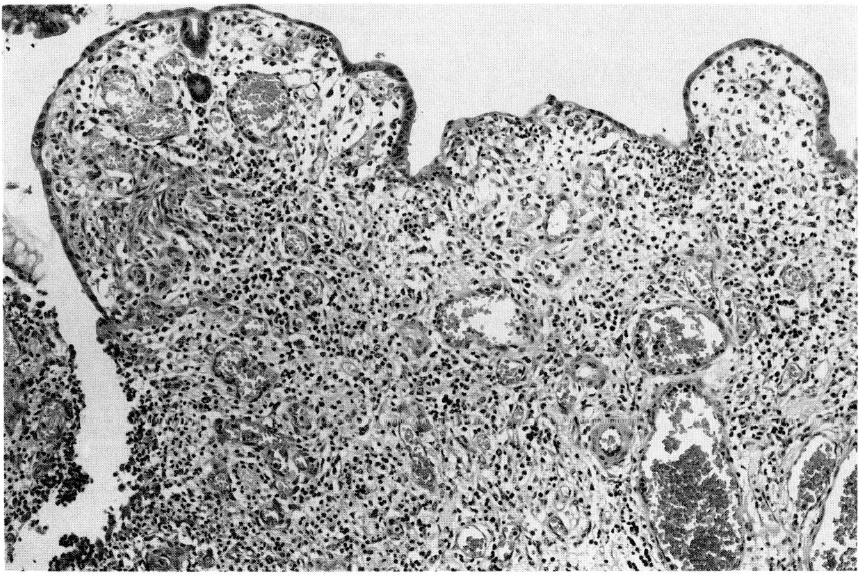

Fig. 4. Granulation tissue and regrowth of the surface epithelium in the reparative phase of ischaemic colitis. HE, × 157.5

determined by the depth of crypt damage that occurs. If the basal epithelium survives, the crypts can regenerate and the mucosa return to normal (DAWSON and SCHAEFER 1971; WHITEHEAD 1976). If damage is more severe, distorted and reduced numbers of crypts are the end result. At first granulation tissue forms and then the epithelium regrows over the surface (Fig. 4). Regeneration of crypts follows most often with fibrosis of the lamina propria, which is the characteristic feature of the reparative and subsequent phases. Its presence allows a distinction to be made from the distorted crypt pattern seen in other causes of inflammatory bowel disease, in particular ulcerative colitis. It is accompanied by capillary proliferation and a mild to moderate mixed inflammatory infiltrate which can include iron-laden histiocytes (MARSTON et al. 1966). The latter are a relatively specific feature of ischaemic damage but not an especially sensitive one in biopsy work.

4.2.3 The Phase of Stricture

Fibrosis, the hallmark of healing after ischaemic damage, involves not only the mucosa but in cases of chronic vascular insufficiency also the muscularis mucosae, submucosa and superficial fibres of the circular muscle. It is the basis for the formation of an ischaemic stricture. This can be the end-point not only of servere disease in which immediate surgery had been avoided, but also recurrent bouts of mild or subclinical disease. This latter

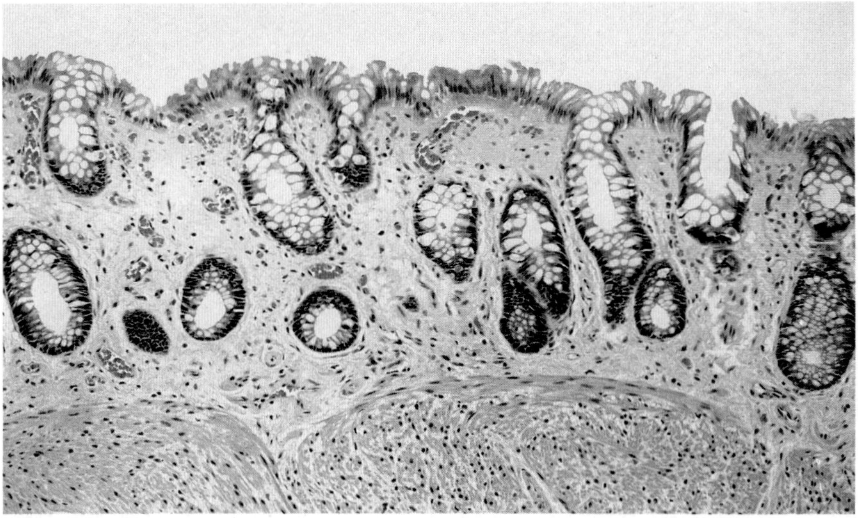

Fig. 5. In the healed phase of ischaemia there is fibrosis of the lamina propria with crypt atrophy and mild telangiectasia. HE, × 157.5

picture is often referred to under the category of evanescent colitis or transient colitis (MARSTON et al. 1966; MILLER et al. 1971; BARCEWICZ and WELCH 1980; HERON et al. 1981). Fibrosis dominates the biopsy picture, inflammation is minimal and the crypt architecture shows varying degrees of distortion (Fig. 5). A van Gieson stain is useful to highlight these features and again, the presence of iron-laden macrophages is a useful diagnostic attribute when present.

5 Difficulties and Differential Diagnoses

The diagnosis is relatively clear-cut when any of the above patterns are also accompanied by an arteritis, obvious primary vascular occlusion or a classical clinical history and colonoscopic picture. In acute but non-gangrenous disease when destruction is limited to the superficial half of the mucosa confusion may arise with pseudomembranous colitis (see below), and very rarely the change in staining quality of the lamina propria may mimic collagenous colitis. The pattern of crypt damage can resemble that seen in infective colitis. However, as discussed below, other parameters in these conditions make confusion unlikely. Problems also arise in the reparative phase, for any healing ulcer can re-epithelialise and will then show crypt distortion, granulation tissue and some fibrosis. However, it will be more focal than that seen in a series of ischaemic biopsies.

5.1 Ulcerative Colitis and Crohn's Disease

To be confident of distinguishing crypt distortion as seen in ulcerative colitis from the pattern in ischaemia all of the other microscopic abnormalities present in the biopsy must be carefully assessed (TALBOT and PRICE 1987) as well as the biopsies from other sites, if colonoscopy was performed. Ischaemic colitis, though it predominates on the left side, is usually patchy and focal mucosal haemorrhages are noted at endoscopy. The inflammatory infiltrate in the ischaemic biopsy seldom reaches the intensity seen in ulcerative colitis and Crohn's disease whilst the unusual pattern of superficial crypt damage seen in the acute stage is unlike anything observed in these latter conditions (Fig. 2). In chronic ischaemia the fibrosis that accompanies the crypt irregularity is distinctive, imparting a dense texture to the lamina propria (Fig. 5). In quiescent atrophic ulcerative colitis the latter often appears empty and hypocellular. Where a pattern of total colitis is seen, ischaemia is an unlikely consideration as such widespread disease of an ischaemic aetiology would almost certainly have precipitated a surgical emergency.

5.2 Mucosal Prolapse Syndrome and Solitary Ulcer

Although this entity is listed under differential diagnosis there are strong arguments for believing the pathologenesis is ischaemic. The term solitary ulcer was applied initially to a lesion on the anterior rectal wall (RUTTER and RIDDELL 1975) but it is now appreciated that the histology can be seen at any site of potential mucosal prolapse (DU BOULAY et al. 1983). Several of the microscopic features of 'prolapse' point to ischaemia based on interference with the blood supply in the mucosa from the shearing stress. Thus there is often an increase in density and eosinophilia of the collagen in the lamina propria, degeneration involving the upper half of the cryptal epithelium and capillary congestion. In addition to the ischaemic features the diagnosis is suggested by the vertically orientated smooth muscle fibres seen in the lamina propria that are in continuity with the muscularis mucosae (Fig. 6). There can also be a variable degree of ulceration. Often the latter is restricted to tiny surface foci between the crypts. These intercryptal erosions or foci of microscopic surface ulceration between adjacent crypts are associated with fibrin, epithelial debris and polymorphs (Fig. 7). They can be seen on the surface of prolapsing piles, on stalked polyps of any variety and on the redundant mucosal folds in diverticular disease. They also have a resemblance to the type 1 lesions of pseudomembranous colitis (see below) (Fig. 8).

On a single biopsy and in the absence of the displaced muscle fibres it can be extremely difficult to separate primary chronic ischaemia from a local focus of mucosal prolapse. However, the sigmoidoscopic, colonoscopic and clinical data usually help resolve the problem with little diffi-

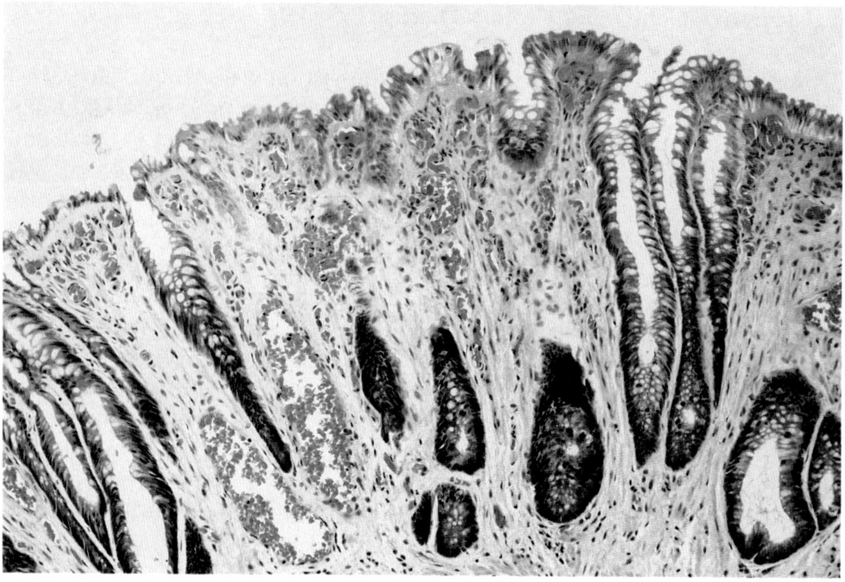

Fig. 6. In this biopsy of the mucosal prolapse syndrome the muscle fibres are well seen running up into the lamina propria. There is telangiectasia, some fibrosis and the crypts show goblet cell depletion. HE, × 157.5

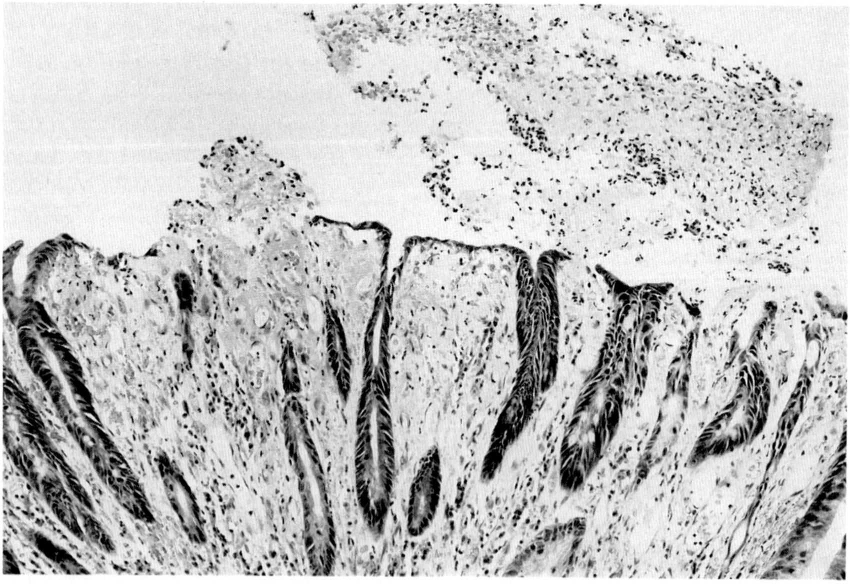

Fig. 7. Intercryptal erosions in mucosal prolapse. Note the crypt degeneration, the opacity of the lamina propria and the absence of significant inflammation. This should be compared with Fig. 8. HE, × 157.5

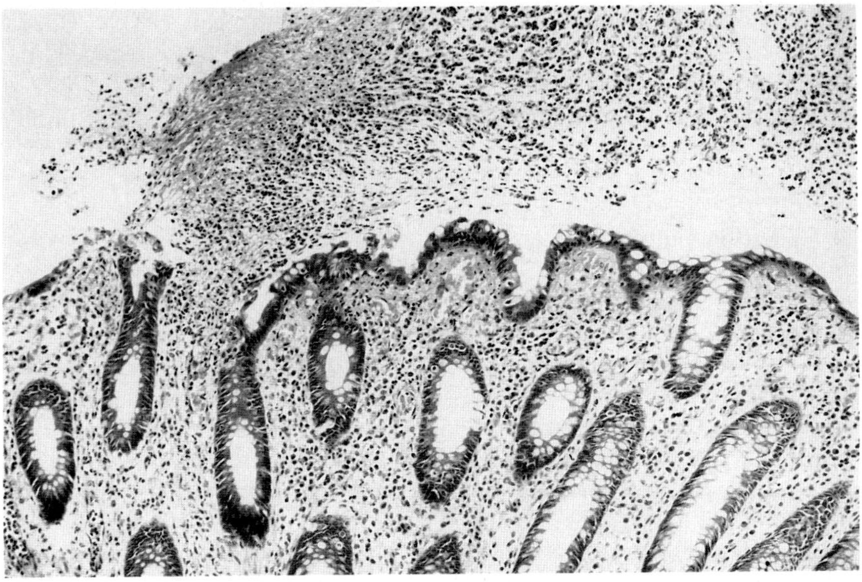

Fig. 8. A type 1 summit lesion in pseudomembranous colitis for comparison with Fig. 7. Although the intercryptal erosion might appear similar here there are more acute inflammatory cells in the lamina propria and the crypts show little abnormality. HE, × 157.5

culty. At the anal margin prolapsing mucosa often presents as a polyp that has been termed an inflammatory cloacogenic polyp (LOBERT and APPELMAN 1981).

5.3 Pseudomembranous Colitis

Prior to the discovery that this condition was due to *Clostridium difficile* (LARSON and PRICE 1977; BARTLETT et al. 1978) it was classified as part of the spectrum of ischaemic bowel disease. The typical type 2 lesions (PRICE and DAVIES 1977) are unlike anything seen in primary ischaemia, though there is a similarity between the type 1 summit lesions (Fig. 8) and the microscopic intercryptal erosions just described in the mucosal prolapse syndrome (Fig. 7). However, the adjacent mucosal changes in these two different conditions makes distinction easy. In pseudomembranous colitis at this stage the mucosa has minimal inflammatory abnormalities, often resemblilng mild forms of infective colitis; in prolapse there is mucosal fibrosis and ramification of muscle fibres within the lamina propria.

As the lesions of pseudomembranous colitis progress, mucosal destruction becomes more complete, with ulceration and inflammatory slough

(PRICE and DAVIES 1977). The ghost outlines of crypts can survive. It is at this stage that the picture is indistinguishable from severe ischaemic colitis. The diagnosis then depends on evaluating other attributes in less affected mucosa, either in a single biopsy or in other biopsy sites if part of a colonoscopic series.

5.4 Radiation Colitis

One of the prime targets of radiation damage is the medium-sized vessel and hence the pathogenesis of radiation-induced colitis is ischaemic. The changes of ischaemic colitis are present but in addition the characteristic bizarre radiation fibroblasts can be seen in the lamina propria and submucosa (BERTHRONG and FAJARDO 1981). They are associated with hyalinisation of the collagen. Telangiectatic capillaries are often prominent in the lamina propria and these too may have a thin cuff of hyalinised eosinophilic collagen (Fig. 9) (HASLETON et al. 1985). The diagnosis of radiation-induced ischaemic colitis rarely presents difficulty and the clinical history provides the strongest initial clue.

5.5 Vasculitis

A vasculitis of the small vessels of the colon can occur during the course of many systemic diseases (Table 2), including Crohn's disease (CAMILLERI et al. 1983; KNUTSON et al. 1968; KUMAR and DAWSON 1972). Gastrointestinal symptoms are rarely the primary presentation and bowel involvement generally becomes manifest during the course of the disease. In one series of patients with rheumatoid arthritis rectal biopsy demonstrated a vasculitis in 40% (TRIBE et al. 1981). In polyarteritis nodosa there is involvement in 40%–70% of cases though colonic involvement is rare. The diagnosis of a systemic vasculitic discorder depends on a biopsy deep enough to show submucosal vessels. It may be necessary to cut levels, for like temporal arteritis, the vasculitis may be focal. The activity of disease at the time of biopsy determines which of the range of features of ischaemia may

Table 2. The causes of colonic vasculitis

Polyarteritis nodosa
Allergic granulomatosis
Rheumatoid arthritis
Systemic lupus erythematosus
Scleroderma
Behçets syndrome
Crohn's disease
Buerger's disease

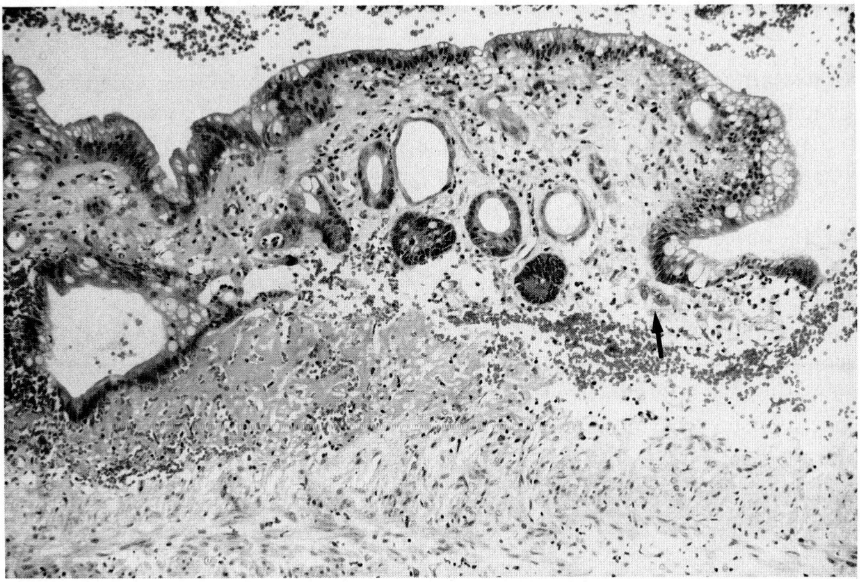

Fig. 9. In this biopsy the opaque hyalinised connective tissue of the lamina propria is well seen with some bizarre radiation fibroblasts (*arrowed*). Some of the crypts illustrate degenerate ischaemic change similar to those in Figs. 1 and 2. HE, × 157.5

be manifest. A Martius scarlet blue stain will help in the identification of fibrin in the walls of involved vessels and an Elastic and van Gieson preparation will demonstrate damaged vessels that may have healed with minimal residual inflammation. A venulitis has been described in systemic lupus erythematosus (HELLILWELL et al. 1985). Buerger's disease is a very rare vasculitic disorder in which colonic disease has been documented as a presenting feature (ROSEN et al. 1985). The characteristic pathology is the presence of mural inflammation in an occluded vessel but with an intact internal lamina. This is in marked contrast to the other causes of vasculiltis. Whilst a challenging diagnosis to make, it is seldom that large enough vessels are sampled in a biopsy.

5.6 Behçet's Syndrome

This multisystem disorder can involve the colon to produce a right-sided ulcerating colitis or a total colitis (SMITH et al. 1973). The picture may resemble ischaemia and a lymphocytic venulitis has been described (LEE 1986). More often the biopsy pattern resembles Crohn's disease (O'CONNELL et al. 1980). If the pattern is ischaemic then it is only with the integration of the clinical data and the history of mucocutaneous ulceration that the diagnosis can be made.

5.7 Collagenous Colitis

In most circumstances collagenous colitis is not likely to be confused with ischaemia. The collagen band, which is usually discrete and subepithelial, points to the correct diagnosis (BOGOMOLETZ et al. 1980 and vide supra) whilst the history of prolonged watery diarrhoea is unlike an ischaemic presentation (KINGHAM et al. 1986). However, occasionally the collagen band appears more diffuse in some foci and can merge into the lamina propria of the upper half of the mucosa. The adjacent regions of the crypts then appear degenerate. Such a picture does have a resemblance to the opaque eosinophilic texture of the superficial lamina propria in ischaemia with its accompanying crypt degeneration (Fig. 10 a, b). The strong staining for collagen, the detection of a more discrete band elsewhere in the biopsy or in other biopsies and the history resolve the problem.

5.8 Drug-Induced Ischaemic Colitis

Vasopressin, ergot, digoxin and antihypertensive drugs can produce vasoconstriction and subsequent ischaemia (RIDDELL 1982). The vascular complications of the contraceptive pill have received much publicity and should certainly be considered if ischaemic changes are recognised in a young female patient (COTTON and THOMAS 1971). The symptomatology is often one of transient attacks of abdominal pain and rectal bleeding. A biopsy may show acute ischaemic damage but recovery has often occurred before arrangements for a biopsy have been made. Recurrent bouts of such attacks can lead to intestinal strictures. Chlorpromazine is a rare cause of ischaemic bowel disease (HAY 1978). It interferes with intestinal motility and can precipitate an obstructive colitis (see below) that is believed to have an ischaemic basis.

5.9 Infective Colitis

The pattern of crypt damage, so-called crypt withering (TALBOT and PRICE 1987), seen in infective colitis has some resemblance to that in the acute ischaemic episode. Thus the cryptal epithelium is degenerate, flattened and hyperchromatic (Fig. 11). The damage is frequently most severe in the superficial half of the mucosa, as in ischaemia (Figs. 1, 2). In general the inflammatory infiltrate, especially the polymorphs seen between the epithelial cells (PRICE et al. 1979), is characteristic and not seen in ischaemia. However, if the inflammation is muted, a diagnostic problem can exist.

Confusion between infection and ischaemia is not too bizarre a concept for in surgical resections there is continuing controversy over the roles of

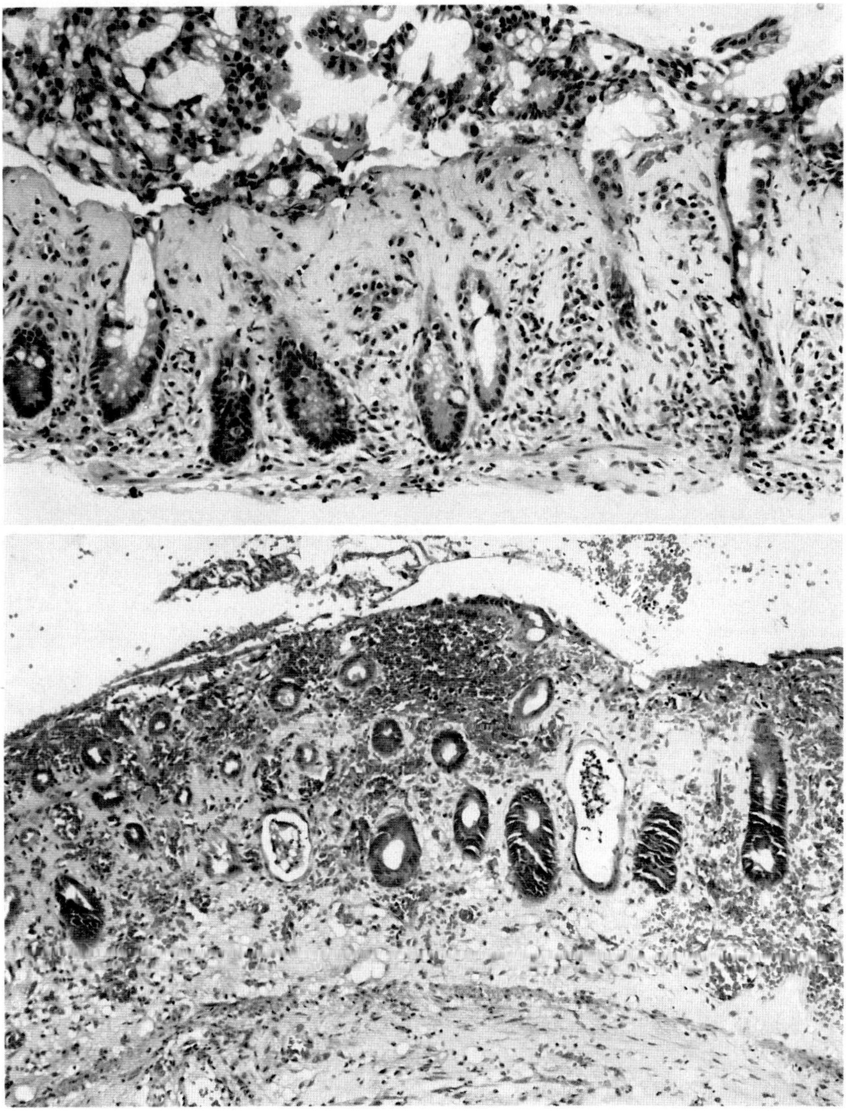

a

b

Fig. 10. a Florid collagenous colitis with an expanded collagen plate occupying two-thirds of the mucosa along with superficial crypt degeneration. This should be compared with Fig. 10b. HE, × 275. **b** A biopsy from a case of acute ischaemic colitis. Towards the right the lamina propria has an opaque eosinophilic texture that can be confused with collagenous colitis (see Fig. 10a). The haemorrhage and the failure to stain for collagen distinguish the biopsy from genuine collagenous colitis. HE, × 157.5

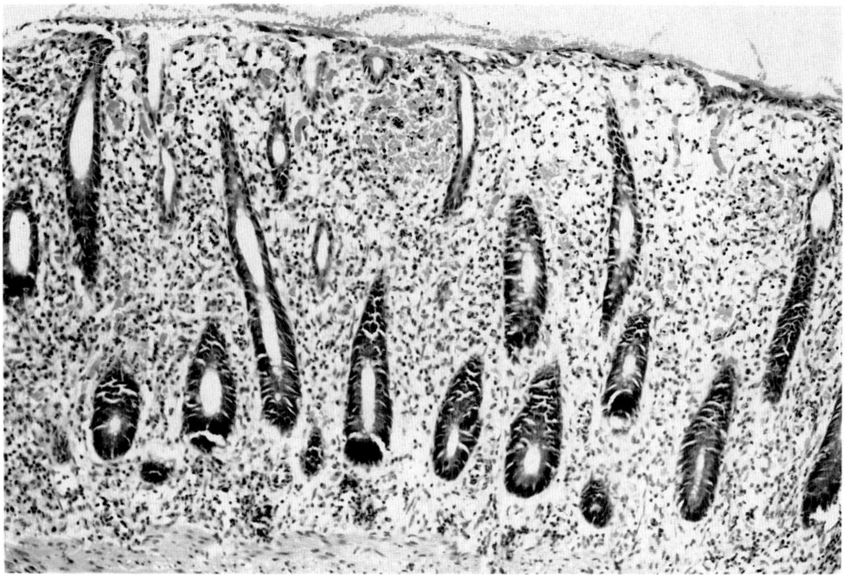

Fig. 11. Infective colitis to demonstrate the crypt withering which can resemble the crypt damage in ischaemia (see Figs. 1, 2 and 7). The acute inflammatory infiltrate and oedematous lamina propria are quite different. HE, × 157.5

infection and ischaemia in the group of conditions that can be loosely termed 'necrotising colitis' (ALSCHIBAJA and MORSON 1977; MARSTON 1986). The ischaemic bowel is susceptible to secondary bacterial infection and conversely some bacterial toxins, such as those of certain *Clostridia* spp., can cause vasoconstriction and hence ischaemic damage (MARSTON 1977).

5.10 Obstructive Colitis

Obstructive colitis is believed to be a form of ischaemic colitis that occurs in 1%–5% of cases proximal to a stenosis or obstruction, of whatever cause. It is usually due to a carcinoma but diverticular disease (FELDMAN 1975), impacted faeces (GEKAS and SCHUSTER 1981) and drugs affecting motility (HAY 1978) may be the cause. The colitis is nearly always seen proximal to the obstruction and separated from it by a zone of normal mucosa. It is seldom a biopsy problem but its importance lies in realising its existence as a pattern of colitis and not making an erroneous diagnosis of Crohn's disease or ulcerative colitis. A biopsy may show the features of the acute phase of ischaemia but may simply show non-specific inflammatory changes in less dramatic cases. The pathogenesis is thought to be via a rise in intraluminal pressure sufficient to produce a fall in intramural blood flow and subsequent ischaemic mucosal damage.

6 Conclusions

Ischaemic colitis in its typical patterns is not a difficult diagnosis to make though the differential problems described here need consideration. In the elderly, who are most at risk it is probably underdiagnosed. It seems most probable that many geriatric patients with biopsies labelled 'non-specific colitis' do have an ischaemic basis for their symptoms and pathology, but it remains proven. A second area in which ischaemia is insufficiently appreciated as the basis for pathology is in mucosal prolapse. Characteristic changes occur relatively commonly as an incidental and focal finding in a wide variety of large bowel problems.

References

Alschibaja T, Morson BC (1977) Ischaemic bowel disease. J Clin Pathol 30 [Suppl 11]:68–77
Barcewicz PA, Welch JP (1980) Ischaemic colitis in young patients. Dis Colon Rectum 123:109–114
Bartlett JG, Moon N, Chang TW, Taylor N, Oderdonk AB (1978) Role of *Clostridium difficile* in antibiotic-associated pseudomembranous colitis. Gastroenterology 75:778–782
Berthrong M, Fajardo LF (1981) Radiation injury in surgical pathology. Part II. Alimentary tract. Am J Surg Pathol 5:153–178
Binns JC, Isaacson P (1978) Age-related changes in colonic blood supply. Their relevance to ischaemic colitis. Gut 19:384–390
Bogomoletz MV, Adnet JJ, Birembaut P, Feydy P, Dupont P (1980) Collagenous colitis: an unrecognised entity. Gut 21:164–169
Brandt L, Boley S, Goldberg L, Mitsudo S, Berman A (1981) Colitis in the elderly. Am J Gastroenterol 76:239–245
Camilleri M, Pusey CD, Chadwick VS, Rees AJ (1983) Gastroinestinal manifestations of systemic vasculitis. Q J Med 52:141–149
Cotton PB, Thomas ML (1971) Ischaemic colitis and the contraceptive pill. Br Med J 3:27–28
Croft RJ, Menon GP, Marston A (1981) Does intestinal angina exist? A critical study of obstructed visceral arteries. Br J Surg 68:316–318
Darsee JR (1979) Cholesterol embolism: the great masquerader. South Med J 72:174–180
Dawson MA, Schaefer JW (1971) The clinical course of reversible ischaemic colitis – observations on the progression of sigmoidoscopic and histological changes. Gastroenterology 60:577–580
Devroede G, Vobecky S, Masse S, Arhan P, Leger C, Duguay C, Hemond M (1982) Ischaemic fecal incontinence and rectal angina. Gastroenterology 83:970–980
Dick AP, Graff R, Gregg D, Peters N, Sarner M (1967) An arteriographic study of mesenteric arterial disease. 1. Large vessel changes. Gut 8:206–220
du Boulay CEH, Fairbrother J, Isaacson PG (1983) Mucosal prolapse syndrome – a unifying concept for solitary ulcer syndrome and related disorders. J Clin Pathol 36: 1264–1268
Feldman PS (1975) Ulcerative disease of the colon proximal to partially obstructive lesions. Dis Colon Rectum 18:601–612
Gekas P, Schuster AM (1981) Stercoral perforation of the colon: case report and review of the literature. Gastroenterology 80:1054–1058
Hasleton PS, Carr N, Schofield PF (1985) Vascular changes in radiation bowel disease. Histopathology 9:517–534

Hay AM (1978) Association between chlorpromazine therapy and necrotizing colitis. Dis Colon Rectum 21:380–382

Helliwell TR, Flook D, Whitworth J, Day DW (1985) Arteritis and venulitis in systemic lupus erythematosus resulting in massive lower intestinal haemorrhage. Histopathology 9:1103–1113

Heron HC, Khubchandani IT, Trimpi HD, Sheets JA, Starik JJ (1981) Evanescent colitis. Dis Colon Rectum 24:555–561

Kingham JGC, Levison DA, Morson BC, Dawson AM (1986) Collagenous colitis. Gut 27:570–577

Knutson H, Lunderquist A, Lunderquist A (1968) Vascular changes in Crohn's disease. AJR 103:380–385

Kumar PJ, Dawson AM (1972) Vasculitis of the alimentary tract. Clin Gastroenterol 1:719–743

Larson HE, Price AB (1977) Pseudomembranous colitis: presence of clostridial toxin. Lancet II:1312–1314

Lee RG (1986) The colitis of Behçet's syndrome. Am J Surg Pathol 10:888–893

Lobert PF, Appelman HD (1981) Inflammatory cloacogenic polyps. A unique inflammatory lesion of the anal transitional zone. Am J Surg Pathol 5:761–766

Margaretten W, McKay DG (1971) Thrombotic ulcerations of the gastrointestinal tract. Arch Intern Med 127:250–253

Marston A (1977) Intestinal ischaemia. Edward Arnold, London, p 81

Marston A (1986) Vascular disease of the gut. Edward Arnold, London, pp 1–15

Marston A, Pheils MT, Lea Thomas, Morson BC (1966) Ischaemic colitis. Gut 7:1–15

May GM, De Weese JA, Rob CG (1963) Haemodynamic effects of arterial stenosis. Surgery 53:513–524

Miller WT, De Poto DW, Scholl HW, Rattensperger EC (1971) Evanescent colitis in the young adult: a new entity? Radiology 100:71–78

O'Connell DJ, Courtney JV, Riddell RH (1980) Colitis of Behçet's syndrome – radiologic and pathologic features. Gastronintest Radiol 5:173–179

Price AB, Davies DRD (1977) Pseudomembranous colitis. J Clin Pathol 30:1–12

Price AB, Jewkes J, Sanderson PJ (1979) Acute diarrhoea *Campylobacter* colitis and the role of rectal biopsy. J Clin Pathol 32:990–997

Reeders JWAJ, Tytgat GNJ, Rosenbusch G, Gratama S (1984) Ischaemic colitis. Martinus Nijhoff, Boston

Renton CJC (1972) Non-occlusive intestinal infarction. Clin Gastroenterol 1:655–674

Riddell RH (1982) The gastrointestinal tract. In: Riddell RM (ed) Pathology of drug induced and toxic diseases. Churchill Livingstone, Edinburgh, pp 516–520

Rosen N, Sommer I, Knobel B (1985) Intestinal Buerger's disease. Arch Pathol Lab Med 109:962–963

Rutter KRP, Riddell RH (1975) The solitary ulcer syndrome of the rectum. Clin Gastroenterol 4:505–530

Scowcroft CW, Sanowski RA, Kozarek RA (1981) Colonoscopy in ischaemic colitis. Gastrointest Endosc 27:156–161

Smith GE, Kime LR, Pitcher JL (1973) The colitis of Behçet's disease: a separate entity? Colonoscopic findings and literature review. Am J Dig Dis 18:987–999

Talbot I, Price AB (1987) Biopsy pathology in colorectal disease. Chapman and Hall, London

Tribe CR, Scott DGI, Bacon PA (1981) Rectal biopsy in the diagnosis of systemic vasculitis. J Clin Pathol 34:843–850

Whitehead R (1971) Ischaemic enterocolitis; an expression of the intravascular coagulation syndrome. Gut 12:912–917

Whitehead R (1976) The pathology of ischaemia of the intestines. Pathol Annu 11:1–52

C Intestinal Spirochaetosis

P. S. TEGLBJÆRG

1 History

Spirochaetes have been noted in human faeces since the end of the last century. Initially they were reported in patients suffering from cholera or infantile diarrhoea (ESCHERICH 1884, 1886), dysentery (DANTEC 1903) or appendicitis (THIROLOIX and DURAND 1911) and an anaerobe spirochaete, *Spirochaeta eugyrata*, was cultured from two symptomatic cases (THIROLOIX and DURAND 1911; HOUGE 1922). Subsequently spirochaetes were reported in the stools of healthy individuals (WERNER 1909; FANTHAM 1916, MACFIE 1917; PARR 1923). Other studies (MAZZA 1930) described the presence of spirochaetes in 9.8% of smears from the appendiceal lumen in patients suspected of having appendicitis, while HURST and VOLLUM (1943) described a case of ulcerative colitis associated with Vincent's organisms. More extensive studies by SHERA (1953, 1962) reported 52 patients in whom Vincent's organisms in faecal smears were associated with colonic symptoms and characteristic sigmoidoscopic appearances described as 'strawberry lesions'. A similar case was described by THOMAS (1956), but no further reports have appeared. Bacteriological culture and further characterisation of the spirochaetes was unsuccessful or incomplete in these early reports, making it difficult to compare the micro-organisms involved.

The attachment of spirochaetes to the surface of the large intestinal mucosa was first described by HARLAND and LEE (1967), who carried out histological and ultrastructural studies and termed the condition 'intestinal spirochaetosis'. In a subsequent study (LEE et al. 1971) they found spirochaetosis in 10/144 (6.9%) rectal biopsies and in 62/790 (7.8%) appendices. No consistent symptom complex could be related to the spirochaetosis. Based on clinical evidence, however, other authors have claimed that the spirochaetes are enteropathogenic, although opinions vary over whether this occurs rarely (GEBBERS et al. 1987) or rather frequently (GAD et al. 1977; CRUCIOLI and BUSUTTIL 1981; DOUGLAS and CRUCIOLI 1981).

In recent years the successful isolation, cultivation and propagation of spirochaetes from stools (TOMPKINS et al. 1981; SANNA et al. 1982) or from rectal biopsy specimens with histologically verified spirochaetosis (HOVIND-HOUGEN et al. 1982) has been reported. The growth characteristics and the morphology of the isolated spirochaetes differ sufficiently from previously isolated treponemes to justify a new designation, and the name *Brachyspira aalborgi* has been proposed for the type species (HOVIND-HOUGEN et al. 1982).

2 Morphology

2.1 Light Microscopy

Live spirochaetes observed with the dark-field technique are short, thin and rather variable in appearance, some being comma shaped whereas others are helical with one or two complete turns. Some show a serpentine swimming type of motility, whereas others may rotate rapidly (HOVIND-HOUGEN et al. 1982; COOPER et al. 1986; JONES et al. 1986). They can be easily identified in hematoxylin-eosin stained sections. At low magnification the brush border of the surface epithelium appears unusually distinct as a dark, blue fringe approximately 3 μm thick. At higher magnifications this fringe is seen to consist of numerous thin sinusoidal micro-organisms

Fig. 1. A section from the superficial part of the colonic mucosa infested with spirochaetes. The spirochaetes appear as a dark fringe covering the surface epithelium (*arrows*). The infestation ceases at the uppermost part of the crypts (*arrowheads*). No inflammatory reaction is observed. Light microscopy, HE, × 240

Fig. 2. A section of the colonic surface epithelium infested with spirochaetes. The sinosoidal spirochaetes are attached end-on to the luminal cell membrane between the microvilli, which appear shorter than normal. *E*, enterocyte; *G*, goblet cell. Electron microscopy, × 8700

Fig. 3. A section of the luminal part of the colonic surface epithelium. The spirochaetes depress the cell membrane, and an electron lucent pit (*P*) is present at the tip of one spirochaete. Electron-dense material (*arrows*) is seen beneath the cell membrane at the point of contact. Nuclear material (*N*) and ribosomes (*R*) are present in the cytoplasm of the spirochaetes. *MV*, microvilli. Electron microscopy, × 50000

Fig. 4. A section of the luminal part of the colonic surface epithelium. Spirochaetes (*arrows*) penetrating into the cytoplasm of the enterocyte (*E*). Electron microscopy, × 8000

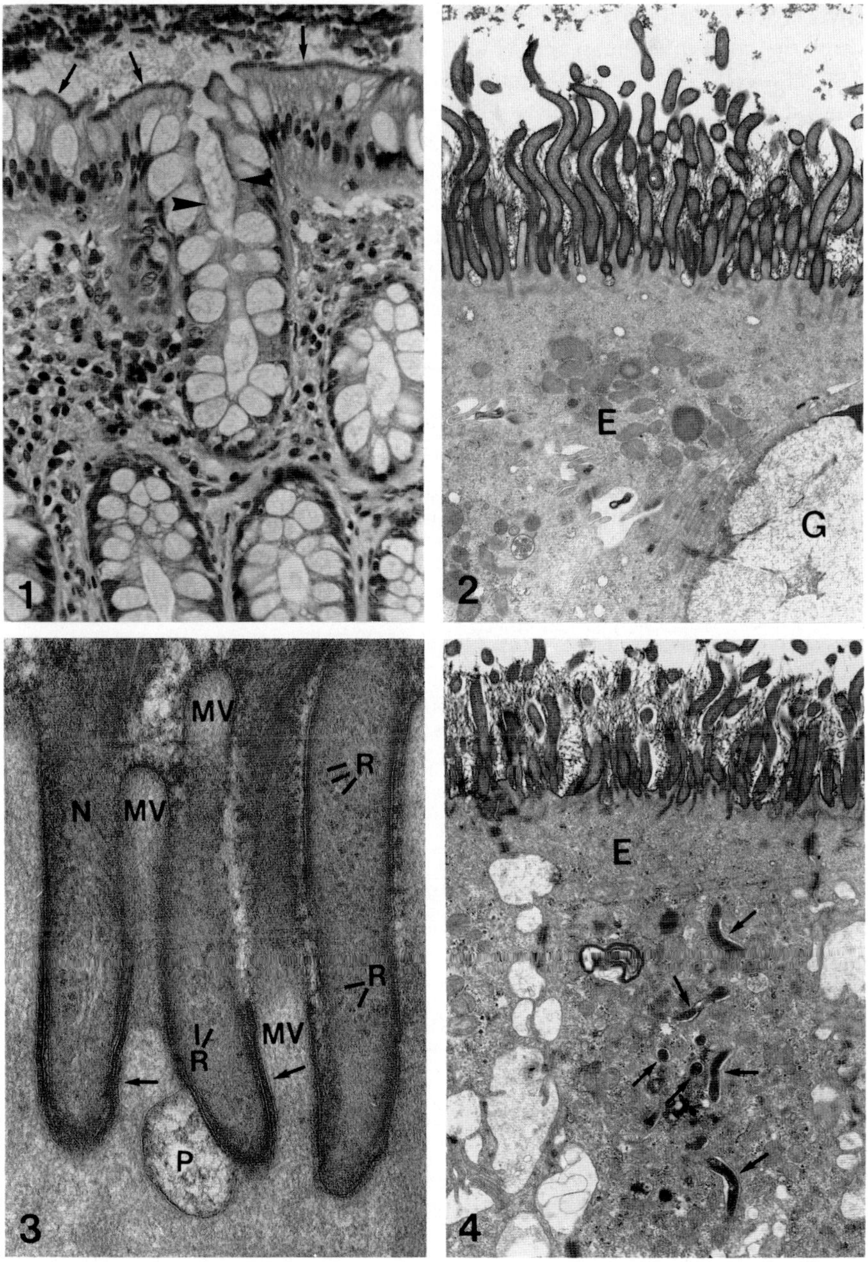

Figs. 1–4

covering the surface of the epithelium, seldom extending more than a short distance into the crypts (Fig. 1) (HENRIK-NIELSEN et al. 1983, 1985; LEE et al. 1971). The epithelial cells harbouring the spirochaetes appear normal, without any morphological signs of damage, and the rest of the mucosa is uninflamed (LEE et al. 1971). Although the spirochaetes are easily demonstrated in hematoxylin-eosin stained sections, silver techniques may produce a more dramatic high contrast staining of the spirochaetes (BURNS 1982; DERVAN 1985). The micro-organisms are Gram-negative.

2.2 Electron Microscopy

Negatively stained spirochaetes are regularly waved with tapered ends. The wavelength is about 2 μm, the maximum width is 0.2 μm, and the organisms are 1.7–6.0 μm long. Four flagella are inserted at each end which wind around the organisms, overlapping in the mid region. The individual flagella consist of a shaft covered by a sheet, and the insertion part possesses a hook and a basal complex. The spirochaetes divide by binary fission of their cytoplasmic membranes (HOVIND-HOUGEN et al. 1982). Variants possessing five flagella at each end (SANNA et al. 1982; COOPER et al. 1986) or being wider than usual (KAPLAN and TAKEUCHI 1979) have been reported.

Ultrastructural examination of infested colonic or appendiceal mucosa usually reveals a forest of spirochaetes attached end-on to the luminal cell membrane between the microvilli. The microvilli themselves appear shorter or even depleted proportional to the density of the attached spirochaetes (Fig. 2) (HOVIND-HOUGEN et al. 1982; GEBBERS et al. 1987; RODGERS et al. 1986). The epithelial surface membrane at the attachment site is usually depressed to form a small electron-lucent pit between the tip of the organism and the cell membrane and a zone of electron-dense material is present just beneath the cell membrane at the point of contact (Fig. 3). The spirochaetes themselves are enveloped by two asymmetric unit membranes, the outer leaflets being slightly wider and more electron dense than the inner leaflets. Ribosomes and nuclear material can be recognised inside the cells. They are most prominent in the central zone, becoming scanty in the tapering ends, although nuclear strands may rarely be observed at the tips of the spirochaetes (HOVIND-HOUGEN et al. 1982). Intracytoplasmic tubules are not seen. The flagella are situated in the periplasmic space: in transverse sections of the middle part of the spirochaetes, they interdigitate.

Scanning electron microscopic studies (TAKEUCHI et al. 1974; GAD et al. 1977; CRUCIOLI and BUSUTTIL 1981; ANTONAKOPOULOS et al. 1982) confirm numerous spiral-shaped micro-organisms attached to the epithelial brush order, all orientated perpendicular to the surface. Their approximate density has been calculated to reach about 1700 organisms/mm^2 (TAKEUCHI et al. 1974).

3 Cultivation

Spirochaetes have been cultured from stool specimens (KAPLAN and TAKEUCHI 1979; TOMPKINS et al. 1981; SANNA et al. 1982; JONES et al. 1986) or from rectal biopsy specimens (HOVIND-HOUGEN et al. 1982; COOPER et al. 1986). They grow under strictly anaerobic conditions in an atmosphere of 5%–10% CO_2/90%–95% H_2 at 37°–38.5°C on pre-reduced trypticase soy agar plates with 5%–10% blood added. The plates can be made selective by adding spectinomycin (400 µg/ml) and polymyxin (5 µg/ml). Some isolates form colonies within 3–5 days (KAPLAN and TAKEUCHI 1979; TOMPKINS et al. 1981; SANNA et al. 1982; COOPER et al. 1986), whereas others (HOVIND-HOUGEN et al. 1982; JONES et al. 1986) grow slower, forming colonies within 2–4 weeks. The spirochaetes ferment glucose, fructose, lactose, maltose, sucrose and mannitol (SANNA et al. 1982) although differences between individual isolates occur indicating that they probably do not represent a homogeneous group (JONES et al. 1986). The enzymatic activity of the spirochaetes has been investigated by HOVIND-HOUGEN et al. (1982) and JONES et al. (1986), the strains published by the latter being enzymatically the most active.

4 Clinical Aspects

Intestinal spirochaetosis occurs worldwide, having been reported from Great Britain (LEE et al. 1971; CRUCIOLI and BUSUTTIL 1981; COTTON et al. 1984; COOPER et al. 1986), France (LESBROS et al. 1981), Switzerland (GEBBERS et al. 1987), Italy (MINIO et al. 1973; SANNA et al. 1982), Scandinavia (GAD et al. 1977; HOVIND-HOUGEN et al. 1982; HENRIK-NIELSEN et al. 1983, 1985; WILLÉN et al. 1985), USA (GEAR and DOBBINS 1968; TAKEUCHI et al. 1974; NEUTRA 1980; SURAWICZ et al. 1987; JONES et al. 1986), USSR (KOVALCHUK and GEBESH 1981), India (MATHAN and MATHAN 1985), South Africa (BURNS and HAYES 1985) and Argentina (MAZZA 1930). Intestinal spirochaetosis occurs in the colon and the appendix, but has never been described in other parts of the gastrointestinal tract.

Information on the prevalence of intestinal spirochaetosis in healthy individuals, who naturally do not present for sigmoidoscopy, is still lacking (ANONYMOUS 1984). The prevalence in larger series of patients with abdominal symptoms necessitating sigmoidoscopy has been 1.9%–6.9% (TAKEUCHI et al. 1974; LEE et al. 1971; HENRIK-NIELSEN et al. 1983). A significantly higher prevalence has been reported among homosexual males attending sexually transmitted disease clinics, among whom the prevalence reaches 30%–36% (MCMILLAN and LEE 1981; SURAWICZ et al. 1987).

The incidence of intestinal spirochaetosis in resected appendices has been reported to be 2.1%–7.6% (LEE et al. 1971; TAKEUCHI et al. 1974; HENRIK-NIELSEN et al. 1985). In normal appendices removed because of suspected acute appendicitis it is 9.8%–12.6% (LEE et al. 1971; HENRIK-NIELSEN et al. 1985), significantly higher than in appendices removed *per occasionem* (1.9%–3.7%) or those with proven acute appendicitis (0.7%–4.4%). The clinical significance of this finding, and the mechanism by which the spirochaetes may cause symptoms mimicking acute appendicitis, remain to be elucidated (HENRIK-NIELSEN et al. 1985).

Most histological studies of intestinal spirochaetosis of the colon and rectum have concluded that the organisms are non-pathogenic. LEE et al. (1971) reported 14 patients in whom no consistent symptom complex could be related to the rectal infestation with spirochaetes. Although so-called spirochaetal dysentery was suspected in two patients with unexplained diarrhoea, in the abscence of a therapeutic trial the pathogenicity of the spirochaetes was not established. TAKEUCHI et al. (1974) were unable to assign any bowel symptom to their four patients with intestinal spirochaetosis. HENRIK-NIELSEN et al. (1983) found 15 cases of intestinal spirochaetosis among 300 patients admitted to a gastrointestinal unit with symptoms requiring sigmoidoscopy. After treatment with neomycin sulphate and bacitracin, which eliminated the spirochaetes in every patient, the original complaints remained unaltered over a follow-up period of 3–4 weeks.

The high prevalence of rectal co-infections in homosexuals makes it difficult to determine the clinical significance of intestinal spirochaetosis in this group (SURAWICZ et al. 1987). McMILLAN and LEE (1981) observed intestinal spirochaetosis in rectal biopsies in 36 of 100 homosexual males, an incidence far in excess of that observed in the heterosexual population. However, they found no convincing evidence that intestinal spirochaetosis should be capable of producing mucosal damage. SURAWICZ et al. (1987) studied 130 homosexual men, 92% of whom had intestinal symptoms. Intestinal spirochaetosis was identified in rectal biopsy specimens from 39. *Neisseria gonorrhoeae* infection was significantly associated with intestinal spirochaetosis. No specific histological abnormality was correlated with intestinal spirochaetosis, and there were no differences in the presence of or type of intestinal symptoms, sigmoidoscopic appearance of the mucosa, type of sexual practice or prior antibiotic use in men with and without intestinal spirochaetosis. TOMPKINS et al. (1981) isolated and cultured spirochaetes from the stools of two homosexuals without intestinal symptoms, and JONES et al. (1986) isolated and cultured a heterogeneous group of spirochaetes from the faeces of 11 homosexuals and were unable to establish any consequence to the human host.

On the other hand there have been a few reports of patients with clinical symptoms in whom the only abnormal feature was the presence of intestinal spirochaetosis. GAD et al. (1977) reported four patients with intestinal spirochaetosis, in whom the spirochaetes were eliminated with neomycin. Symptomatic relief was reported by one patient with alternating constipation and diarrhoea. In another report (KAPLAN and TAKEUCHI 1979), a non-treponemal spirochaete was isolated from the stools of a homosexual man with a chronic purulent rectal discharge. Rectal biopsies, however, were normal and did not reveal mucosa-associated spirochaetes. DOUGLAS and CRUCIOLI (1981) and CRUCIOLI and BUSUTTIL (1981) published studies on 13 patients with intestinal spirochaetosis. Treatment with metronidazole eliminated the spirochaetes, but the symptomatic relief achieved must be regarded as questionable. COTTON et al. (1984) reported four patients with intestinal spirochaetosis complaining of persistent or intermittent diarrhoea and colicky abdominal pains for 3–12 weeks. Most of the patients became asymptomatic after non-specific treatment, although metronidazole appeared to be specific. COOPER et al. (1986) carried out microbiological and electron microscopy studies on rectal biopsy specimens and faecal samples from eight practising homosexual males and five heterosexual controls. Rectal spirochaetosis was present in five of the eight homosexual men. They found a generalised loss of microvilli in the rectal mucosa of homosexual men compared with heterosexuals of similar ages. This loss of microvilli was accentuated in all of the men with spirochaetosis, and was most pronounced in those with the greatest degree of spirochaetal infestation of the mucosa, suggesting a possible mechanism whereby the organisms exert a pathogenic effect through the blockade of passive absorption. Both patients with a high degree of mucosal infestation by spirochaetes had symptoms of proctitis that subsided when treatment with metronidazole was started.

Spirochaetosis of the large intestine in which the spirochaetes penetrated and multiplied in the affected coloncytes in a patient with dysentery was reported by KOVALCHUK and GEBESH (1981). A similar patient with a 10-week history of diarrhoea was reported by RODGERS et al. (1986). Electron microscopy disclosed numerous spirochaetes adherent to the luminal cell membrane, inducing blunting or destruction of microvilli, and in the cytoplasm of colonocytes. Both the spirochaetosis and the symptoms disappeared on treatment with metronidazole. GEBBERS et al. (1987) reported two patients presenting with mild intestinal symptoms, in whom rectal spirochaetosis was the only morphological abnormality diagnosed by light microscopy. Electron microscopy revealed spirochaetes within epithelial cells and in subepithelial macrophages. In addition, numerous partially degranulated intra-epithelial mast cells and a marked increase in the proportion of plasma cells within the lamina propria that stained immunohistochemically with antibodies against IgE was observed. Mucosal penetration of the spirochaetes was suggested to be responsible for this unusual immune response. In one patient treatment with metronidazole eliminated the spirochaetes and resulted in symptomatic relief.

Pentetration of spirochaetes into the colonocytes and the subepithelial macrophages is not always associated with clinical symptoms, however. The phenomenon was reported in asymptomatic patients by MINIO et al.,

(1973) and Takeuchi et al. (1974) and in a patient with symptomatic Crohn's disease (Antonakopoulos et al. 1982) in whom the colonic epithelium was heavily infested with spirochaetes, often penetrating the epithelial cells or located in occasional macrophages in the lamina propria and even within the occasional Schwann cell. To summarise, there have been only six reported cases in whom intestinal symptoms could convincingly be related to intestinal spirochaetosis (Gad et al. 1977; Kovalchuk and Gebesh 1981; Cooper et al. 1986; Rodgers et al. 1986; Gebbers et al. 1987). A breaching of the mucosal barrier has been established in three of these, resulting in penetration of spirochaetes into the host tissues (Fig. 4). A similar spectrum of intestinal spirochaetal infestation is seen in animals: in mice and monkeys mucosal invasion is absent, and the spirochaetes are non-pathogenic, while in pigs swine dysentery is associated with mucosal invasion (Harris and Kinyon 1974). Serological characterisation of the spirochaetes has not yet been published, and it is not known whether the organisms induce any antibody response in the human host. However, the possibility of stimulating the immune system is present when spirochaetal antigens are taken up by macrophages.

5 Conclusions

The human colon and appendix may harbour unique strains of cultivatable mucosa-associated spirochaetes. At present it is unknown whether these are of one or more types. The route of infection remains obscure. Considerable disagreement exists about the pathological importance of spirochaetosis. Further work is needed to determine whether the organisms are harmless commensals or opportunistic pathogens requiring initial host cell damage as a prerequisite to colonisation and infection, as is suggested by the high prevalence among homosexuals. The mechanism of adherence to eukaryotic cell surfaces, the intercellular replicative cycle of the micro-organisms, the pathophysiology and the relation between the spirochaetes and the human immune system require investigation.

References

Anonymous (1984) Intestinal spirochaetes. Lancet I:720

Antonakopoulos G, Newman J, Wilkinson M (1982) Intestinal spirochaetosis: an electron microscopic study of an unusual case. Histopathology 6:477–488

Burns PA (1982) Staining intestinal spirochaetes. Med Lab Sci 39:75–77

Burns DG, Hayes MM (1985) Rectal spirochaetosis – symptomatic response to metronidazole and mebendazole. S Afr Med J 68:335–336

Cooper C, Cotton DKW, Hudson MJ, Kirkham N, Wilmott FEW (1986) Rectal spirochaetosis in homosexual men: characterisation of the organism and pathophysiology. Genitourin Med 62:47–52

Cotton DKW, Kirkham N, Hicks DA (1984) Rectal spirochaetosis. Br J Vener Dis 60:106–109

Crucioli V, Busuttil A (1981) Human intestinal spirochaetosis. Scand J Gastroenterol 70 [Suppl]:177–179

Dantec le M (1903) Dysenterie spirillaire. C R Soc Biol (Paris) 55:617

Dervan P (1985) Stain for spirochaetes (letter). Hum Pathol 16:1079

Douglas JG, Crucioli V (1981) Spirochaetosis: a remediable cause of diarrhoea and rectal bleeding? Br Med J 283:1362

Escherich T (1884) Klinisch-therapeutische Beobachtungen aus der Cholera-Epidemie in Neapel. Artzl Intell-Bl 31:561–564

Escherich T (1886) Beiträge zur Kenntnis der Darmbakterien. Münch Med Wochenschr 33:815–833

Fantham HB (1916) Observations of *Spirochaeta eugyrata*, as found in human faeces. Br Med J I:815–816

Gad A, Willén R, Furugård K, Fors B, Hradsky M (1977) Intestinal spirochaetosis as a cause of longstanding diarrhoea. Ups J Med Sci 82:49–54

Gear EV, Dobbins WO (1968) Rectal biopsy. A review of its diagnostic usefulness. Gastroenterology 55:522–544

Gebbers J-O, Ferguson DJP, Mason C, Kelly P, Jewell DP (1987) Spirochaetosis of the human rectum associated with an intraepithelial mast cell and IgE plasma cell response. Gut 28:588–593

Harland WA, Lee FD (1967) Intestinal spirochaetosis. Br Med J 3:718–719

Harris DL, Kinyon M (1974) Significance of anaerobic spirochetes in the intestines of animals. Am J Clin Nutr 27:1297–1304

Henrik-Nielsen R, Orholm M, Pedersen JO, Hovind-Hougen K, Teglbjærg PS, Thaysen EH (1983) Colorectal spirochetosis: clinical significance of the infestation. Gastroenterology 85:62–67

Henrik-Nielsen R, Lundbeck FA, Teglbjærg PS, Ginnerup P, Hovind-Hougen K (1985) Intestinal spirochetosis of the vermiform appendix. Gastroenterology 88:971–977

Houge MJ (1922) *Spirochaeta eugyrata*. A note on its life history and cultivation. J Exp Med 36:617–626

Hovind-Hougen K, Birch-Andersen A, Henrik-Nielsen R, Orholm M, Pedersen JO, Teglbjærg PS, Thaysen EH (1982) Intestinal spirochetosis: morphological characterization and cultivation of the spirochete *Brachyspira aalborgi* gen. nov. sp. nov. J Clin Microbiol 16:1127–1136

Hurst A, Vollum RL (1943) Ulcerative colitis caused by Vincent's organisms. Guy's Hosp Rep 92:118–120

Jones MJ, Miller JN, George WL (1986) Microbiological and biochemical characterization of spirochetes isolated from the feces of homosexual males. J Clin Microbiol 24:1071–1074

Kaplan LR, Takeuchi A (1979) Purulent rectal discharge associated with a nontreponemal spirochete. JAMA 24:52–53

Kovalchuk VK, Gebesh VV (1981) A case of spirochetosis of the large intestine with intracellular localization of bacteria. Arkh Patol 43:59–62

Lee FD, Kraszewski A, Gordon J, Howie JGR, McSeveney D, Harland WA (1971) Intestinal spirochaetosis. Gut 12:126–133

Lesbros F, Mallet-Guy Y, Berger F (1981) La spirochétose intestinale. Arch Anat Cytol Pathol 29:249–251

Macfie JWS (1917) The prevalence of *Spirochaeta eugyrata* in Europeans and natives in the Gold Coast. Lancet I:336–340

Mathan MM, Mathan VI (1985) Rectal mucosal morphologic abnormalities in normal subjects in southern India: a tropical colonopathy? Gut 26: 710–717

Mazza S (1930) Espiroquetosis appendiculares. Pren Med Argent 17:464–468

McMillan A, Lee FD (1981) Sigmoidoscopic and microscopic appearance of the rectal mucosa in homosexual men. Gut 22:1035–1041

Minio F, Tonietti G, Torsoli A (1973) Spontaneous spirochete infestation in the colonic mucosa of healthy men. Rendic Gastroenterol 5:183–195

Neutra MR (1980) Prokaryotic-eukaryotic cell junctions: attachment of spirochetes and flagellated bacteria to primate large intestinal cells. J Ultrastruct Res 70: 186–203

Parr LW (1923) Intestinal spirochetes. J Infect Dis 33:369–383

Rodgers FG, Rodgers C, Shelton AP, Hawkey CJ (1986) Proposed pathogenic mechanism for the diarrhea associated with human intestinal spirochetes. Am J Clin Pathol 86:679–682

Sanna A, Dettori G, Grillo R, Rossi A, Chiarenza D (1982) Isolation and propagation of a strain of treponema from the human disgestive tract – preliminary report. L'Igiene Moderna 77:287–297

Shera AG (1953) A syndrome associated with intestinal spirochaetosis. J Clin Pathol 6:327–328

Shera AG (1962) Specific granular lesions associated with intestinal spirochaetosis. Br J Surg 50:68–77

Surawicz CM, Roberts PL, Rompalo A, Quinn TC, Holmes KK, Stamm WE (1987) Intestinal spirochetosis in homosexual men. Am J Med 82:587–592

Takeuchi A, Jervis HR, Nakazawa H, Robinson DM (1974) Spiral-shaped organisms on the surface colonic epithelium of the monkey and man. Am J Clin Nutr 27:1287–1296

Thiroloix J, Durand A (1911) Spirochétémie au cours d'une appendicite aigue. Hémo et séroculture. Isolement et culture du parasite. Emploi du 606. Arrét de la septicémie. Bul Mem Soc Med Hosp III 31:653–662

Thomas GK (1956) "Strawberry lesion" of the recto-sigmoid. Br Med J 2:209–211

Tompkins DS, Waugh MA, Cooke EM (1981) Isolation of intestinal spirochaetes from homosexuals. J Clin Pathol 34:1385–1387

Werner H (1909) Über Befunde von Darmspirochäten beim Menschen. Zentralbl Bakteriol Parasitenkd Infektionskr Hyg Abt 1 Orig Reihe A 52:241–243

Willén R, Carlén B, Cronstedt J, Willén H (1985) Intestinal spirochaetosis of the colon diagnosed with colono-ileoscopy and multiple biopsies. Endoscopy 17:86–88

D Biopsy Diagnosis of Hirschsprung's Disease and Related Disorders

P. U. HEITZ and P. KOMMINOTH

1 Introduction

An impaired regulation of motor functions of the intestine often causes the passage of the bowel contents to be impeded. The coordination of intestinal activity is effected by an extrinsic and intrinsic enteric nervous system, the organisation of which is highly complex (MEIER-RUGE 1974; WEINBERG 1975; ELLIOTT and LAWRENSON 1981). In 1888 the Danish physician Hirschsprung described two patients with severe constipation caused by congenital megacolon. The history of the elucidation of the pathogenesis of Hirschsprung's disease and the introduction of enzyme histochemical methods as diagnostic tools have been described in detail elsewhere (EHRENPREIS 1970; MEIER-RUGE 1974).

Several disorders of intestinal innervation are recognised at present, collectively called 'dysganglionoses' by some authors (MEIER-RUGE 1983). The term 'Hirschsprung's disease' should be applied only to aganglionosis of a short segment of the colon; other disorders should be defined according to the type of impaired innervation and the extent thereof. In contrast to the variety of morphological forms of abnormal intestinal innervation, the symptoms are very similar, usually consisting of severe constipation and abdominal protrusion. The abnormally innervated part of the intestine (most often the colon) behaves as a functional stenosis, caused by permanent contraction of the longitudinal muscle layers, without peristalsis, and the colon proximal to the stenosis is markedly dilated (secondary megacolon, MEIER-RUGE 1968).

In the following discussion we attempt to demonstrate that the morphological basis of clinical Hirschsprung's disease may be more complex than previously realised.

2 Normal Innervation of the Large Intestine

The very complex development, morphology (Fig. 6a) and physiology of normal innervation of the intestine have been repeatedly described previously (MEIER-RUGE 1974; WEINBERG 1975). Therefore only a brief account is given here, considering mainly the practical aspects.

It is difficult to detect neuronal bodies and nerve fibres in the intestinal wall, especially in the neonate, using conventional stains. The application of enzyme histochemistry for visualisation of acetylcholinesterase and lactate dehydrogenase, or of immunohistochemistry for localisation of 'neurone-specific' enolase or of the calcium binding cytosolic protein S-100, is necessary (HALL and LAMPERT 1985; TAGUCHI et al. 1985). Only a relatively small number of fine cholinergic nerve fibres can be seen in the normal intestine using the reaction for acetylcholinesterase (Fig. 1); neuronal cell bodies occur singly or in small groups. The histochemical reaction for lactate dehydrogenase and the immunohistochemical reaction for neurone-specific enolase are appropriate for the visualisation of neuronal bodies, while the localisation of protein S-100 permits the visualisation of Schwann cells and paraganglionic satellite cells. It is important to realise that while the myenteric and submucosal plexuses extend distally as far as the internal anal sphincter, the number of neuronal bodies decreases in the the distal rectum (MEIER-RUGE 1985). Conversely, the density of cholinergic nerve fibres increases distally (MEIER-RUGE 1974). These facts must be taken into consideration for the diagnosis of biopsies taken near the anus.

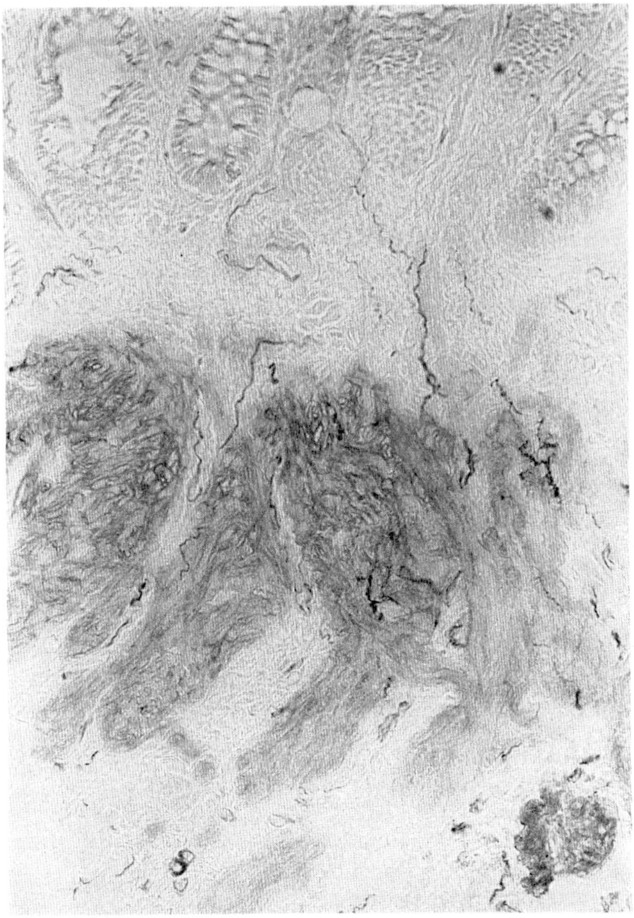

Fig. 1. Normal innervation of the human colon. Fine meandering cholinergic nerve fibres are present in the submucosa, muscularis mucosae (*centre*) and mucosa. Small groups of cholinergic neurones are present in the submucosa (*bottom*). Enzyme histochemical reaction for acetylcholinesterase, × 200

3 Biopsy Technique, Transport and Processing of Specimens

3.1 Biopsy Technique

Two techniques of intestinal biopsy are established: In a *suction biopsy* (or partial-thickness biopsy) only the mucosa and (at least some of) the submucosa can be examined (DOBBINS and BILL 1965). The technique is fast and simple, and can be carried out in neonates without general anaesthesia. A diagnosis can often be made, provided the biopsy measures at least 3–5 mm in diameter and 1–2 mm in depth, using appropriate techniques. In contrast, a *full-thickness biopsy* contains all layers of the intestinal wall, but can only be obtained after general anaesthesia.

In our opinion suction biopsies should be done first if a disorder of intestinal innervation is suspected. For Hirschsprung's disease biopsies should be taken at intervals of 1 cm, beginning immediately proximal to the linea dentata, the last biopsy being taken from normal appearing intestine if possible. This procedure prevents overlooking so-called ultra-short segment Hirschsprung's disease and, if subsequent surgical resection is performed, avoids excision of too short an intestinal segment. Full-thickness biopsies, or surgical specimens, are needed for a precise diagnosis of the various other disorders of intestinal innervation (see Sect. 5).

3.2 Transport

For enzyme histochemical investigations the biopsies should be sent to the laboratory by special mail in humid Petri dishes on ice (not on dry ice!) in a Dewar flask. The time interval between excision and processing in the laboratory should be kept as short as possible. In our experience a delay exceeding 8–10 h is detrimental to the enzyme histochemical visualisation of acetylcholinesterase and lactate dehydrogenase. Optimal conventional fixation should be ensured for subsequent immunohistochemical investigations.

3.3 Histochemistry

Conventional histology, using tinctorial stains, is not reliable for making a precise diagnosis. The introduction of enzyme histochemistry during the 1950s and 1960s (KAMIJO et al. 1953; NIEMI et al. 1961; MEIER-RUGE 1968; BENNETT et al. 1968; GARRETT et al. 1969) was a great improvement, and enzyme histochemical reactions are now widely used (WAKELY and MCADAMS 1984). The tissue samples are quenched in melting isopentane (2-methyl-butane) at −160°C or liquid nitrogen, and cut in a cryostat (10–12 μm) perpendicular to the surface of the mucosa. One section is stained with haemalum and eosin, and 6–24 sections stained with histochemical techniques for acetylcholinesterase (E. C. 3.1.1.7; KARNOVSKY and ROOTS 1964) and for lactate dehydrogenase (E. C. 1.1.1.27; HESS et al. 1958; MEIER-RUGE 1982) in order to minimise sampling errors.

Deparaffinised sections (5 μm) of biopsies fixed in buffered formaldehyde (4%) and embedded in paraffin are incubated with antisera to neurone-specific enolase, synaptophysin or protein S-100 applying the unlabelled antibody enzyme method (STERNBERGER 1986) or avidin biotin-peroxidase complex technique (GUESDON et al. 1979), using appropriate controls.

3.4 Artefacts

The histochemical reactions must be carried out by an experienced technician and interpreted by an experienced pathologist. Non-specific reactions for acetylcholinesterase occur in the smooth muscle fibres of the muscularis mucosae, in lymphoid follicles, in oedema fluid, in traumatised tissue, and in small haemorrhagic foci. False-negative results may occur in biopsies from neonates in whom the enzyme activity may be insufficient to be detected by the techniques currently used (BLISARD and KLEINMAN 1986).

3.5 Enzyme Histochemistry Versus Immunohistochemistry

We consider the enzyme histochemical processing of intestinal biopsies most appropriate for the diagnosis of disorders of innervation if handling, transport and processing of tissue are appropriate and fast, if the technician is skilful and experienced, and if the pathologist is experienced and aware of possible artefacts.

The advantage of immunohistochemistry for protein S-100, neurone-specific enolase and synaptophysin is its feasibility on fixed specimens. On the other hand, precise diagnosis of the various disorders is more difficult, and less specific than diagnosis based on enzyme histochemistry. Very extensive immunohistochemical investigations, using a battery of antibodies not yet readily available, may improve the sensitivity of this technique in the future.

4 Own Experience

We have investigated 2688 suction biopsies and surgical samples from 677 patients for diagnostic purposes. The biopsies were taken either to investigate suspected aganglionosis (621 patients) or to assess the remaining colon after surgery for disorders of colonic innervation (56 patients). Clinical suspicion of abnormal innervation based, on symptoms of dilatation of the colon and/or impedance of passage of bowel contents due to contraction of a colonic segment, could be confirmed by suction biopsy in 110 of 621 patients (17.7%). The various diagnoses made are shown in Table 1. Ninety patients had classical Hirschsprung's disease, with aganglionosis confined to a segment of colon, and this diagnosis made on suction biopsy was confirmed subsequently in surgical samples from 22. Aganglionosis of the entire colon was found in two patients, and in one further case this was combined with neuronal dysplasia of the appendix. Other diagnoses included hypoganglionosis (six patients), neuronal dysplasia or hyperganglionosis (four patients), absence of extrinsic and intrinsic innervation

Table 1. Morphological diagnosis in 621 patients with clinically suspected Hirschsprung's disease

	Females	Males	Total
1. Aganglionosis (segment of the colon)	20	70	90
2. Aganglionosis, probable	1	–	1
3. Aganglionosis of the entire colon	1	1	2
4. Aganglionosis of the colon combined with neuronal dysplasia of the appendix	–	1	1
5. Hypoganglionosis	1	5	6
6. Hypoganglionosis, probable	1	–	1
7. Neuronal dysplasia (hyperganglionosis)	3	1	4
8. Absence of extrinsic and intrinsic innervation (small and large intestine)	3	–	3
9. Absence of extrinsic and intrinsic innervation of the small intestine combined with aganglionosis of the entire colon	–	1	1
10. Lack of intrinsic innervation (segment of the colon)	–	1	1
11. No morphological diagnosis	3	6	9
12. 'Normal' innervation	207	295	502
Total	240	381	621

of the small and large intestines (three patients), absence of small intestinal innervation combined with aganglionosis of the entire colon (one patient) and absence of intrinsic innervation in the presence of extrinsic nerves in a segment of the colon (one patient). A diagnosis could not be reached in the first biopsy from 9 of the 621 patients (1.6%). In two patients (0.32%) a false-negative diagnosis was corrected in subsequent biopsies.

In 56 patients with an established diagnosis of disordered innervation, who had undergone surgery 1–20 years previously, the innervation of the residual colon was investigated. In 19 patients a normal innervation was found, whereas in 27 patients an aganglionic segment remained. One patient had aganglionosis of the entire colon, three patients had persistent hypoganglionosis, one patient had persistent neuronal dysplasia (hyperganglionosis) and in five patients the findings were equivocal.

Our experience indicates that approximately 80% of patients with clinical features suggesting disordered intestinal innervation have no demonstrable morphological abnormality, and biopsy confirmation is obviously essential before surgery is undertaken. Moreover, since residual aganglionic segments seem to be common in patients who have undergone surgery, better pre- or peroperative delineation of the affected zone with multiple biopsies is to be recommended.

5 Morphology and Classification of Abnormal Intestinal Innervation (Dysganglionoses)

5.1 Diseases of the Intrinsic Innervation of the Colon

5.1.1 Aganglionosis of the Colon (Fig. 6b)

Aganglionosis (Fig. 2) is defined by a lack of neurones of the submucosal plexus (Meissner's plexus) and myenteric plexus (Auerbach's plexus), combined with hyperplasia of cholinergic nerve fibres in the circular muscle layer, muscularis mucosae and mucosa with a high activity of acetylcholinesterase (MEIER-RUGE and MORGER 1968; MEIER-RUGE 1974). In biopsies taken proximal to the left colonic flexure, the diagnosis of aganglionosis can be made if absence of submucosal neuronal bodies alone can be demonstrated, because hyperplasia of cholinergic nerve fibres is often lacking.

In our experience aganglionosis of a segment of the colon is by far the most common form of abnormal enteric innervation. It is much commoner in males than in females (see below), usually presenting before the age of 5 years, and often during the first month of life. The aganglionic segment can be rather long, short or ultra-short (REHBEIN et al. 1969; MEIER-RUGE 1985; BLISARD and KLEINMAN 1986; SELDENRIJK et al. 1986). An extreme variant is Zuelzer-Wilson's disease (see below; ZUELZER and WILSON 1948; MEIER-RUGE et al. 1972; IKEDA and GOTO 1986).

It is of interest that an aganglionosis was found to persist after surgery in 27 out of 56 patients in our series. It is well recognised that the aganglionic segment is often more extensive than the macroscopically constricted segment of large bowel, and intra-operative frozen sections may be valuable in identifying the upper level of aganglionosis. Moreover, the extent of aganglionosis is also apparently greater than the hyperplasia of cholinergic nerve fibres detected in a biopsy containing only the mucosal layer: we have observed a transitional zone, confirming the previously report by HAMOUDI et al. (1982).

5.1.2 Hypoganglionosis of the Colon (Fig. 6c)

Hypoganglionosis is characterised by a decreased number of intrinsic neuronal bodies and cholinergic nerve fibres. Rare neuronal bodies occur in the submucosa, but groups of neurones are lacking (MEIER-RUGE 1974). Hypoganglionosis may occur as an isolated condition or combined with aganglionosis.

This variant is uncommon, except in the transitional zone between an aganglionotic and a normal segment in Hirschsprung's disease. In our opinion the diagnosis should not be made unless extensive quantitative

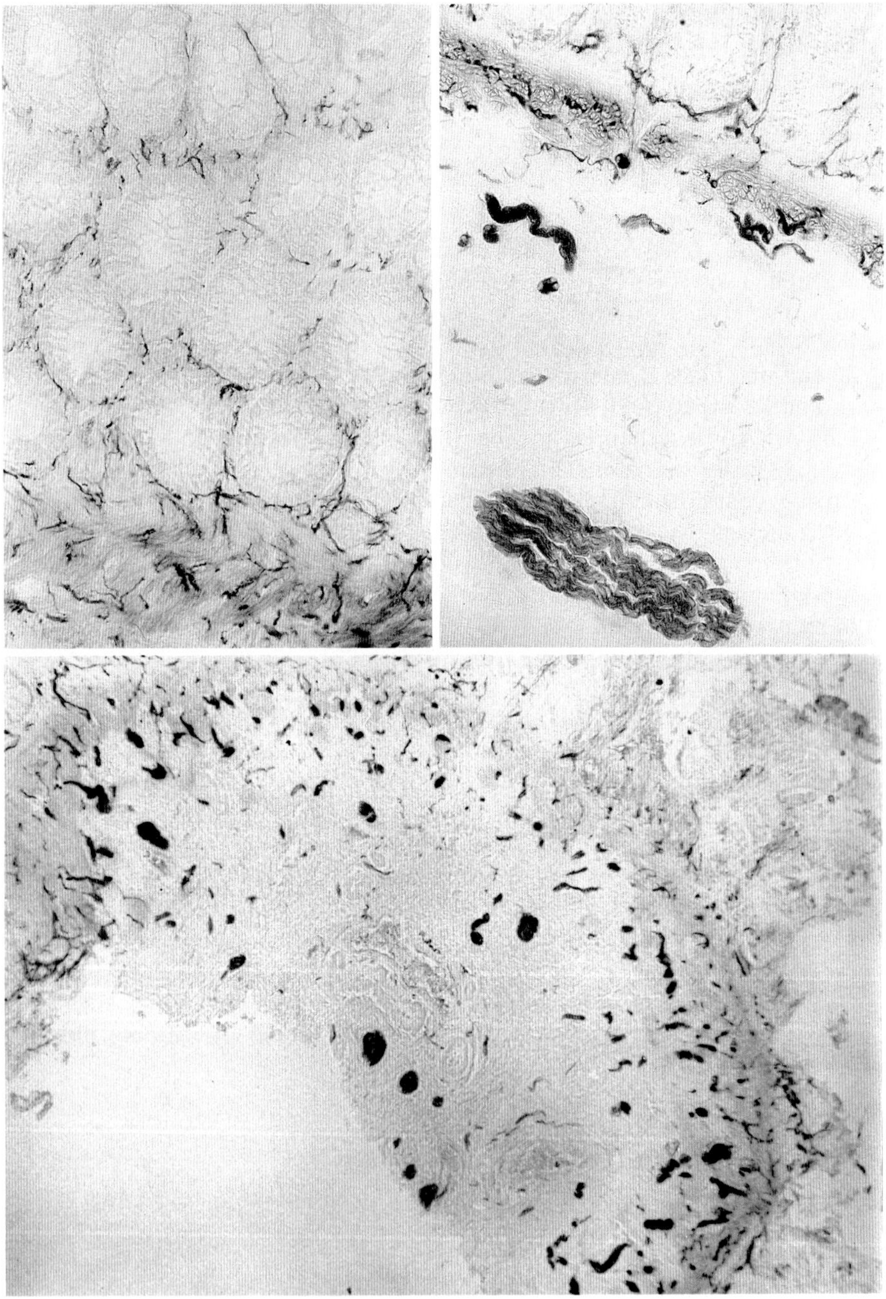

a b c

Fig. 2a–c. Aganglionosis of the colon of a 7-day-old girl. Enzyme histochemical reaction for acetylcholinesterase. **a** A large number of hypertrophic cholinergic nerve fibres are seen in the muscularis mucosae (*bottom*) and surrounding the crypts of the mucosa. × 200. **b** Prominent bundles of cholinergic nerve fibres are present in the submucosa. × 100. **c** Bundles of cholinergic nerve fibres are seen in the submucosa and muscularis mucosae, without neuronal bodies. × 200

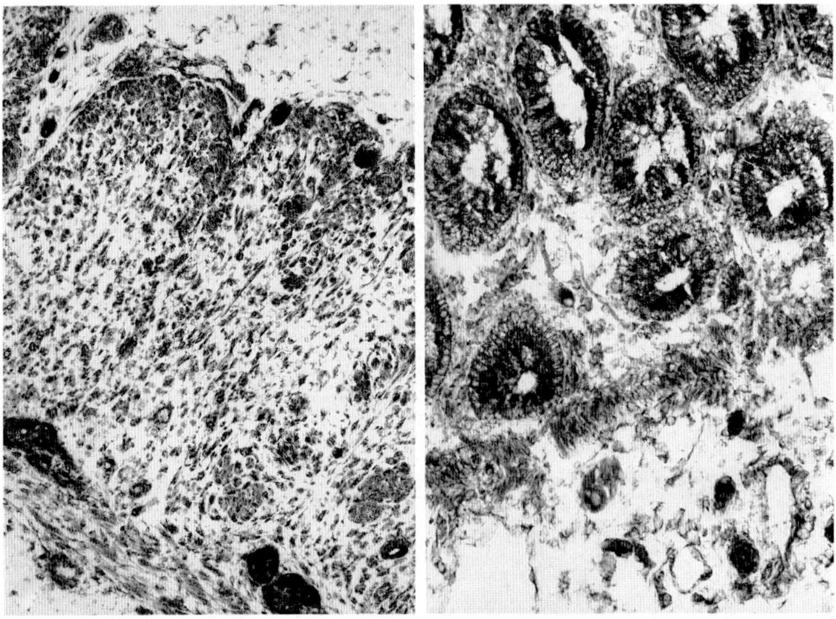

Fig. 3 a, b. Neuronal dysplasia (hyperganglionosis) of the colon of a 4-month-old boy. **a** Large number of cholilnergic nerve fibres (*black*) running through the circular muscle layer, and large number of neuronal bodies (*large black dots*) between the circular and longitudinal muscle layers and at the border between the circular muscle layer and submucosa (*top*). Enzyme histochemical reaction for acetylcholinesterase, × 100 **b** Three groups of neuronal bodies in the submucosa (*bottom right*) and single neuronal body present in the mucosa (*centre*) Enzyme histochemical reaction for lactate dehydrogenase, × 100

analyses can be carried out, e.g. on three or more full-thickness biopsies (MEIER-RUGE 1974). The clinical symptoms resemble those of aganglionosis.

5.1.3 Neuronal Dysplasia (Hyperganglionosis) of the Intestine (Fig. 6 d)

Neuronal dysplasia or hyperganglionosis (GARRETT and HOWARD 1981) (Fig. 3) clinically resembles aganglionosis. In our experience a short segment of neuronal dysplasia is often combined with aganglionosis. Neuronal dysplasia not associated with other disorders is apparently uncommon. Segmental and disseminated forms can occur (SCHAERLI and MEIER-RUGE 1981; FADDA et al. 1983). The condition is characterised by hyperplasia of cholinergic nerve fibres in the circular muscle layer, submucosa and mucosa, and hyperplasia of neuronal bodies in both intramural nerve plexuses (Fig. 3 a). Neuronal bodies may be associated with nerve fibres in the mucosa (Fig. 3 b) and small groups of neurones present within the muscle layers (Fig. 3 a) are sometimes striking.

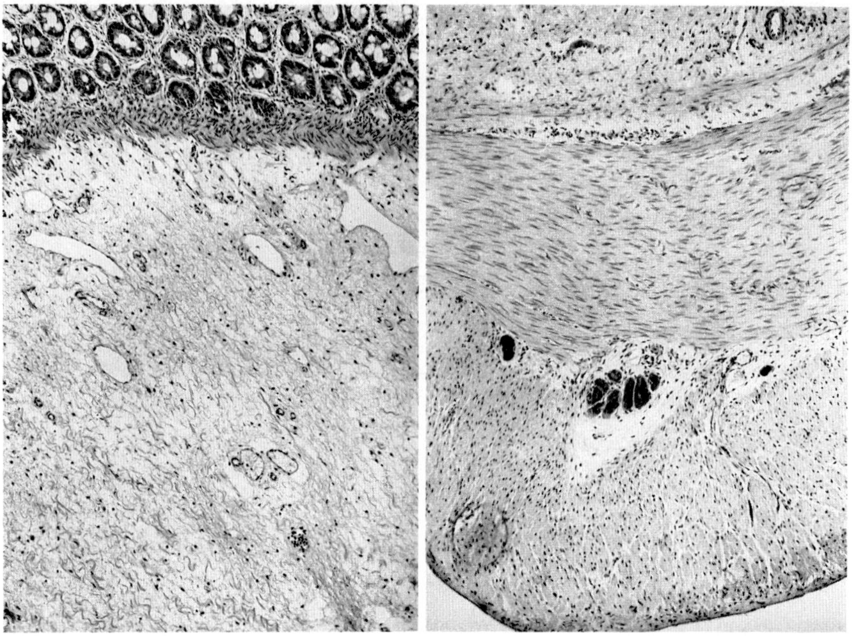

a b

Fig. 4a, b. Absence of intrinsic innervation of the colon in the presence of extrinsic innervation in an 8-month-old boy. **a** Absence of nerve fibres in the mucosa, muscularis mucosae and submucosa. Immunocytochemical reaction for protein S-100, × 100. **b** Presence of bundles of cholinergic nerve fibres between the circular and longitudinal muscle layers and cholinergic nerve fibres running through the longitudinal muscle layer (*bottom right*). Enzyme histochemical reaction for acetylcholinesterase, × 100

The diagnosis of neuronal dysplasia cannot be made reliably on biopsies containing only intestinal mucosa, and the full thickness of the bowel wall should be assessed.

5.1.4 Absence of Intrinsic Innervation of the Colon (Fig. 6e)

This type of abnormal innervation is very uncommon. The symptoms in our patients were identical to those of aganglionosis. Intrinsic neuronal bodies in the colonic wall are absent. An extremely small number of intrinsic nerve fibres may be found (Fig. 4a), while large bundles of extrinsic cholinergic nerve fibres penetrate as far as the zone between the longitudinal and circular muscle layers (Fig. 4b). This lesion may occur as an isolated condition or in combination with absence of innervation of the small intestine (RUDIN et al. 1986a).

5.2 Diseases of Intrinsic and Extrinsic Innervation of the Intestine

5.2.1 Absence of Innervation of the Intestine (Fig. 6f)

A diagnosis of absence of innervation of the intestine can only be made on surgical samples that include all layers of the intestinal wall. It is a rare condition which, due to the frequently extensive absence of innervation, is often incompatible with life, in contrast to the diseases mentioned above.

We have observed four patients. In three we were unable to find nerve fibres or neuronal bodies either in the entire colon, or in part of the small intestine (Fig. 5a–c) while in the fourth a lack of innervation of the small intestine distal to the duodenum was combined with aganglionosis of the entire colon (Fig. 5d). The detailed findings in these patients and a review of the literature were given by RUDIN et al. (1986a, b).

5.3 Extent of the Diseases

All types of abnormal innervation of the intestine probably occur either as segmental or diffuse diseases.

6 Symptoms and Clinical Diagnosis

The symptoms of the various types of abnormal innervation of the intestine are similar, although not identical. In classical aganglionosis there is a short stenosis of the distal colon and rectum, distension of the colon proximal to the stenosis, constipation and massive abdominal distension. More extensive involvement, such as a long segment of aganglionosis or a widespread defect of innervation of the small intestine and the colon, causes vomiting and a slowdown of faecal transit in the colon. Sometimes there is early, severe and repeated vomiting and passage of meconium may even occur. Roentgenograms generally show a narrow colon and signs of ileus of the small intestine. Peristalsis is weak or absent. This contrasts with classical aganglionosis.

The clinical diagnosis of abnormal innervation of the intestine is based on the clinical picture of chronic constipation or ileus and abdominal protrusion, an X-ray examination and/or enema disclosing a contracted segment of the colon with proximal dilatation, and manometric examination of the rectum.

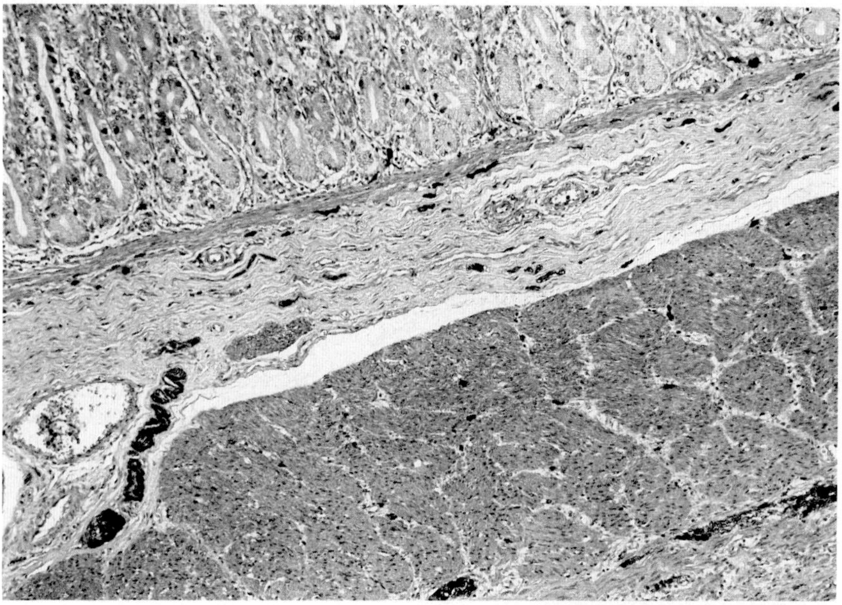

a

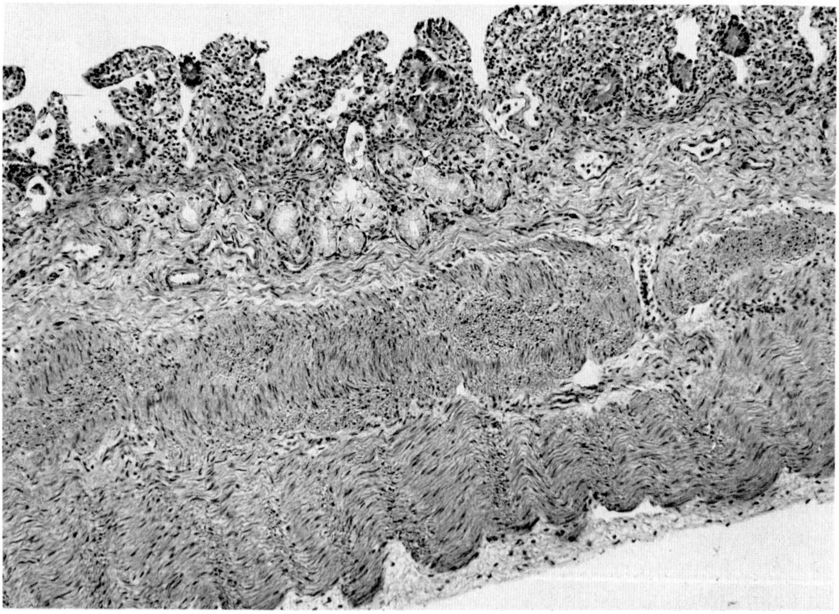

b

Fig. 5 a–d. Absence of intrinsic and extrinsic innervation in the small intestine, and aganglionosis in the colon in a 4-month-old boy. **a** Presence of nerve fibres and neuronal bodies (*black*) in the wall of the antrum of the stomach. Neurone-specific enolase, × 100. **b** Lack of neuronal bodies and nerve fibres in the wall of the duodenum. Neurone-specific enolase, × 100. **c** Absence of cholinergic nerve fibres in the mucosa (*top right*), muscularis mucosae (*top right*), submucosa (*center*) and circular muscle layer (*bottom left*). Enzyme histochemical reaction for acetylcholinesterase. × 100. **d** Typical picture of aganglionosis in the colon with a large number of bundles of cholinergic nerve fibres in the submucosa and muscularis mucosae, and large single fibres in the mucosa. Absence of neuronal bodies. Enzyme histochemical reaction for acetylcholinesterase, × 100

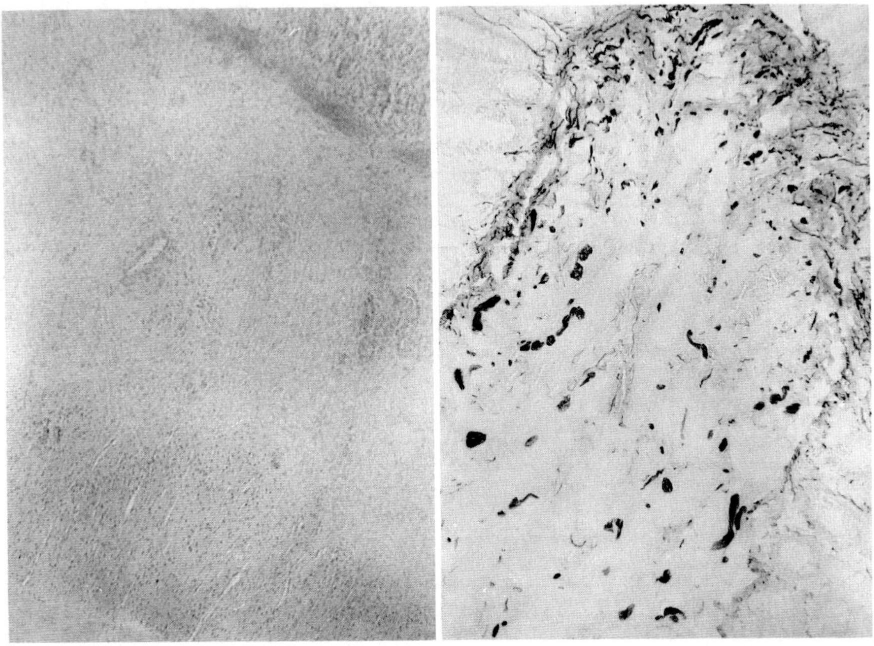

c d

7 Incidence, Sex Ratio and Genetics

Different authors have estimated aganglionosis of a short colonic segment to occur in 1/10000 to 1/30000 (BODIAN and CARTER 1963) or 1/5000 to 1/8000 (BLISARD and KLEINMAN 1986) live births. The long segment variant of the disease (i.e. a contracted segment expanding proximal to the rectosigmoid) comprises approximately 10% of all cases of aganglionosis (EHRENPREIS 1970; MEIER-RUGE 1972).

The estimation of the incidence of the various forms of abnormal intestinal innervation varies considerably. The incidence of an ultra-short segment has been estimated at 10% of all aganglionoses, or 6.8% of all abnormal intestinal innervations (MEIER-RUGE 1985). The incidence of an aganglionosis of the entire colon has been indicated as 6%–14.9% of all aganglionoses (IKEDA and GOTO 1986). This is at variance with our experience. Neuronal dysplasia (or hyperganglionosis) has been said to be as common as aganglionosis (FADDA et al. 1983). We cannot confirm this finding, if neuronal dysplasia unassociated with other disorders is considered (see Sect. 5.1.3).

The male/female ratio in classical (short) segment aganglionosis is 3–4:1 (MEIER-RUGE 1974; ZIEGLER et al. 1984). The ratio drops progressively in aganglionosis affecting longer segments, and is approximately 1:1 in aganglionosis of the entire colon (BODIAN and CARTER 1963; MEIER-

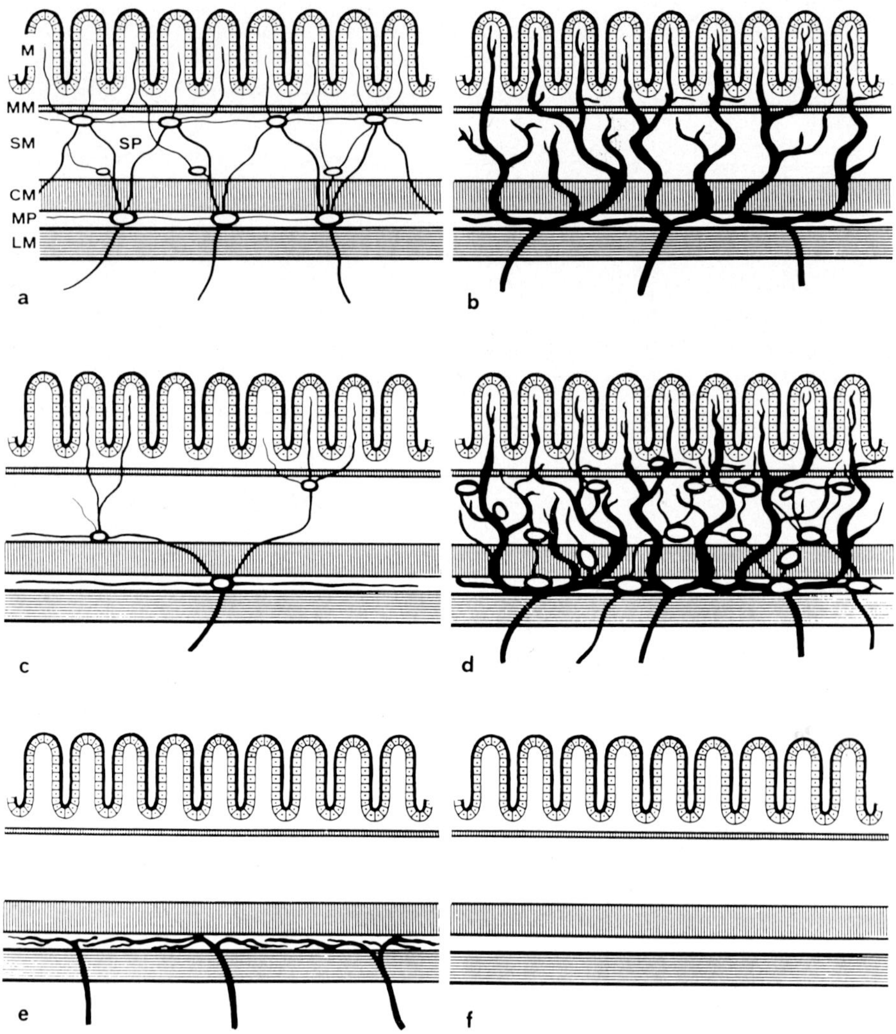

Fig. 6a–f. Schematic drawing of the innervation and its disturbances in the human intestine. **a** Normal innervation of the colon. Presence of groups of neurones in the submucosal plexus (*SP*) and in the myenteric plexus (*MP*) with interconnecting nerve fibres. *M*, mucosa; *MM*, muscularis mucosae; *SM*, submucosa; *CM*, circular muscle layer; *LM*, longitudinal muscle layer. **b** Aganglionosis of the colon. Absence of neuronal bodies, along with a large number of bundles of intrinsic cholinergic nerve fibres penetrating into the mucosa. **c** Hypoganglionosis. Small number of neuronal bodies and nerve fibres. **d** Neuronal dysplasia (hyperganglionosis). Presence of large bundles of intrinsic nerve fibres combined with a large number of neuronal bodies occurring singly or in groups in the myenteric plexus, within the circular muscle layer, in the submucosa and occasionally in the mucosa. **e** Absence of intrinsic innervation in the presence of extrinsic innervation of the colon. Cholinergic extrinsic nerve fibres are penetrating through the longitudinal muscle layer and forming bundles between the circular and longitudinal muscle layers. Note absence of neuronal bodies. **f** Absence of extrinsic and intrinsic innervation. Lack of nerve fibres and neuronal bodies in the entire wall of the small and/or large intestine

RUGE 1974). The sex ratio of patients with absence of intestinal innervation has been estimated at approximately 1:1 (RUDIN et al. 1986a).

Among 207 patients suffering from classical aganglionosis (short segment) only six patients were siblings (BODIAN and CARTER 1963). The length of the aganglionic segment was in general constant in members of the same family. The risks of the illness occurring in children from families with aganglionosis is estimated to be 1:20 for males and 1:100 for females. For aganglionosis affecting a long segment, the risk is estimated to be 1:10, independent of sex. In contrast, eight siblings from four families have been reported among 16 patients suffering from a partial defect or absence of the enteric nervous system. The total number of children in the affected families is 27. An analysis of these families suggests autosomal-recessive inheritance of the disease (RUDIN et al. 1986a). This is in agreement with the results published by another group (MACKINNON and COHEN 1977). Absence of the enteric nervous system is probably not linked to aganglionosis affecting a short segment but is possibly connected to the long segment variant or to Zuelzer-Wilson's disease, as patients suffering from a combination of aganglionosis of the entire colon with absence of innervation of the small intestine have been described (RUDIN et al. 1986b).

8 Pathogenesis

8.1 Primary Forms of Abnormal Innervation

The extrinsic parasympathetic innervation of the intestine begins to develop during the 5th and 6th week after conception (OKAMOTO and UEDA 1967). The proliferation of extrinsic parasympathetic nerves of the sacral root S2–S4 continues until the end of the 7th week. Neuroblasts of the vagus nerve migrate into the intestinal wall from the 7th to the 12th week. According to one hypothesis this migration proceeds in the cranial-caudal direction, beginning in the oesophagus and stomach. By the end of the 8th week neuroblasts are found in the colon down to the left curvature and after 12 weeks the entire colon is innervated. The neuroblasts subsequently form intrinsic plexuses. It is proposed that aganglionosis of the short distal colonic segment is caused by a late defect of neuroblast migration (YNTEMA and HAMMOND 1954; MEIER-RUGE 1974). On the other hand, absence of innervation of the intestine could result from an earlier event, occurring during the 5th or 6th week, that prevents the development of both extrinsic innervation and intrinsic plexuses.

Other workers have described migration of neuroblasts proceeding from both ends of the embryonic intestine ('dual origin and gradient theory', TAM and LISTER 1986). In addition, influences of the microenvironment (LE DOUARIN 1981) and of trophic substances (BURNSTOCK 1981; HENDRY et al. 1981) have been stressed recently. Finally, intra-uterine intestinal ischaemia or infections could cause defects of innervation.

8.2 Secondary Forms of Abnormal Innervation

Ischaemia, infections (viruses, Chagas, disease), severe necrotising colitis, and drugs can cause neuronal destruction.

9 Conclusions

The diagnosis of the five forms of abnormal innervation of the intestine requires morphological analysis of biopsies by a pathologist who is familiar with their histological and histochemical features and with the benefits and limitations of the techniques applied. The diagnosis must be precise because it governs management, usually curative surgery, and gives prognostic information in at least one of the diseases which is often incompatible with life. Current understanding allows the following conclusions to be drawn:

1. Several biopsies should be taken at defined distances (interval 1 cm), beginning at the linea dentata in order to determine the extent of the lesion and to recognise lesions present in a very short segment of the colon.
2. The anatomical site of a biopsy must be taken into consideration when making a diagnosis (see Sect. 5.1.1).
3. A suction biopsy should contain the mucosa, muscularis mucosae and parts of the submucosa. In our opinion a biopsy containing mucosa only often fails to give a precise diagnosis of the various lesions.
4. A precise diagnosis on the basis of tinctorial stains cannot be reached.
5. Diagnosis based on enzyme histochemical reactions for acetylcholinesterase and lactate dehydrogenase has been shown to be safe, provided an experienced technician processes and an experienced pathologist examines the specimens. Time and costs for this procedure can be saved by optimising aliquoting and storage of the reagents. A disadvantage of this procedure is the necessity of a fast transport on ice of the tissue: enzyme histochemical reactions should be carried out within 10 hours.
6. At least six sections per biopsy should be examined.
7. The diagnosis can also be made using immunocytochemical methods, which can be applied to formaldehyde-fixed specimens. Using antisera or antibodies raised against protein S-100, neurone-specific enolase or synaptophysin, a diagnosis can be reached (HALL and LAMPERT 1985;

TAGUCHI et al. 1985). In addition, antibodies reacting with biogenic amines, peptides or choline acetyltransferase can be applied to define the type of neuronal bodies and nerve fibres. In our experience the diagnosis based on cryostat sections and enzyme histochemistry is faster and more reliable than immunohistochemistry performed on fixed specimens.

8. It is important to use techniques well established in a given laboratory to reach a precise diagnosis because of its implications for the treatment of the patient.
9. It should be borne in mind that a transition zone exists between the abnormally and normally innervated segments which should be resected at surgery, because otherwise functional intestinal obstruction may persist.

It has been claimed that the lesions of aganglionosis show an evolution with age. Although we have been unable to confirm a systematic distinction of types of disordered innervation depending on the age of the infant as described recently (DE BRITO and MAKSOUD 1987), the possibility of evolution of lesions with time needs further investigation.

Acknowledgement. The authors gratefully acknowledge the expert technical assistance of Mrs. M. Kasper.

References

Bennett A, Garrett JR, Howard ER (1968) Adrenergic myenteric nerves in Hirschsprung's disease. Br Med J I:487–489

Blisard KS, Kleinman R (1986) Hirschsprung's disease: a clinical and pathologic overview. Hum Pathol 17:1189–1191

Bodian M, Carter CO (1963) A family study of Hirschsprung's disease. Ann Hum Genet 26:261 271

Burnstock G (1981) Current approaches to development of the autonomic nervous system: clues to clinical problems. In: Elliott K, Lawrenson G (eds) Development of the autonomic nervous system. Ciba Foundation Symposium 83. Pitman Medical, London, pp 1–18

De Brito IA, Maksoud JG (1987) Evolution with age of the acetylcholinesterase activity in rectal suction biopsy in Hirschsprung's disease. J Pediatr Surg 22:425–430

Dobbins WO, Bill AH (1965) Diagnosis of Hirschsprung's disease excluded by rectal suction biopsy. N Engl J Med 272:990–993

Ehrenpreis T (1970) Hirschsprung's disease. Year Book Medical, Chicago, pp 57–58

Elliott K, Lawrenson G (1981) Development of the autonomic nervous system. Ciba Foundation Symposium 83. Pitman Medical, London

Fadda B, Maier WA, Meier-Ruge W, Schaerli A, Daum R (1983) Neuronale intestinale Dysplasie. Eine kritische 10-Jahresanalyse klinischer und bioptischer Diagnostik. Z Kinderchir 38:305–311

Garrett JR, Howard ER (1981) Myenteric plexus of the hind-gut: developmental abnormalities in humans and experimental studies. In: Elliott K, Lawrenson G (eds) Development of the autonomic nervous system. Ciba Foundation Symposium 83. Pitman Medical, London, pp 326–354

Garrett JR, Howard ER, Nixon HH (1969) Histochemical diagnosis of Hirschsprung's disease. Lancet II:436

Guesdon JL, Ternynck T, Avrameas S (1979) The use of avidin-biotin interaction in immunoenzymatic techniques. J Histochem Cytochem 27:1131–1139

Gullotta F, Straaten G (1977) Hirschsprungsche Krankheit mit gleichzeitiger Aganglionose und sogenannter neuronaler Kolondysplasie. Z Kinderchir 20:42–49

Hall CL, Lampert PW (1985) Immunohistochemistry as an aid in the diagnosis of Hirschsprung's disease. Am J Clin Pathol 83:177–181

Hamoudi AB, Reiner CB, Boles ET jr, McClung HJ, Kerzner B (1982) Acetylthiocholinesterase staining activity of rectal mucosa. Arch Pathol Lab Med 106:670–672

Hendry IA, Hill CE, Bonyhady RE (1981) Interactions between developing autonomic neurons and their target tissues. In: Elliot K, Lawrenson G (eds) Development of the autonomic nervous system. Ciba Foundation Symposium 83. Pitman Medical, London, pp 194–212

Hess R, Scarpelli DG, Pearse AGE (1985) The cytochemical localization of oxidative enzymes. II. Pyridine nucleotide-linked dehydrogenases. J Biophys Biochem Cytol 4:753–760

Hirschsprung H (1888) Stuhlträgheit Neugeborener in Folge von Dilatation und Hypertrophie des Colon. Jb Kinderheilk 27:1–7

Ikeda K, Got S (1986) Total colonic aganglionosis with or without small bowl involvement: an analysis of 137 patients. J Pediatr Surg 21:319–322

Kamijo K, Hiatt RB, Koelle FB (1953) Congenital megacolon. A comparison of the spastic and hypertrophied segments with respect to cholinesterase activities and sensitivities to acetylcholine, DFP and the barium ion. Gastroenterology 24:173–185

Karnovsky MJ, Roots L (1964) A "direct-coloring" thiocholine method for cholinesterase. J Histochem Cytochem 12:219–221

Le Douarin NM (1981) Plasticity in the development of the peripheral nervous system. In: Elliott K, Lawrenson G (eds) Development of the autonomic nervous system. Ciba Foundation Symposium 83. Pitman Medical, London, pp 19–50

Mackinnon AE, Cohen SJ (1977) Total intestinal aganglionosis. Arch Dis Child 52:898–899

Meier-Ruge W (1968) Das Megacolon. Virchows Arch [A]344:67–85

Meier-Ruge W (1972) Fortschritte in der Diagnostik des aganglionären Segments. Pädiatr Pädol 2:55–64

Meier-Ruge W (1974) Hirschsprung's disease: its aetiology, pathogenesis and differential diagnosis. In: Grundmann E, Kirsten WH (eds) Current topics in pathology, vol 59. Springer, Berlin Heidelberg New York, pp 131–179

Meier-Ruge W (1982) Diagnosis of Hirschsprung's disease, morphological diagnosis. In: Holschneider AM (ed) Hirschsprung's disease. Hippokrates, Stuttgart; Thieme-Stratton, New York, pp 62–71

Meier-Ruge W (1983) Zur Pathogenese anorektaler Anomalien und Dysganglionosen. In: Hofmann-v. Kap-herr S (eds) Anorektale Fehlbildungen. Gustav Fischer, Stuttgart, pp 19–22

Meier-Ruge W (1985) Der ultrakurze Morbus Hirschsprung. Ein bioptisch zuverlässig objektivierbares Krankheitsbild. Z Kinderchir 40:146–150

Meier-Ruge W, Morger R (1968) Neue Gesichtspunkte zur Pathogenese und Klinik des Morbus Hirschsprung. Schweiz Med Wochenschr 98:209–214

Meier-Ruge W, Hunziker O, Tobler H-J, Walliser C (1972) The pathophysiology of aganglionosis of the entire colon (Zuelzer-Wilson syndrome). Beitr Pathol 147:228–236

Niemi M, Kouvalainen K, Hjelt L (1961) Cholinesterase and monoamine oxidase in congenital megacolon. J Pathol Bateriol 82:363–366

Okamoto E, Ueda T (1967) Embryogenesis of intramural ganglia of the gut and its relation to Hirschsprung's disease. J Pediatr Surg 2:437–443

Rehbein F, Halsband H, Hofmann S (1969) Hirschsprungsche Krankheit mit langem engen Segment. Dtsch Med Wochenschr 14:708–716

Rudin C, Jenny P, Ohnacker H, Heitz PU (1986a) Absence of the enteric nervous system in the newborn: presentation of three patients and review of the literature. J Pediatr Surg 21:313–318

Rudin C, Jenny PM, Fliegel CP, Ohnacker H, Heitz PU (1986b) Zuelzer-Wilson-Syndrom bei fehlender Darminnervation. Z Kinderchir 41:287–292

Schaerli AF, Meier-Ruge W (1981) Localized and disseminated forms of neuronal intestinal dysplasia mimicking Hirschsprung's disease. J Pediatr Surg 16:164–170

Seldenrijk CA, van der Harten HJ, Klueck P, Tibboel D, Moorman-Voestermanns K, Meijer CJLM (1986) Zonal aganglionosis. Virchows Arch [A]410:75–81

Sternberger LA (1986) Immunocytochemistry, 3rd edn. John Wiley, New York

Taguchi T, Tanaka K, Ikeda K (1985) Immunohistochemical study of neuron specific enolase and S-100 protein in Hirschsprung's disease. Virchows Arch [A]405:399–409

Tam PKH, Lister J (1986) Development profile of neuron-specific enolase in human gut and its implications in Hirschsprung's disease. Gastroenterology 90:1901–1906

Wakely PE jr, McAdams AJ (1984) Acetylcholinesterase histochemistry and the diagnosis of Hirschsprung's disease: a 3 1/2 year experience. Pediatr Pathol 2:35–46

Weinberg AG (1975) Hirschsprung's disease – a pathologist's view. In: Rosenberg HS, Bolande RP (eds) Perspectives in pediatric pathology, vol 2. Medical Publishers, Chicago, pp 207–239

Yntema CL, Hammond WS (1954) The origin of intrinsic ganglia of trunk viscera from vagal neural crest in chick embryo. J Comp Neurol 101:515–541

Ziegler HW, Heitz PU, Kasper M, Spichtin HP, Ulrich J (1984) Aganglionosis of the colon. Morphologic investigations in 524 patients. Pathol Res Pract 178:543–547

Zuelzer WW, Wilson JL (1948) Functional intestinal obstruction on a congenital neurogenic basis in infancy. Am J Dis Child 75:40–64

E Malignant Polyps – Pathological Factors Governing Clinical Management[1]

P. HERMANEK

1 Introduction

The idea that colorectal carcinoma arises from dysplasia is widely accepted nowadays. Within the framework of this dysplasia-carcinoma sequence, there are different morphological presentations which range from mild dysplasia to obvious invasive and metastasising carcinoma (Fig. 1). The stepwise transitions have not yet been uniformly named, so that up to now different clinical conclusions can still be drawn from the same histological findings.

The commonest form of dysplasia in the colon and rectum manifests itself macroscopically as a polyp, in other words, as a circumscribed lesion which projects from the mucosa into the lumen. When such polyps are found in the colon and rectum, one must consider the possibility that they may be neoplastic polyps (adenomas, polypoid dysplasias) in which carcinoma may have already developed. This has diagnostic and therapeutic consequences which can often be assessed in differing ways.

---

[1] This paper is dedicated to Prof. Dr. KURT ELSTER, a pioneer in the field of modern gastroenterological pathology, on the occasion of his 70th birthday.

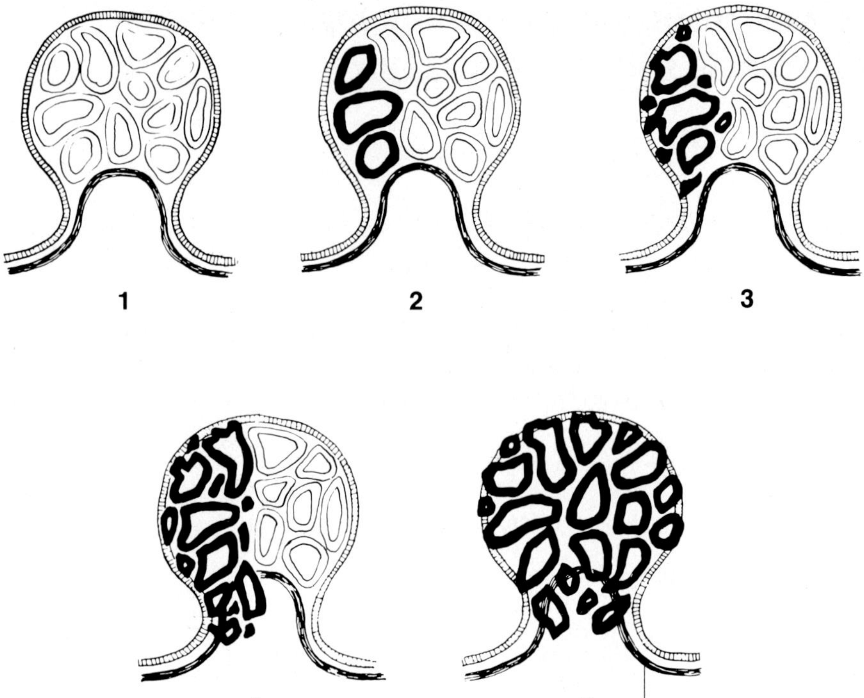

Fig. 1. Dysplasia-carcinoma sequence. *Thick black lines*: epithelial structures with cellular features of malignancy. *1*, Adenoma with mild or moderate dysplasia (low grade dysplasia); *2*, adenoma with severe dysplasia, type a (carcinoma in situ, pTis, intra-epithelial neoplasm, high grade dysplasia); *3*, adenoma with severe dysplasia, type b (intramucosal carcinoma, pTis) (lesion with invasion of the lamina propria, but without potential for metastasis); *4*, adenoma with invasive carcinoma (invasion of the submucosa, pT1); *5*, adenocarcinoma with invasion of the submucosa only (pT1)

2 Nomenclature of the Dysplasia-Carcinoma Sequence

Dysplasia is defined as an unequivocal neoplastic epithelial alteration without invasive growth (Fig. 1/1 and 1/2). It is characterised by cytological atypia, aberrant differentiation and disorganised architecture (MORSON et al. 1985). One can, depending on the extent of deviation from the normal, make a distinction between mild, moderate and severe dysplasia, whereby severe dysplasia corresponds to carcinoma in situ or intra-epithelial neoplasia.

When a neoplasm in the colon or rectum has invaded at least the submucosa and therefore has metastatic potential (Fig. 1/4, 1/5, 2), it can be considered a carcinoma in a biological and clinical sense. These lesions are termed invasive carcinomas (MORSON and SOBIN 1976).

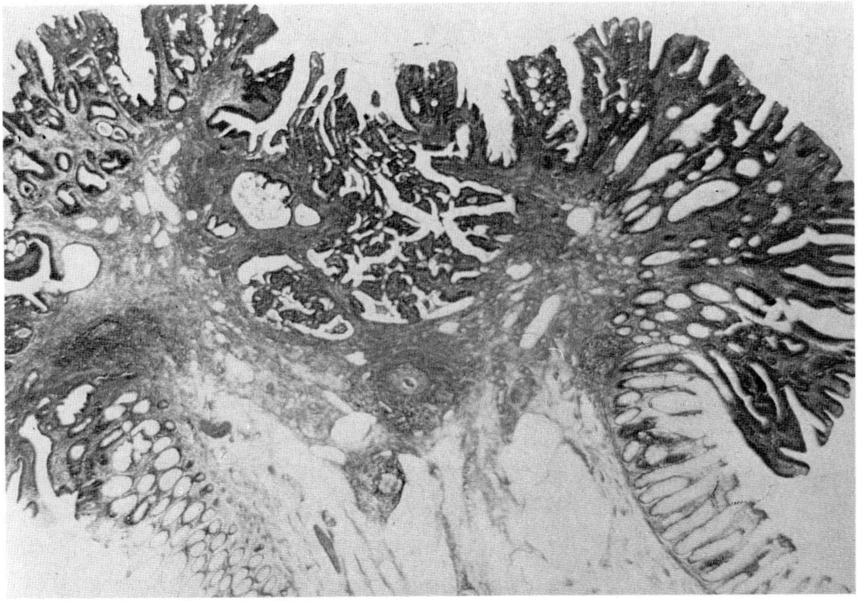

Fig. 2. Malignant polyp: Adenoma with adenocarcinoma removed by endoscopic polypectomy. The carcinoma is limited to the submucosal zone of the head of polyp and has been removed completely

Between dysplasia and carcinoma as defined above, we find an intermediate step: a neoplasm which shows invasive growth into the lamina propria or between fibres of the muscularis mucosae, but does not reach the submucosa (Fig. 1/3). According to clinical experience, lymph node metastasis is not to be expected in these 'mucosal' or 'intramucosal' carcinomas (FENOGLIO-PREISER 1985) because, according to FENOGLIO et al. (1973), lymphatic vessels are found only at the level of and below the crypt bases. This explanation is not entirely tenable, however, because in pathological conditions lymph vessels containing tumour cells can be demonstrated between the mucosal crypts (Fig. 3). Nevertheless, the irrefutable fact remains that in 'mucosal carcinomas' metastasis does not take place and local excision of the lesion with a small margin of clearance represents adequate treatment. According to the new pTNM Classification (UICC 1987), such lesions, as well as adenomas with severe dysplasia, are classified as in situ carcinomas. We do not use this nomenclature in order to avoid confusion and overtreatment; we routinely name all of these lesions adenomas with severe dysplasia. In compiling statistics on the results of therapy for colorectal carcinoma, one should only include tumours which have invaded at least the submucosa.

The dysplasias from which the carcinomas arise develop in rare cases from chronic inflammations (mostly ulcerative colitis, rarely Crohn's disease or schistosomiasis). They very rarely develop within non-neoplastic

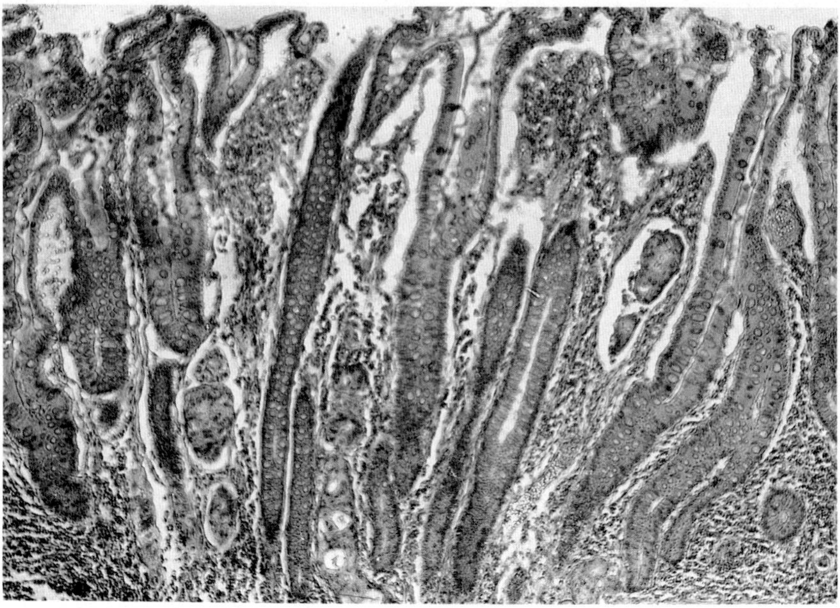

Fig. 3. Tumour cells within lymphatic vessels between the crypts (at a level higher than the lowest portion of the crypts). Patient with advanced invasive adenocarcinoma with extensive lymphatic spread

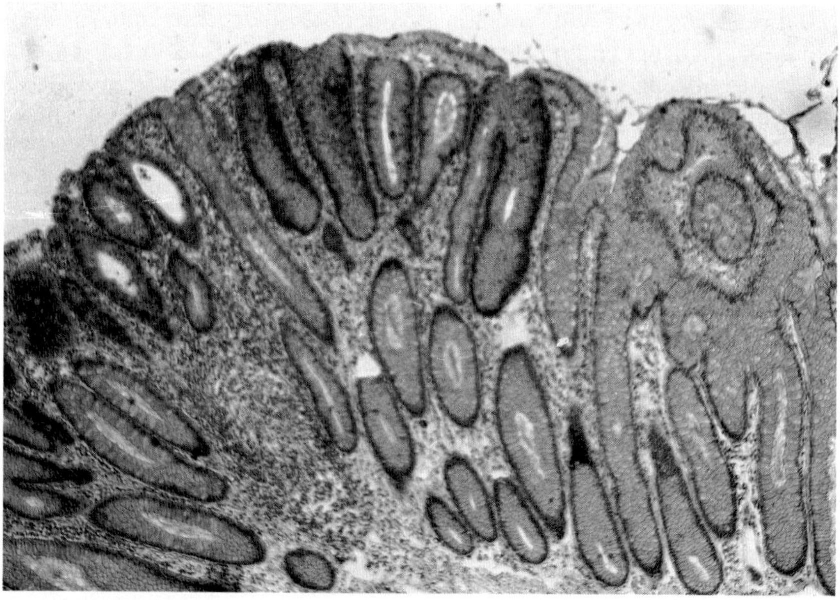

Fig. 4. So-called flat adenoma. Some crypts with dysplastic epithelium, without significant projection from the mucosa into the lumen

Table 1. Different manifestations of adenomas

Numer	Solitary Multiple Polyposis (> 100) = adenomatosis	
Macroscopic appearance	Flat Polypoid: sessile semi-pedunculated pedunculated	
Histological type	Tubular Tubulovillous Villous	
Grade of dysplasia	Mild Moderate	low
	Severe	high

polyps such as Peutz-Jeghers, juvenile or hyperplastic polyps or those following uretero-sigmoidostomy. The great majority of dysplasias develop in non-inflamed mucosa, namely as a focal change which can be termed an adenoma. These adenomas have a variety of characteristics. Table 1 shows the different possibilities in number, macroscopic and histological type and degree of dysplasia. By far the commonest type is a carcinoma which develops in a solitary or in one of multiple polypoid adenomas. 'Flat adenomas' (Fig. 4) remain relatively uncommon; they are difficult to recognise at endoscopy, except in cases of melanosis coli, in which the adenomas stand out as non-pigmented areas. Carcinoma can also develop in flat adenomas and give rise to what has been described in the literature as 'carcinoma de novo'.

3 Definition of Malignant Polyps

The concept of malignant polyps has been accorded different meanings in the literature (FORDE 1987). Sometimes it is used to describe adenomas with severe dysplasia, sometimes invasive carcinomas, sometimes it is even used to include both lesions. In the following, a malignant polyp shall be considered *a carcinoma which has invaded the submucosa and which is discovered during microscopic examination of an endoscopically removed polyp.*

This definition encompasses the common cases in which carcinoma develops in a polypoid adenoma, as well as the considerably rarer cases in which a polyp formation is completely formed of invasive carcinoma. These cases are sometimes termed polypoid carcinomas. However, here one must emphasise that the evidence for residual adenoma is not of independent prognostic significance for the biological and clinical behaviour.

Table 2. Frequency of invasive carcinoma in adenomas. Dependence on size, macroscopic and histological type of adenoma. ERCRP (Erlangen Registry of Colorectal Polyps) 1978–1984. a) Total results (endoscopically and surgically removed adenomas, adenomas as incidental findings during colorectal surgery). b) Only endoscopically removed adenomas

Adenoma groups	Frequency of carcinoma			
	a)		b)	
Histological type				
Tubular	180/4894	(3.7%)	27/3165	(0.9%)
Tubulovillous	307/1605	(19.1%)	45/ 975	(4.6%)
Villous	203/ 384	(52.9%)	5/ 98	(5.1%)
Size				
≤ 5 mm	1/3039	(0.03%)	0/2112	(0%)
6–10 mm	14/1508	(0.9%)	9/1055	(0.9%)
11–20 mm	87/1164	(7.5%)	39/ 840	(4.6%)
21–30 mm	114/ 386	(29.5%)	20/ 204	(9.8%)
31–40 mm	111/ 224	(49.6%)	1/ 42	(2.4%)
> 40 mm	347/ 472	(73.5%)	4/ 28	(14.3%)
Unknown	16/ 90	(17.8%)	4/ 57	(7.0%)
Macroscopic appearance				
Sessile	45/1280	(3.5%)	32/ 943	(3.4%)
Semi-pedunculated	37/ 984	(3.8%)	12/ 560	(2.1%)
Pedunculated	605/4540	(13.4%)	33/2688	(1.2%)
Unknown	3/ 79	(3.8%)	0/ 47	(0%)
Total material	690/6883	(10.0%)	77/4238	(1.8%)

The majority of malignant polyps are carcinomas in which invasion is limited to the submucosa. This includes carcinomas which are defined as pT1 tumours according to the UICC pTNM Classification, and which are often designated as early colorectal carcinomas (HERMANEK and GALL 1986; MORSON 1985). There are also other early colorectal carcinomas which do not present as endoscopically resectable polyps, and rarely malignant polyps may lie on top of more deeply infiltrating carcinomas.

The probability that an invasive carcinoma has already developed in an adenoma depends on the size of the adenoma as well as on its macroscopic and histological type (Table 2) (HERMANEK et al. 1983) and on the degree of dysplasia in the adenoma (MUTO et al. 1975).

4 Diagnosis

Forceps biopsies from polyps of the colon and rectum allow diagnosis of neoplastic or non-neoplastic lesions. Here one must always emphasise that when neoplastic epithelium is found in a forceps biopsy, further differentiation is impossible, and especially that the presence of an invasive car-

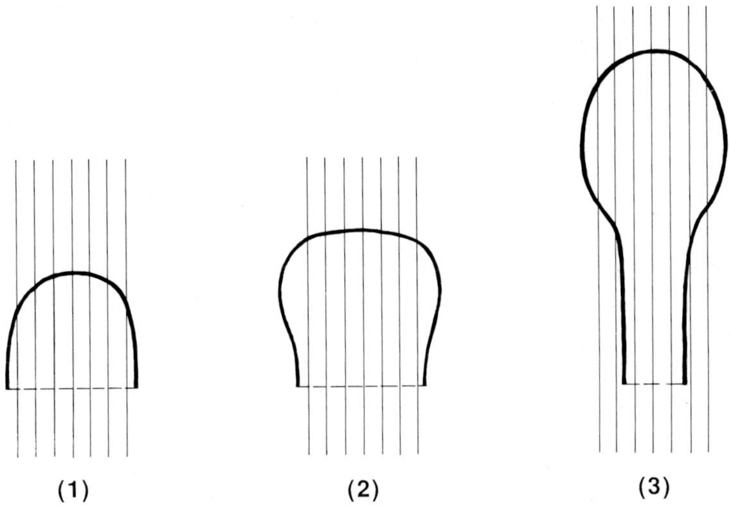

Fig. 5. Histological methods in colorectal polyps. Direction of sectioning: (*1*) sessile, (*2*) semipedunculated, (*3*) pedunculated polyp

cinoma in the submucosa cannot be excluded; this is because forceps biopsies do not include the submucosa. When dysplasia is found in forceps biopsies from polypoid lesions we therefore always include the following sentence in the pathology report: "A definitive assessment of the biopsied polypoid growth is only possible after the microscopic examination of the completely removed lesion."

The procedure of choice for making a definitive diagnosis of neoplastic polyps is endoscopic polypectomy using a diathermy snare. Experienced endoscopists can remove polyps with bases of 15–20 mm in one piece. This is important for the pathologist's assessment because only when the polypoid growth has been removed whole and not piecemeal is it possible to say whether or not the adenoma and/or carcinoma has been completely excised (Morson 1985).

Polyps which have been removed with a diathermy snare should, as a rule, be immediately fixed in formalin. In the case of sessile or semipedunculated polyps, where the diameter of the resection area is small, we recommend that the base be marked before fixation by perpendicularly inserting a pin or by Indian ink. In this fashion, the pathologist can later easily recognise the resection area, a feat which is otherwise difficult, if not impossible, because after fixation the resection area often retracts and is covered by the surrounding polypoid mucosa.

In processing polyps for histology, precise orientation of the specimen is necessary during embedding so that the direction of sectioning is perpendicular to that of the resection line; only in this fashion can one make an assessment of the completeness of the removal of the adenoma or carcinoma. It is therefore essential to identify the resection area (base or stalk) and to embed polyps carefully as shown in Fig. 5.

Definite assessment of whether or not there is a small carcinoma in an adenoma, and whether the adenoma and/or the carcinoma within it has been completely removed, requires the preparation of step sections (not serial sections). Only then can one confidently write the histology report (BLUNDELL and EARNEST 1980; HERMANEK 1983).

5 Pathologist's Report on the Histological Assessment of Excised Polyps

The histology report on an excised polyp should include all of the statements listed in Table 3. Using these, the clinician can appropriately plan further therapeutic procedures.

For the assessment of adequacy of excision, microscopic identification of the eosinophilic coagulation necrosis caused by the diathermy snare at the resection area is of decisive importance. We speak of incomplete excision when the tumour growth in this area reaches the resection line. If tumour lies in the area of diathermy, but does not reach the resection line, or when the malignant polyp has been sent in several pieces, and topographical orientation of the specimen is uncertain (LIPPER et al. 1983), we say that excision is doubtfully complete even when the endoscopist believes that removal was complete.

Information on the histological type and the degree of differentiation of malignant polyps is considered important by all authors. In our material the majority were ordinary adenocarcinomas and mucinous adenocarcinomas were rare, forming only 4.4% (6/137). Grading should be done according to DUKES and BUSSEY's method (1958), where cellular arrangement is taken into consideration (Fig. 6). A disorganisation of glands and single cells at the advancing front of the tumour alone do not warrant grade 3. The majority of tumours having these features are well or moderately differentiated carcinomas. According to four large studies (COOPER 1983; MORSON et al. 1984; HAGGITT et al. 1985; CRANLEY et al. 1986), the percentage of poorly differentiated carcinoma in malignant polyps was 5% (11/220); our own study showed 7.3% (10/137).

The significance of invasion of lymphatic vessels is still a controversial issue. It is of decisive importance to assess lymphatic invasion carefully, because according to our own experience, this diagnosis is too often made. Shrinkage during embedding causes formation of spaces around tumour nests which are incorrectly diagnosed as lymphatic vessel invasion. The diagnosis of lymphatic vessel invasion can only be made when clumps of tumour cells can be found in channels which are unequivocally lined with endothelium (Fig. 7).

With regard to consideration of further therapeutic procedures in the event of carcinoma, we began to differentiate between low risk and high the risk cases in 1977 (HERMANEK 1977). This gives the clinician some idea

Table 3. Reporting excised polyps

1. Histological classification[a]:	Non-neoplastic polyp Neoplastic epithelial polp: adenoma adenoma with carcinoma[b] carcinoma Neoplastic polyp of other type (i.e. carcinoid tumour, leiomyoma etc.)
2. Adequacy of removal[c]:	Incomplete Doubtfully complete Complete
3. In the case of carcinoma (with or without adenoma):	
a) Histological type[a]	Adenocarcinoma Mucinous adenocarcinoma Signet-ring cell carcinoma Undifferentiated carcinoma Other
b) Histological grading[d]	G1 well differentiated G2 moderately differentiated G3 poorly differentiated G4 undifferentiated
c) Invasion of lymphatics	Yes No
d) Summary of assessment of risk of lymph node metastases being already present:	
High risk	Poorly differentiated (G3) or undifferentiated (G4) and/or microscopically demonstrated invasion of lymphatic vessels
Low risk	All other forms

[a] Corresponds to the WHO Classification (MORSON and SOBIN 1976.

[b] Only neoplastic proliferations with invasion at least into the submucosa are considered carcinomas.

[c] In polyps in which adenomatous as well as carcinomatous structures are present, one should state for each portion whether the lesion has been completely removed or not.

[d] In the event that there are different degrees of differentiation, the classification should be made according to the most unfavourable degree; signetring cell and undifferentiated carcinomas are classified as G4.

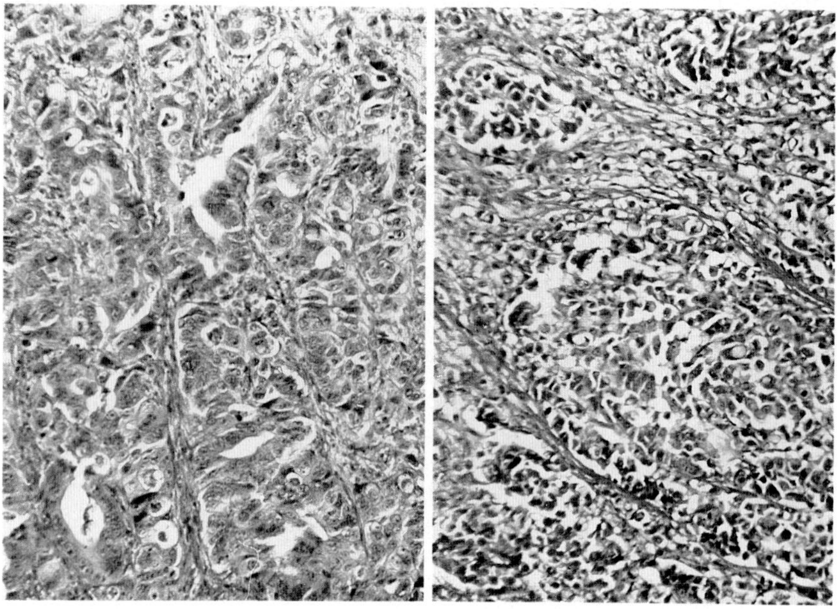

Fig. 6. Poorly differentiated adenocarcinoma

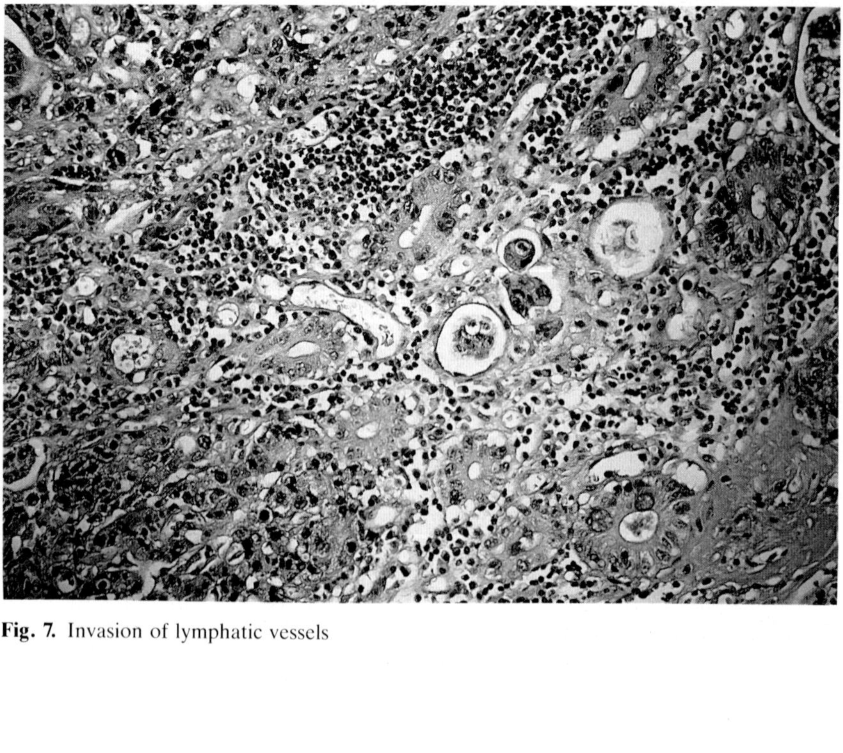

Fig. 7. Invasion of lymphatic vessels

of the risk of lymph node metastases being present at the time of excision of the polyp.

Some authors consider that other statements on the polypectomy specimen are relevant in planning further therapy. These include: macroscopic type (sessile, semi-pedunculated, pedunculated), histological type of residual adenoma (tubular, tubulovillous, villous), subdivision of the depth of invasion and invasion of veins. We are of the opinion that all of these categories are of no clinical significance (see below).

6 Clinical Consequences

Therapeutic procedures following excision of a malignant polyp should be planned in the first instance according to whether or not the carcinoma was completely removed during polypectomy.

6.1 Procedure in the Event of Complete Removal of Carcinoma

The titles of two publications illustrate the range of opinion on this topic: "Endoscopic Polypectomy: Inadequate Treatment for Invasive Colorectal Carcinoma" (COLACCHIO et al. 1981) and "Hands Off Cancerous Large Bowel Polyps" (RIDDELL 1985). A comprehensive overview of differing opinions in the English literature can be found in WILCOX et al. (1986). There is an ever increasing tendency not to recommend further major surgery following complete endoscopic removal of a malignant polyp. Some surgeons share this opinion (DE COSSE 1984; GALL and SCHEELE 1986).

If the carcinoma in a malignant polyp has been completely removed, the major concern of the clinician is whether or not regional lymph node metastases are present, because clearance of such deposits is the only rationale for major surgery. Unfortunately, even with modern imaging techniques, reliable evaluation of the status of regional lymph nodes is impossible. Metastases from completely removed malignant polyps, as a general rule, are small and only involve a few lymph nodes. In our own 13 cases, in which lymph node metastases were found at radical surgery following excision of a malignant polyp, the largest diameter of involved lymph nodes in seven patients was 5 mm or less, greater than 5–10 mm in three patients, and greater than 10 mm in only three patients.

The most reliable method for evaluating the risk of lymph node metastases is at present the histological evaluation of the primary tumour. At St. Mark's Hospital in London, only poor differentiation of the carcinoma is considered to indicate high potential for lymph node metastasis. Since 1977, we in Erlangen have also considered histological evidence of lymphatic vessel invasion as a marker of high metastatic risk; this agrees with the

Table 4. Microscopic findings in polypectomy specimens related to subsequent major surgery specimens. (1) Dept. of Surgery and Dept. of Medicine, Univ. of Erlangen, 1969–1986; (2) Institute of Pathology, Bayreuth, 1982–1987 (Prof. Dr. M. STOLTE, unpublished data)

Findings in polypectomy specimens	Findings in subsequent surgical specimens	
	Incidence of regional lymph node metastasis	
A) Judgement of the risk of regional lymph node metastasis having already taken place	(1)	(2)
Low risk	2/41 = 5%	2/42 = 5%
High risk	11/41 = 27%	5/18 = 27%
	Incidence of residual carcinoma in the intestinal wall	
	(1)	(2)
B) Adequacy of removal		
Complete	0/36 = 0%	0/35 = 0%
Doubtfully	1/11 = 9%	–
Incomplete	13/35 = 37%	21/34 = 60%

Note: The percentage of high risk cases is higher in Erlangen (1) because in the last 10 years, patients with low risk tumours have undergone major surgery only in the relatively rare event of incomplete polypectomy.

opinions of many American authors (SHATNEY et al. 1974; WOLFF and SHINYA 1975; STEARNS 1978; WITT and WINAWER 1981; LIPPER et al. 1983; CHRISTIE 1984; FENOGLIO-PREISER 1985; RIDDELL 1985). We have not yet observed undifferentiated carcinoma or signet ring cell carcinoma within malignant polyps, but we have introduced these cases into the concept of low and high risk (see page 284).

Other factors discussed in the literature appear to us to be of no relevance – we base this opinion on examinations of resected specimens following classical surgery. Besides depth of infiltration only the grade of differentiation and histologically proven invasion of lymphatic vessels show an independent influence on the incidence of lymph node metastases (HERMANEK and GIEDL 1988). The subdivision of the level of invasion (1–4, corresponding to the head, neck or base of the polyp and the submucosa of the gut wall according to HAGGITT et al. 1985) and the macroscopic type of the malignant polyp (whether pedunculated, semi-pedunculated or sessile), while related to the likelihood of complete removal, have no certain influence on the incidence of lymph node metastases (COOPER 1983; MORSON et al. 1984; CRANLEY et al. 1986). The same holds true for the presence or absence of residual benign adenoma in malignant polyps

(COOPER 1983; LIPPER et al. 1983; MORSON et al. 1984; HAGGITT et al. 1985; RIDDELL 1985; CRANLEY et al. 1986) or the histological type of such a residual adenoma (CRANLEY et al. 1986). Proof of invasion of veins indicates a higher risk for haematogenous distant metastases, but is of no value in predicting lymph node metastases (RIDDELL 1983).

The data compiled in Table 4 A demonstrate that assessment of the grade of differentiation and lymphatic vessel invasion are of value in selecting patients for major surgery following excision of a malignant polyp. Our own findings, as well as those from the Bayreuth Institute of Pathology, where histological assessment was carried out by independent pathologists (Prof. Dr. Stolte and Dr. Eydt), are shown. The nearly identical results demonstrate that the recommendations made on the basis of histological assessment are reproducible. Nevertheless, histological parameters only provide an estimate of risk and the possibility that in a small proportion of unoperated cases lymph node metastases may remain behind must be considered. We have estimated this risk to be about 3%–5% (HERMANEK and GALL 1986; HERMANEK and GIEDL 1988).

6.2 Procedure in the Event of Incomplete or Doubtfully Complete Removal of Carcinoma

There is a general consensus that further surgery is necessary when the pathologist finds tumour at the resection line of an excised malignant polyp; this also holds true even when the endoscopist thinks the lesion has been completely removed. This is illustrated in the following case report:

H. J., a 54 year-old female, underwent endoscopic polypectomy by an experienced endoscopist who was of the opinion that the lesion was completely removed. Histology showed an adenoma with moderately differentiated adenocarcinoma, reaching the resection line. Because the endoscopist was convinced that he had resected through healthy tissue, numerous biopsies from the polypectomy region were taken. No tumour tissue was found at microscopy. At the insistence of an external pathologist and the author (who was asked for a second opinion on this case), the patient was referred to the Department of Surgery of the University of Erlangen, where a low anterior resection was performed. Beneath the regenerated intact mucosa, at the polypectomy site, we found residual tumour in the submucosa of the resection specimen; its greatest dimension was 1.8 mm.

This case illustrates that any attempt to prove or rule out possible residual tumour by means of forceps biopsies is futile. Planning therapy on the basis of endoscopy results instead of on histology reports of the polypectomy specimen is to be strongly discouraged.

Clinical management following a pathologist's report of doubtfully complete removal of a malignant polyp is more troublesome. We have been cautious in such cases and have recommended further surgery, tailored according to the age and operative risk of the individual patient.

Table 4 B shows the results of employing the above policy for incompletely excised malignant polyps at two centres, with reference to the presence of residual tumour in the subsequent resection specimen. The fact that residual tumour was not found in the gut wall after incomplete removal, in every case, can be explained by the fact that during polypectomy the underlying gut wall also receives diathermy current and that the resulting millimetre-wide necrosis destroys any residual tumour present. However, the presence of residual tumour in about a third of the cases after incomplete polypectomy supports the view that further operation is indicated in such cases.

Many years ago, we recommended classical radical surgery, i.e. removal of the site of the primary tumour with wide margins of clearance and en bloc removal of the regional lymph nodes for all cases with 'incomplete removal' or 'doubtfully incomplete removal' of malignant polyps. On the basis of our own experience with limited treatment of early colorectal carcinoma over the past few years (HERMANEK and GALL 1986), and similar reports from other centres (LOCK et al. 1978; KILLINGBACK 1985; WHITEWAY et al. 1985), we now increasingly discuss the use of local surgical excision for low risk type malignant polyps which have been incompletely removed. According to the site of the lesion, one can perform transanal disc excision, segmental resection or tubular resection (GALL 1982). Important criteria for this are the individual's operative risk and the necessity to avoid a permanent colostomy.

6.3 Selection Criteria for Major Surgery Following Removal of Malignant Polyps

Table 5 summarises the treatment policy carried out in the Department of Surgery and the Department of Medicine at the University of Erlangen. This plan is followed in many other institutions in Germany and other German-speaking countries. Two important conditions are necessary for its success:

1. The histological analysis of the polypectomy specimens must be technically perfect (with optimal orientation) and careful (with step sections).
2. The patient must be willing to participate in a closely monitored follow-up programme. The purpose of this is to diagnose and treat any local recurrences at an early stage and thus achieve good results. Follow-up endoscopies are necessary for this; in the first year these should be performed every 3 months, and in the second year every 6 months.

The success of the policy is shown by the follow-up results from our patients who underwent endoscopic polypectomy only. The data summarised in Tables 6 and 7 as well as similar reports from other institutions support the current opinion that endoscopic polypectomy alone can be considered the procedure of choice in carefully selected patients with

Table 5. Therapeutic procedures in malignant polyps

Histological diagnosis on polypectomy specimen: adenocarcinoma

Adequacy of removal?

- Incomplete/doubtfully incomplete
  - Low risk → Surgical local excision (or classical cancer surgery)
  - High risk → Classical cancer surgery
- Complete
  - High risk → Classical cancer surgery
  - Low risk → No further surgery

malignant polyps (Wolff and Shinya 1975; Gillespie et al. 1979; Muto et al. 1980; Rossini et al. 1982; Christie 1984; Morson et al. 1984; Frei 1985; Cranley et al. 1986). One must recognise that even in appropriately selected patients there is a small (but not significantly increased) risk that endoscopic therapy alone will leave behind lymph node metastases in a small portion of cases (3%–5%) (see Sect. 6.1). This risk must be weighed against the risk of major surgery, especially in elderly patients in whom classical radical operation carries a significant surgical mortality. One must also consider the effect on the quality of life of a permanent colostomy in the case of carcinomas of the lower rectum. All of these factors should be discussed with the patient before agreeing a course of management.

The treatment of patients with malignant polyps is an example of how modern clinical oncology continuously seeks to tailor treatment for the individual patient. In planning therapy, the pathologist plays an important

Table 6. Reliability of criteria for recommending major surgery after endoscopic removal of malignant polyps (Dept. of Surgery and Dept. of Medicine, Univ. of Erlangen, 1969–1986)

Recommendation for major surgery	Number of patients	Positive findings on specimens of further major surgery: residual tumour in intestinal wall and/or regional lymph node metastasis
No	9	0
Yes	70	24 = 34%
Doubtful	8	1 = 13%

Table 7. Follow-up of patients with malignant polyps (Dept. of Surgery, Univ. of Erlangen, 1969–1985/31. 12. 1987)

Recommendation according to the findings on polypectomy specimens	Further major surgery after polypectomy	Number of patients	5-year survival rate (age-corrected with 95% confidence interval)	Median survival time (months)	Local recurrence or local residual tumour	Curative reoperation of local recurrence	Surgical mortality	Cancer deaths
No further surgery	Not performed	45	95 ± 16%	Undef.	1 (2%)	–	–	1 (2%)
	Performed	4	(100%)[a]	137.5	–	–	–	–
Further surgery	Performed	45	100 ± 1%	Undef.	1 (2%)	1 (2%)	1 (2%)	2 (4%)
	Not performed	10	(27%)[a]	30.0	5 (50%)	–	–	5 (50%)

[a] Unreliable because of the small number of patients.

role, and in order to achieve optimal results, a close and trusting cooperation between gastroenterologists, surgeons and pathologists is of decisive importance.

References

Blundell CR, Earnest DL (1980) A caution concerning conservative management of colonic polyps containing invasive carcinoma. Gastrointest Endosc 26:54–55

Christie JP (1984) Malignant colon polyps – cure by colonoscopy or colectomy? Am J Gastroenterol 79:543–547

Colacchio TA, Forde KA, Scantlebury VP (1981) Endoscopic polypectomy. Inadequate treatment for invasive colorectal carcinoma. Ann Surg 194:704–707

Cooper HS (1983) Surgical pathology of endoscopically removed malignant polyps of the colon and rectum. Am J Surg Pathol 7:613–623

Cranley JP, Petras RE, Carey WD, Paradis K, Sivak MV (1986) When is endoscopic polypectomy adequate therapy for colonic polyps containing invasive carcinoma? Gastroenterology 91:410–427

De Cosse JJ (1984) Malignant colorectal polyp. Gut 25:433–436

Dukes CE, Bussey HJR (1958) The spread of rectal cancer and its effect on prognosis. Br J Cancer 12:309–320

Fenoglio CM, Kaye GI, Lane N (1973) Distribution of human colonic lymphatics in normal, hyperplastic and adenomatous tissues. Gastroenterology 64:51–66

Fenoglio-Preiser CM (1985) The distribution of large intestinal lymphatics: relationship to risk of metastasis from carcinomas of the large intestine. In: Fenoglio-Preiser CM, Rossini FP (eds) Adenomas and adenomas containing carcinoma of the large bowel: advances in diagnosis and therapy. Cortina International, Verona; Raven, New York, pp 7–14

Forde KA (1987) The "malignant colon polyp". A critique and opinion. Surg Endosc 1:55–58

Frei JV (1985) Endoscopic large bowel polypectomy. Adequate treatment of some completely removed, minimally invasive lesions. Am J Surg Pathol 9:355–359

Gall FP (1982) Die tubuläre Rectum- und Colonresektion. Chirurg 53:489–494

Gall FP, Scheele J (1986) Maligne Tumoren des Rektums. In: Gall FP, Hermanek P, Tonak J (eds) Chriurgische Onkologie. Springer, Berlin Heidelberg New York, pp 520–580
Gillespie PE, Chambers TJ, Chan KW, Doronzo F, Morson BC, Williams CB (1979) Colonic adenomas – a colonoscopic survey. Gut 20:240–245
Haggitt RC, Glotzbach RE, Soffer EE, Wruble LD (1985) Prognostic factors in colorectal carcinomas arising in adenomas; implications for lesions removed by endoscopic polypectomy. Gastroenterology 89:328–336
Hermanek P (1977) On the diagnosis of colorectal polyps. Beitr Pathol 161:203–205
Hermanek P (1983) Polypectomy in the colorectum. Histological and oncological aspects. Endoscopy 15:158–161
Hermanek P, Gall FP (1986) Early (microinvasive) colorectal carcinoma. Pathology, diagnosis, surgical treatment. Int J Colorect Dis 1:79–84
Hermanek P, Giedl J (1988) Neues aus der chirurgischen Pathologie des kolorektalen Karzinoms. Wien Med Wochenschr 138:292–296
Hermanek P, Frühmorgen P, Guggenmoos-Holzmann I, Altendorf A, Matek W (1983) The malignant potential of colorectal polyps. A new statistical approach. Endoscopy 15:16–20
Killingback MJ (1985) Indications for local excision of rectal cancer. Br J Surg 72:54–56
Lipper St, Kahn LB, Ackermann LV (1983) The significance of microscopic invasive cancer in endoscopically removed polyps of the large bowel. Cancer 52:1691–1699
Lock MR, Cairns DW, Ritchie JK, Lockhart-Mummery HE (1978) The treatment of early colorectal cancer by local excision. Br J Surg 65:346–349
Morson BC (1966) Precancerous and early malignant lesions of the large intestine. Br J Surg 55:725–731
Morson BC (1985) Histological criteria for local excision. Br J Surg 72:S 53–54
Morson BC, Sobin LH (1976) Histological typing of intestinal tumours. International histological classification of tumours No. 15. WHO, Geneva
Morson BC, Bussey HJR, Samoorian S (1977) Policy of local excision for early cancer of the colorectum. Gut 18:1045–1050
Morson BC, Whiteway JE, Jones EA, Macrae FA, Williams CB (1984) Histopathology and prognosis of malignant colorectal polyps treated by endoscopic polypectomy. Gut 25:437–444
Morson BC, Jass JR, Sobin LH (1985) Precancerous lesions of the gastrointestinal tract. A histological classification. Bailliere Tindall, London
Muto T, Bussey HJR, Morson BC (1975) The evolution of cancer of the colon and rectum. Cancer 36:2251–2270
Muto T, Kamiya J, Sawada T et al. (1980) Colonoscopic polypectomy in diagnosis and treatment of early carcinoma of the large intestine. Dis Colon Rectum 23:68–75
Riddell RH (1985) Hands off "cancerous" large bowel polyps. Gastroenterology 89:432–441
Rossini FP, Ferrari A, Spandre M, Coverlizza S (1982) Coloscopic polypectomy in diagnosis and management of cancerous adenomas: an individual and multicentric experience. Endoscopy 14:124–127
Shatney CH, Lober PH, Gilbertsen VA, Sosin H (1974) The treatment of pedunculated adenomatous colorectal polyps with focal cancer. Surg Gynecol Obstet 139:845–850
Stearns Jr MW (1978) Benign and malignant neoplasms of colon and rectum. Diagnosis and management. Surg Clin North Am 58:605–618
UICC TNM Classification of malignant tumours, 4th edn (1987) Hermanek P, Sobin LH. Springer, Berlin Heidelberg New York, pp 47–49
Whiteway J, Nicholls RJ, Morson BC (1985) The role of surgical local excision in the treatment of rectal cancer. Br J Surg 72:694–697
Wilcox GM, Anderson PB, Colacchio TA (1986) Early invasive carcinoma in colonic polyps. A review of the literature with emphasis on the assessment of the risk of metastasis. Cancer 57:160–171
Witt TR, Winawer SJ (1981) Cancer in a colonic polyp, or malignant colonic adenomas – is polypectomy sufficent? Gastroenterology 81:625–626
Wolff WI, Shinya H (1975) Definitive treatment of "malignant" polyps of the colon. Ann Surg 182:516–525

Prognostic Factors in Colorectal Cancer

J. R. JASS

1 Introduction

This account will describe the role of the histopathologist in the management of patients with colorectal cancer. The contributions of the pathologist fall into three areas: the interpretation of biopsies, particularly of the rectum, the management of early cancer and the reporting of surgical specimens of advanced rectal cancer. Information provided by the pathologist may not only determine the likely prognosis but also demonstrate the need for further treatment. Conventional methods of pathological examination do have their limitations. New techniques may provide important insight into the biological behaviour of malignant cells. This review will include a critical account of the value of immunohistochemistry, molecular biology and flow cytometry.

2 Role of Rectal Biopsy

Rectal biopsy has three aims: confirmation of the diagnosis of malignancy, histological typing of the malignant tumour and histological grading of malignancy. A clinically suspicious lesion should receive a definitive tissue diagnosis, particularly when it is located in the rectum. Failure to do so may result in an unnecessary rectal excision. A number of conditions can mimic rectal cancer clinically, histologically or both. They include solitary rectal ulcer syndrome, oleogranuloma, barium granuloma, endometriosis and, most importantly, benign adenoma. There is a danger of diagnosing small crushed incision biopsies from the surface of an adenoma as cancer. Furthermore reactive changes at the site of the incision biopsy may be interpreted as focal malignancy when the whole polyp is later excised. The pathologist should therefore discourage incision biopsies and state a strong preference for total excisional biopsy whenever this is feasible. Three findings assist in the diagnosis of malignancy: the cytology and architecture of the neoplastic epithelium, invasion by neoplastic epithelium across the line of the muscularis mucosae into the submucosa and a desmoplastic reaction around the invading epithelium. Neoplastic epithelium confined to the mucosa has no metastatic potential and therefore does not need to be treated by radical surgery.

Colorectal tumours may occasionally be secondary to malignant growths in adjacent organs invading the bowel directly from without (e.g. prostate) or by haematogenous spread from a distant site. Most signet-ring cell carcinomas of the rectum are gastric secondaries. Clearly if the pathologist suspects a secondary tumour this must be carefully confirmed or refuted before surgical removal of the bowel can be countenanced. Leukaemic deposits as well as primary or secondary lymphoma may mimic primary undifferentiated carcinoma and neuroendocrine (oat cell) carcinoma. Non-keratinising small cell squamous cell carcinoma and melanoma of the anal canal may both present as rectal tumours and cause diagnostic difficulties. These differential diagnoses are of considerable clinical importance since surgical treatment of leukaemia, lymphoma, squamous cell carcinoma of the anus and neuroendocrine carcinoma (REDMAN and PAZDUR 1987) of the rectum would be inappropriate. Mucinous carcinoma of the rectum is more likely to show extensive local spread and lymph node involvement than non-mucinous carcinoma (SASAKI et al. 1987) (Table 1). This finding may warn against restorative surgery when the choice of anterior resection or rectal excision is finely balanced.

Table 1. Relationships between histological type of rectal carcinoma and other pathological variables (after SASAKI et al. 1987)

Pathological variables	Histological type		
	Adenocarcinoma	Mucinous Ca[a]	Signet-ring Ca
Involved lymph nodes	50%	65%	91%
Extensive local spread	30%	48%	78%
Diffuse infiltration	25%	38%	93%
Poor differentiation	9%	40%	100%

[a] > 75% of tumour volume composed of mucus.

Table 2. Relationships between histological grade of carcinoma and spread (after DUKES and BUSSEY 1958)

	Extensive local spread	Lymph node spread
Low	16%	30%
Average	22%	47%
High	51%	81%

Histological features used for grading colorectal cancer include: tubule configuration, loss of cellular polarity and variation in nuclear size and shape (JASS et al. 1986). Tubule configuration is the most important variable in the subjective assessment of grade of malignancy. The classical studies of DUKES and BUSSEY (1958) demonstrated important relationships between grade, the extent of local spread and the risk of lymph node metastasis (Table 2).

The discovery of a high grade tumour in a rectal biopsy should warn against an attempt at restorative surgery because of the increased risk of incomplete removal and local recurrence. Conversely the report of low grade tumour might encourage the surgeon to resect a bulky tumour whose size and attachment to adjacent structures might be due merely to fibrosis and inflammation. In practice the grading of malignancy is subjective (THOMAS et al. 1983). Overgrading may occur when biopsies are small and crushed and undergrading may be a consequence of tumour heterogeneity. Clinical assessment provides the mainstay of surgical decision making, but the grade of malignancy may influence management in some borderline cases.

3 Early Colorectal Cancer

The term 'early' as applied to a gastrointestinal tumour cannot be equated with a specific pathological stage of the disease, but serves to identify cancers that are judged on *clinical* grounds to be curable. The usual morphological definition is a cancer that has not spread in direct continuity beyond the submucosa, regardless of the presence of lymph node metastases. Although knowledge of lymph node metastasis is an extremely valuable source of prognostic information, the clinician cannot know the lymph node status preoperatively. Early colorectal cancer differs from other forms of early gastrointestinal malignancy in that it is frequently treated and cured by local means alone. Early colorectal cancer presents in one of four ways: malignant adenoma (usually a pedunculated adenoma with a focus of malignancy), polypoid carcinoma, large sessile adenoma (usually villous) with a focus of malignancy and small ulcerating cancer (Fig. 1). The first two are treated by snare polypectomy. The endoscopist may or may not have suspected a diagnosis of malignancy. Large sessile adenomas of the rectum may be treated by submucous excision and the diagnosis of cancer is often unsuspected preoperatively. The small ulcerating cancer of the rectum is always diagnosed and subjected to rigorous clinical assessment prior to surgical removal.

Although early colorectal cancer presents and is treated in a variety of ways, the broad policy of management is the same. This policy was forged from a study of radical operation specimens which demonstrated important relationships between direct spread in continuity, tumour grade and lymph node involvement. Out of a total of 2084 rectal cancers treated by radical surgery, 46 were limited to the submucosa. Five of these were associated with lymph node metastases, but three of the five were poorly differentiated tumours. Thus only 2/43 (4.7%) early, non-poorly differentiated rectal cancers treated by radical surgery were accompanied by nodal metastases (MORSON 1966).

The small ulcerating cancer of the lower rectum presents an interesting dilemma to the clinician. Local excision will obviate the need for a colostomy and is associated with less morbidity and lower perioperative mortality. On the other hand the technique of removing a disc of rectal wall bearing a small cancer contravenes all the laws of bowel cancer surgery. Theoretically the patient is placed at risk of local recurrence due to implantation of viable tumour cells into the perirectal fat. More importantly cure may be compromised by leaving behind tumour in lymphatics and lymph nodes. Nevertheless by adhering to a strict policy, 24 carefully selected patients have been safely managed by curative local excision performed at St. Mark's Hospital (WHITEWAY et al. 1985). This number is small, but early rectal cancer is likely to be detected with increasing frequency as screening becomes more widely adopted. An ulcerating cancer may be a candidate for curative local excision if it is small, mobile and accessible

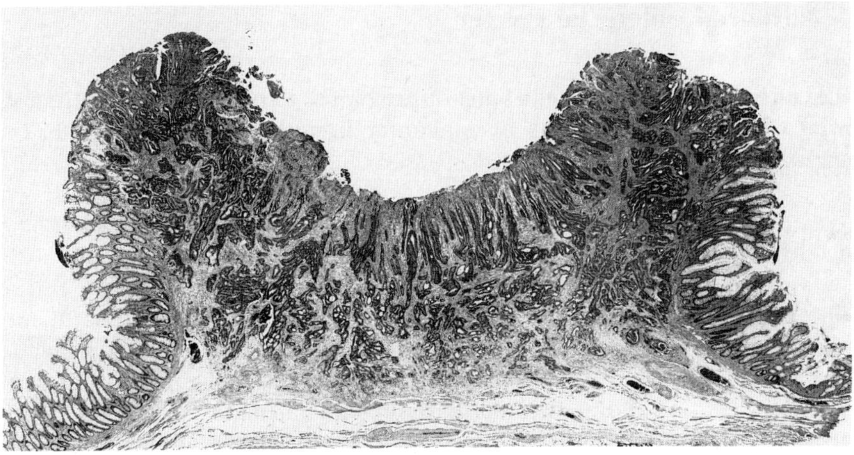

Fig. 1. Early, small ulcerating adenocarcinoma of the rectum. The tumour invades the superficial submucosa. There is no residual adenomatous tissue. HE, × 15

and, for the reasons given above, not found to be poorly differentiated. In addition there should be no palpable retrorectal lymph nodes. The latter may seem somewhat stringent, but it is in fact unusual to find large *reactive* nodes in association with a small cancer. Intrarectal ultrasound will probably assume considerable importance in the assessment of early rectal cancer. Following disc excision, the histopathologist must again ensure that the tumour is not poorly differentiated as well as demonstrate that excision is complete and that tumour does not extent beyond the external muscle coat of the rectum. It should be stressed that the risk of lymph node metastasis does not become excessive until tumours traverse the bowel wall and penetrate the perirectal fat. There is no information on the significance of lymphatic or venous invasion, mainly because this is so rarely seen in specimens of early colorectal cancer.

Of the 24 patients treated by curative local excision, the above criteria were met in 19 and additional radical surgery was therefore not indicated (WHITEWAY et al. 1985). Sixteen were alive and well at 5 years with no evidence to tumour recurrence. Three died of unrelated conditions. The histological criteria were not met in five patients and further surgery was therefore dictated by the policy. No residual cancer was found, but two patients died with distant metastases and the remainder were alive and well at 5 years. This small series indicates that local excision is safe, providing that a strict policy is adhered to. The theoretical risk of local recurrence by implantation of tumour cells appears to be unfounded, at least in this small selected series. The study invites the interesting suggestion that if an early colorectal cancer cannot be cured by local excision, then it cannot be cured at all.

4 Advanced Colorectal Cancer

It is unsatisfactory to provide a list of prognostic variables without attempting to justify their adoption or explaining how they may be derived in a standardised manner.

4.1 Macroscopic Features, Dissection and Spread of Cancer

The fresh surgical specimen should be sent to the pathology department, where it is opened along the antimesenteric border and preliminary measurements are taken. Specimens removed after hours should be refrigerated at 4° C and submitted to the pathology department at the earliest opportunity. By measuring the transverse diameter of the tumour and the bowel circumference at the midpoint of the growth, the % involvement of the bowel circumference can be calculated. The specimen should be pinned onto a cork mat and immersed in formalin for 24 h, unpinned and fixed for a further 24 h. The precise anatomical location of the tumour may not be obvious and clinical guidance should always be provided. The gross appearance of the tumour is related to prognosis (WOOD and WILKIE 1933). Protuberant tumours have the best prognosis, followed by well circumscribed ulcerating growths. The least favourable outcome is associated with diffusely infiltrating cancers. Small, stricturing tumours are included in the latter category. The presence of adenomas may have a favourable influence upon outcome that is independent of stage and grade (KRONBORG et al. 1986). The risk of metachronous neoplasia is increased when adenomas are present.

4.1.1 Local Spread

Dissection will be greatly facilitated by the use of a knife with a heavy handle and a long, razor-sharp blade. The tumour should be sliced transversely into blocks of tissue that are 3–4 mm thick and which include the deep margin of surgical excision. With careful examination it may be possible to judge whether or not the tumour is confined to the bowel wall and to measure the extent of any extramural spread as well as the minimum clearance at the deep surgical margin. It is unnecessary to submit all this tissue for histological examination. Samples should be selected which include the point of maximum spread and the minimum deep clearance. It is preferable to make a gross inspection of multiple slices and to select one with care (Fig. 2) than to trim off three random samples of tumour mechanically. Macroscopic examination may also reveal extramural venous invasion, tumour deposits that are discontinuous with the main growth and lymph nodes deep to the tumour. These will require histological study. The deep surgical margin may be coated with Indian ink to ensure that it is

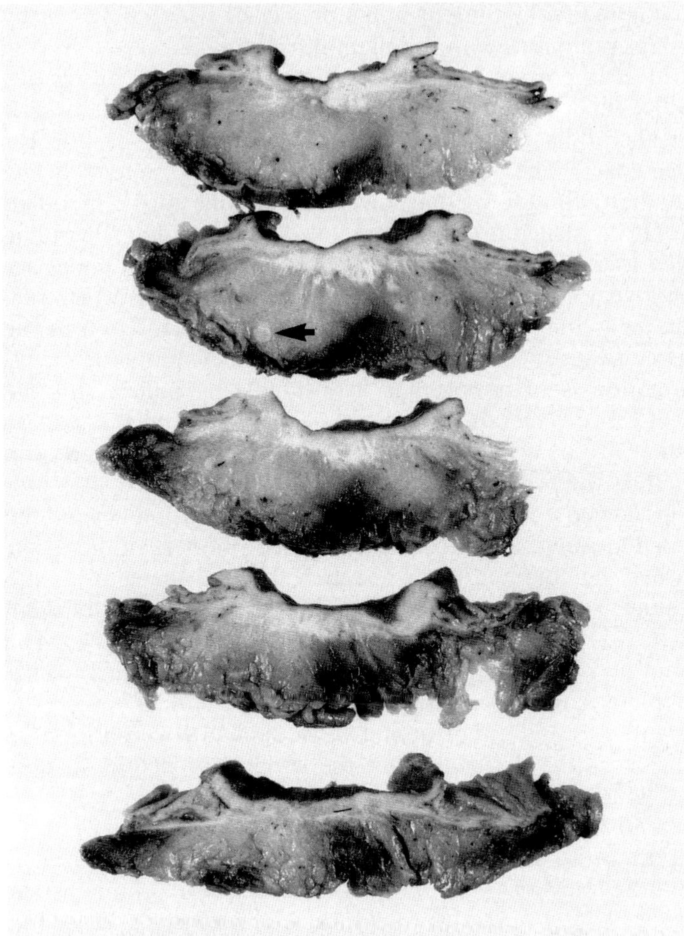

Fig. 2. Tissue sections through an ulcerating carcinoma which include perirectal fat and the deep excision margin. The second block from the top should be selected for histological examination because there is a tumour deposit close to the deep margin of excision (*arrow*). Although discontinuous with the main growth, this deposit did not appear to be within a lymph node

incorporated within the histological section. Macroscopic measurements should be confirmed microscopically since fibrosis may be mistaken for cancer and gross measurements may overestimate the extent of local spread. If destroyed by tumour the location of the outer edge of the bowel may be estimated by simple extrapolation.

Probably the most important fact that needs to be recorded by the pathologist is whether or not the deep excision margin is involved by tumour. If it is involved the operation should be defined as non-curative (QUIRKE et al. 1986). The deep excision margin may be involved through direct spread in continuity, by tumour in lymphatics or lymph nodes or by tumour deposits discontinuous with the main growth.

The second most important item concerns the level of spread in relation to the bowel wall. A tumour is defined as being limited to the wall if it extends no further than the outer edge of the muscularis propria (or external muscle coat). The upper rectum is covered anteriorly by peritoneum, but the definition of the bowel wall should not be modified by the presence of this structure. This is true also for the colon. Providing a cancer is limited to the wall (as defined above) and that lymph nodes are not invaded, the 5-year cure is virtually 100% (see below). It is worth noting whether tumour is limited to the submucosa in order to confirm the relationship between extent of local spread and risk of lymph node metastasis. This information is of importance in rationalising policies for the local treatment of cancer (see above). Neoplasms confined to the mucosa have not been shown to be capable of metastasis and the vast majority can be accommodated by the term 'adenoma'.

Tumours of the lower rectum are infraperitoneal. Extension beyond the bowel wall may lead to invasion of adjacent organs. Tumours of the upper anterior rectum may be confined to or penetrate beyond the serosa, with or without invasion of adjacent organs. Despite involvement of adjacent organs, complete excision en bloc may have been achieved. The pathologist should always endeavour to show whether or not excision is complete. Incomplete removal, histologically confirmed spread beyond the serosa or in distant sites and either operative or spontaneous perforation of the bowel all justify the designation of the surgical procedure as non-curative.

Extent of spread beyond the bowel wall should be measured (CHAN et al. 1985; QUIRKE et al. 1986) as this may be of prognostic importance. Simple extrapolation may be used when the muscularis propria is destroyed by tumour. Direct spread into adjacent organs such as vagina, bladder and prostate should be recorded. It is unnecessary to examine the proximal and distal resection margins at the microscopic level unless the margins are close (< 3 cm) to the tumour or the cancer shows either a highly infiltrative pattern of growth or extensive vascular or lymphatic permeation.

4.1.2 Lymph Node Spread

Lymph node spread is the most important pathological prognostic variable in patients undergoing curative surgery for rectal cancer (JASS et al. 1987). All lymph nodes which drain the segment of bowel harbouring a cancer should be dissected out and subjected to histological examination. Again, a knife with a long, razor-sharp blade should be used to cut sections through the well-fixed mesentery at 1 mm intervals (Fig. 3). A small scalpel will be far less effective. The harvest of lymph nodes, the number of

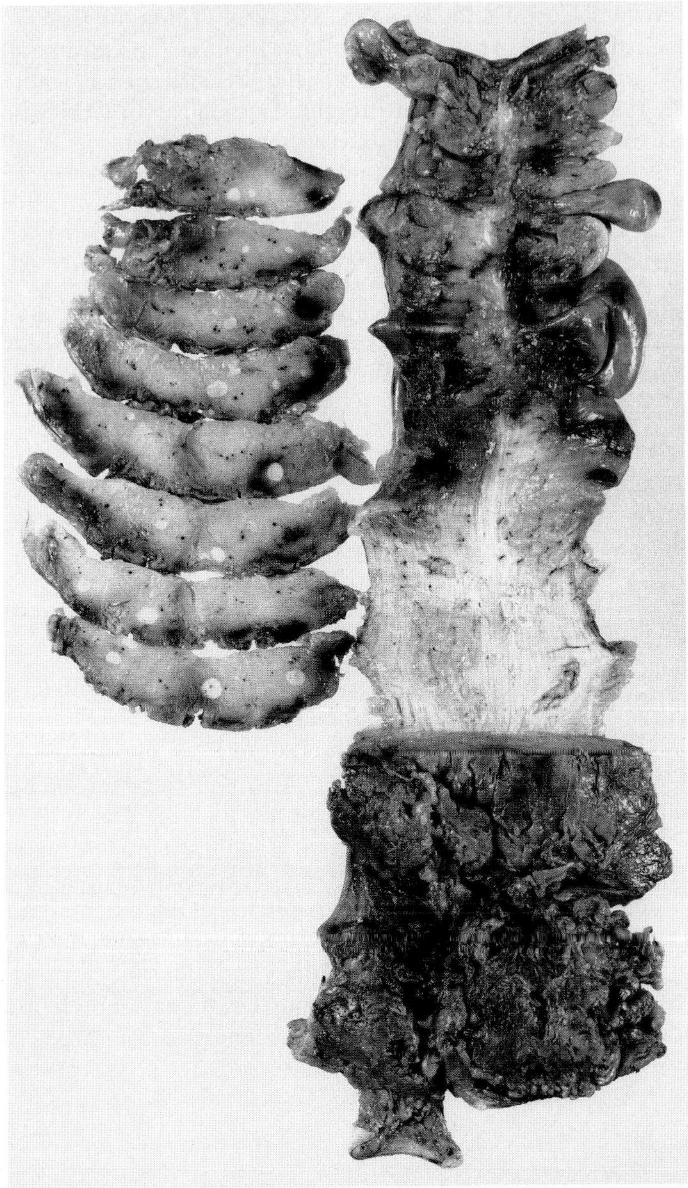

Fig. 3. A sample of tissue sections taken through a well-fixed mesorectum. At least 20 lymph nodes can be counted

nodes containing metastatic tumour and the presence of tumour in a lymph node at the limit of lymphatic dissection should be recorded. A single section through the centre of each node has been the method of sampling at St. Mark's Hospital for 60 years. Nodules of tumour that are discontinuous with the main growth may be found within the extramural fat without any signs of a residual lymph node (Fig. 2). The clinical significance of this observation is unknown at present. Permeation of lymphatic or perineural spaces should be recorded (Knudsen et al. 1983).

4.1.3 Venous Spread

Venous spread has been found to confer no independent prognostic information in the presence of other pathological variables (Jass et al. 1987). The assessment is somewhat subjective and it is recommended that only invasion of extramural veins with muscular walls should be recorded. This observation may be important in individual cases.

4.1.4 Distant Spread

Histological proof should be obtained when this is feasible.

4.2 Histological Characteristics

4.2.1 Tumour Type

Most colorectal cancers are adenocarcinomas. Mucinous carcinomas secrete large amounts of mucus and account for about 10% of cases. Other types are rare and include signet-ring cell, large cell undifferentiated, small cell undifferentiated, squamous, adenosquamous and carcinoid tumours. Tumour typing, at least into adenocarcinoma, mucinous carcinoma and signet-ring cell carcinoma, appears to confer no important independent prognostic information in the presence of other pathological variables (Sasaki et al. 1987). However, tumour typing may be of considerable importance in understanding the aetiology and histogenesis of large bowel cancer and for this reason should continue to be recorded.

4.2.2 Differentiation

Architecture or tubule configuration is the most important indicator of grade of differentiation (Jass et al. 1986). The presence of irregularly folded, distorted and often small tubules or the absence of any attempts at tubule formation should be the essential hallmarks of poorly differentiated cases (Fig. 4a). All other tumours (approximately 80%) should be recorded as 'other' (Fig. 4b). This recommendation reflects the subjective nature of grading and poor levels of interobserver agreement (Thomas et al. 1983). Tumours are frequently heterogeneous (see below) but in view

a

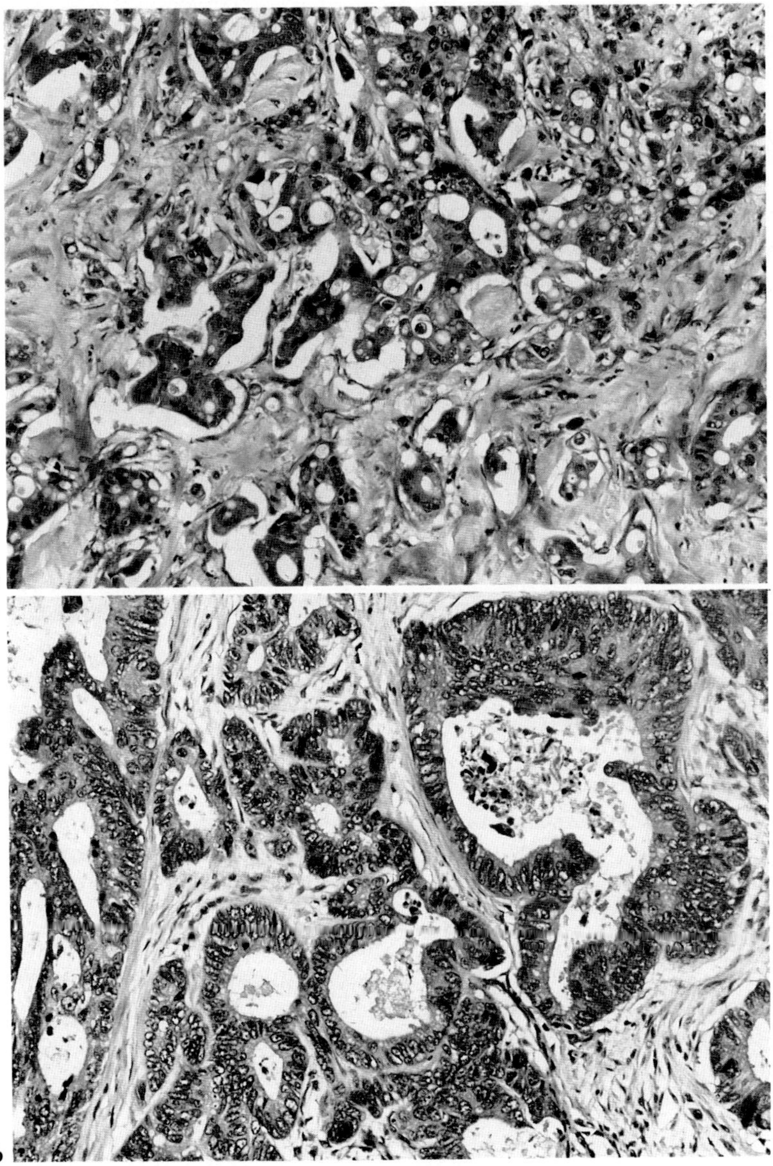

b

Fig. 4a, b. Poorly differentiated adenocarcinoma (**a**) showing irregular clumps of cells as compared to a moderately differentiated adenocarcinoma (**b**). HE, × 75

of the concept of the selection of clones of increasing malignancy it is logical to grade by the worst area rather than by the predominant pattern.

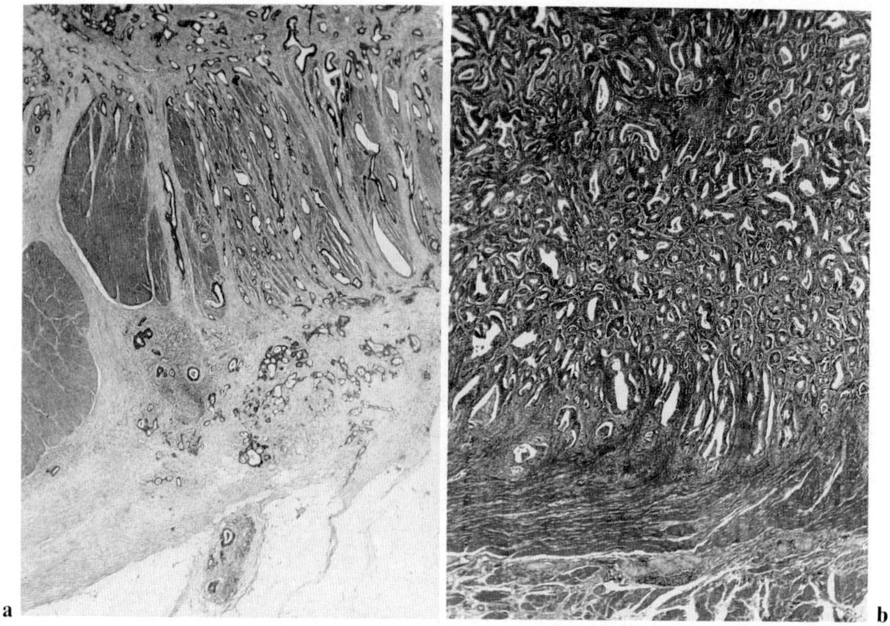

Fig. 5 a, b. Diffusely infiltrating adenocarcinoma (**a**) as compared to an expanding tumour (**b**) HE, × 10

4.2.3 Invasive Margin

About 25% of rectal tumours invade in a diffusely infiltrative manner, appearing to dissect between normal structures in a seemingly effortless fashion that is usually unopposed by any form of inflammatory response (Fig. 5 a, b). This can often be appreciated readily by the gross inspection of tumour slices at the time of dissection since the margins of such growths are difficult to define macroscopically as well as microscopically. This is a most unfavourable feature and a tumour should not be described as diffusely infiltrating unless the pathologist has no doubts about the veracity of the designation. Diffusely infiltrating tumours are often but by no means always poorly differentiated.

4.2.4 Lymphocytic Infiltration

The presence of an inflammatory mantle at the advancing edge of a tumour confers an excellent prognosis that is at least partly independent of other pathological variables (JASS 1986). Eosinophils, neutrophils and plasma cells as well as lymphocytes are often represented within the mantle, which follows the contour of the invasive margin of the tumour. This is most easily appreciated when the invasive margin is well circumscribed (Fig. 6 a, b). When the tumour is less well circumscribed, the cellu-

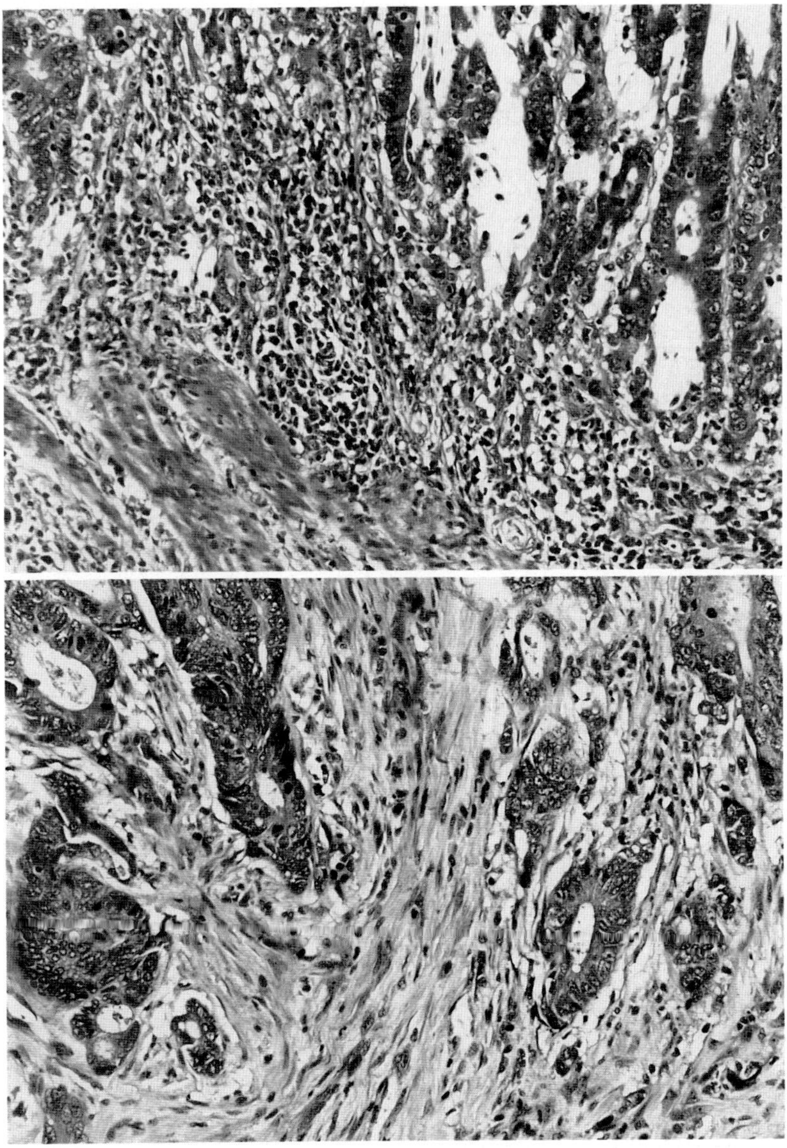

a

b

Fig. 6a, b. Conspicuous peritumoral lymphocytic infiltration (**a**) as compared to scanty infiltration (**b**). HE, × 75

lar stroma occurs as a cap at the apex of each advancing tongue. This inflammatory lamina may resemble the normal lamina propria and its presence may indicate the persistence of the normal interactive network that links intestinal epithelium and mucosa-associated lymphoid tissue. This would in turn indicate the preservation of a high level of functional differentiation and thereby account for the excellent prognosis. The finding characterises about 25% of rectal cancers and is more frequent in the earlier stages of the disease (JASS 1986). Cancers are often well differentiated but the finding is also typical of well circumscribed, large cell undifferentiated tumours (reminiscent of medullary carcinoma of the breast). It is not necessary to observe enormous numbers of lymphocytes; rather it is the presence of a delicate cellular stroma that *includes* lymphocytes that is important. This should be present at the deepest point of tumour. Doubtful cases should be excluded if the excellent prognostic significance of the observation is to be maintained.

4.3 Prognostic Classification

It is important to distinguish between curative and non-curative operations and this requires close liaison between surgeon and pathologist. If an operation has not been curative this does not necessarily mean that the patient is doomed. Thus in some instances the situation may be salvaged by offering some form of adjuvant therapy such as postoperative pelvic irradiation for an incompletely excised rectal cancer. Non-curative procedures should therefore be grouped separately and the reason or reasons for this designation should be stated. When the surgeon believes that tumour has been left within the patient, histological confirmation should be obtained whenever this is feasible. Suspected distant metastases or residual tumour within the bed of the primary growth should be biopsied accordingly. Operations should also be regarded as non-curative if there has been spontaneous or operative perforation of the bowel, carrying the theoretical risk of dissemination of tumour cells into the peritoneal cavity. When cancer is not removed en bloc as, for example, when iliac or para-aortic nodes are biopsied separately and found to contain tumour, it must be assumed that microscopic disease has been left behind. Finally the pathologist must confirm that the specimen has been completely excised at the deep excision margin as described above.

Unfortunately about 50% of patients undergoing 'curative' surgery for large bowel cancer ultimately die with distant metastases. FINLAY and MCARDLE (1986) showed that the usual explanation will be the presence of established but clinically occult hepatic metastases at the time of surgery. This conclusion was based on the use of a highly sensitive computerised tomographic scan of the liver. All long-term deaths due to distant metastases were correctly predicted by a positive liver scan. There were some false-positive cases, indicating the practical limitations of their approach. However, the biological and clinical implications of the study are of great importance. If FINLAY and MCARDLE (1986) are correct then the prognosis of patients undergoing curative surgery can be derived only by the *detection* of clinically occult hepatic metastases. Unfortunately, as noted above, the attainment of 100% sensitivity compromises specificity and the accurate detection of occult liver metastases must await the development of improved scanning methods. However, there is another approach to this problem which stems from their suggestion that cancers may be divisible according to the possession of a high or low metastatic potential. Thus the biological properties of the tumour and the character of its interaction with the host might be exploited to *predict* the presence of occult hepatic metastases. This exciting possibility highlights the inadequacy of traditional staging classifications which are anatomically based. They may indicate how far the tumour has spread within the *specimen*, but one needs to know how far the tumour has progressed within the *patient*. This is of more than academic interest. It may be more beneficial to treat patients by liver perfusion with cytotoxic drugs, a potentially hazardous procedure, when there is a high likelihood of liver involvement.

It should be possible to develop an improved prognostic classification by identifying those biological or pathological features of a tumour that have important and independent relationships with cancer-related death. According to the evidence cited above such variables should in effect be predicting the presence of occult hepatic metastases (assuming that the patient has undergone 'curative' surgery). It should be pointed out that the published attempt at this exercise (JASS et al. 1987) is deficient in that histological examination of the deep excision line was not performed with the stringency advocated above. This may have resulted in the failure to exclude a small number of non-curative cases. Furthermore only rectal cancers were studied. Four of the eight variables subjected to Cox regression analysis were shown to influence survival independently in a series of 379 patients undergoing 'curative' surgery for rectal cancer (JASS et al. 1987). These will now be discussed.

4.3.1 Lymph Node Invasion

The number of positive lymph nodes (0, 1–4, > 4) was the most important predictive variable. Only just over 10% of patients with no positive lymph nodes died as a result of cancer (Fig. 7). The likelihood of a cancer-related death increased in register with the number of affected nodes, becoming high when the total exceeded four (Fig. 7). One may in turn infer that distant metastasis becomes more likely with increasing numbers of affected lymph nodes. The fact that there is not an exact relationship between nodal and distant metastasis is not surprising since the mechanism of spread will often be different. For example the extension of a tongue of tumour via a lymphatic into an adjacent lymph node may not require and therefore indicate the acquisition of a high metastatic potential. More active methods of spread may be implicated in cases with multiple nodal metastases and such examples would signal the acquisition of a more aggressive phenotype. Although the study of lymph node spread has traditionally been regarded as a static indicator of extent of spread, it is likely that the exercise could be extended to provide important information about the biological behaviour of the tumour. Additional attention could

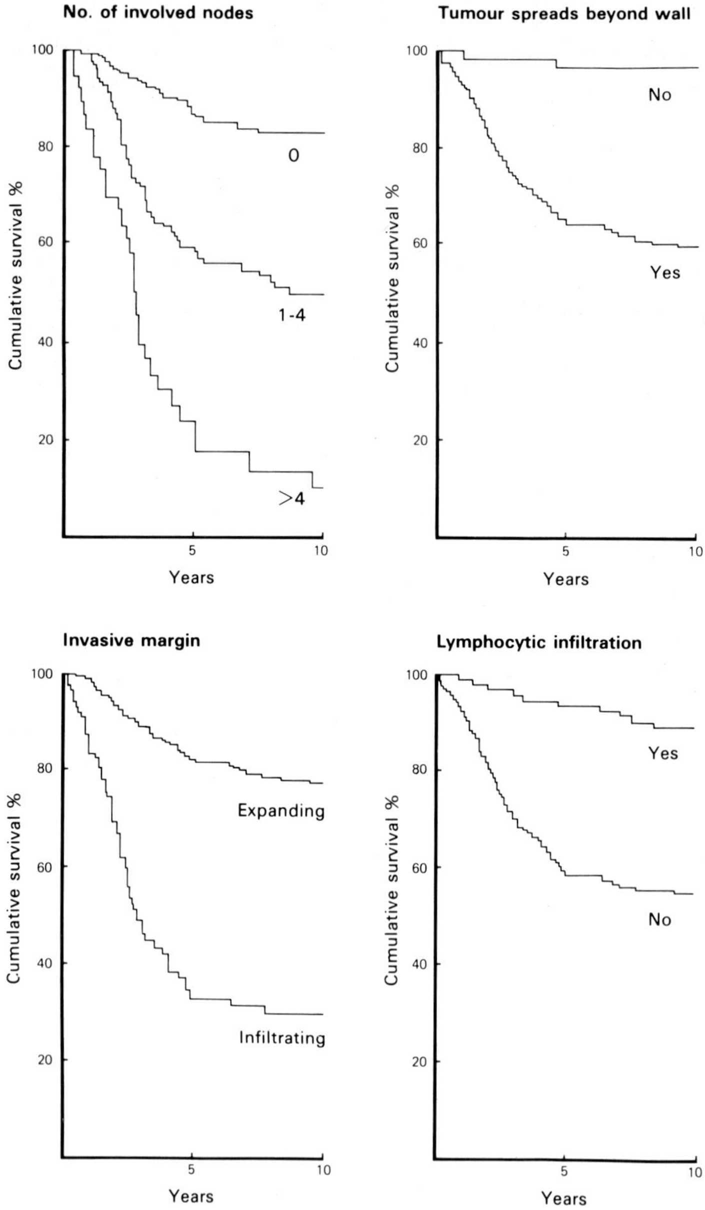

Fig. 7. Survival curves for a series of 379 'curative' operations for rectal cancer and four independent variables

be placed on the histopathology of lymph node deposits, noting features such as stromal reaction, invasion of capsule, extent of replacement and reactivity of residual nodel tissue.

4.3.2 *Extent of Direct Spread*

Five-year survival approaches 100% for rectal cancers in which direct spread in continuity is limited to the bowel wall (extending no further than the muscularis propria or externa) (Fig. 7). This includes cancers with lymph node metastases, but relatively few lymph node positive cases are associated with tumours that are otherwise limited to the bowel wall. It is important to ensure that the predictive usefulness of this variable is not diluted by accepting amongst the intramural group equivocal cases or tumours showing extramural spread that is limited to within veins. The prognostic model was not improved by stratifying cases with extramural spread as slight and moderate versus extensive (JASS et al. 1987). Although this had been only a subjective assessment made at the time of the original dissection, one might have expected cases with extensive spread to have been more prone to incomplete removal and therefore to local recurrence. It is possible that a proportion of these advanced tumours were removed from the analysis by virtue of the surgeon believing excision to have been incomplete and the operation to have been non-curative. In addition the local recurrence rate at St. Mark's Hospital is low. It is unlikely that the extent of extramural spread will in future be shown to influence survival in patients undergoing curative surgery if the deep excision margin is examined carefully and involvement is deemed to identify operations as non-curative. Although direct spread in continuity has been a central component of all staging systems, its predictive value is not as great as one might have supposed. The effect of the exercise is to identify a small group of patients, perhaps 15% in a typical series, as having an excellent prognosis. No useful information is provided for the remaining 85% of patients (Fig. 7).

4.3.3 *Character of Invasive Margin*

This exercise identified a group of patients, 25% of the total, as having a poor prognosis (Fig. 7). Similar survival curves were produced for grade of differentiation, but a smaller proportion of cancer (15%) were graded as poorly differentiated. The superior prognostic power of the assessment of the invasive margin (aided by the simplicity and reproducibility of the exercise) ousted differentiation in the Cox regression analysis. The utility of the exercise now seems to be well founded (QUIRKE et al. 1987; SCOTT et al. 1987b).

Table 3. Scoring of prognostic variables (after JASS et al. 1987)

	Score
Number of lymph nodes with metastases:	
0	0
1–4	1
5 or more	2
Tumour confined to bowel wall:	
Yes	0
No	1
Character of invasive margin:	
Expanding	0
Infiltrating	1
Peritumoral lymphocytic infiltrate:	
Yes	0
No	1

Table 4. Derivation of prognostic groups from total pathological scores (after JASS et al. 1987)

Group	Total score
I	0–1
II	2
III	3
IV	4–5

4.3.4 Peritumoral Lymphocytic Infiltration

This exercise identified a group of patients, (25% of the total) with over a 90% chance of cure (Fig. 7) and was shown to be of independent value (JASS et al. 1987). Its importance has been stressed by others also (ZHOU et al. 1983; CARLON et al. 1984; SVENNEVIG et al. 1984). However, some workers have found that the potential usefulness of the exercise is limited by the paucity of tumours that can be identified as having a marked lymphocytic infiltrate (SCOTT et al. 1987b). As described above, assessment depends more upon the character of the stroma at the invading margin of the growth than the density of the lymphocytic infiltrate. The absence of the feature is not helpful.

The above variables have differing strenghts. Some, such as limitation of tumour to the bowel wall and lymphocytic infiltration, identify patients with an excellent prognosis. Others, namely five or more positive lymph nodes and diffuse infiltration, are markers of a poor outcome. A cumulative prognosis for the individual patient may be calculated by entering the coded variables into the Cox proportional hazards regression model (COX 1972). However, it is very much simpler and only slightly less accurate to produce integer scores for each variable that reflect the computed regression coefficients (Table 3). The total score for each patient is converted into a prognostic group as shown in Table 4. The superiority of this prognostic classification over the Dukes classification has been demonstrated (JASS et al. 1987).

4.4 Tumour Heterogeneity

The exsistence of tumour heterogeneity is firmly established. Not only may histopathology appearances vary from one part of a tumour to another, but the cancer may include subpopulations of vells which differ in antigenic expression, growth rate and DNA content (ARENDS et al. 1985; HART and FIDLER 1981). It is likely that the behaviour ot the tumour will be determined by the most poorly differentiated component, but this has not been subjected to detailed study. It should be appreciated that malignant epithelium at the ulcerated surface and deep advancing edge of the tumour may appear relatively disorganised. This should be ignored. Tiny foci of less differentiated epithelium may also be unimportant. Somehow the pathologist must decide if a small area of less differentiated tumour has become sufficiently established to influence the course of the disease.

The problems engendered by tumour heterogeneity have probably been overstated. Thus the demonstration of structural or functional heterogeneity may not necessarily be associated with important clinical sequelae. For example it is known that a single tumour may yield several cell lines in vitro having different metastatic potential. However, such studies do not prove that metastases established in vivo are derived from special populations of cells with a high metastatic potential. In fact most studies have shown that the cells in metastases are indistinguishable from those in the primary growth (ALEXANDER 1983; WEISS et al. 1983). The establishment of a metastasis is probably a random event (albeit reflecting the overall biological characteristics of the primary tumour) and not the result of the evolution of an aggressive subclone. Cells with the ability to metastasise are derived from transient compartments of the tumour and not from a fixed subclone. This means that small tissue samples will often be representative of the overall biological aggressiveness of the tumour. This has been illustrated in a recent detailed study of the distribution of tumour DNA as measured by flow cytometry (see below). This study showed that the majority of colorectal carcinomas are homogeneous with respect to DNA ploidy (SCOTT et al. 1987a).

5 New Techniques

It is important to achieve a clearer understanding of the cellular mechanisms that allow tumour cells to spread and colonise distant sites. This information will not only help to provide an index of biological aggressiveness, but may also lead to the development of treatment strategies based on the neutralisation of selected properties of tumour cells. Structural and functional differences between normal and cancer cells can now be demonstrated by a variety of powerful techniques. Each of these utilises a bewildering and ever-increasing multitude of probes. As often as not, a particular probe will uncover a difference between normal and tumour cells and this finding will form the basis of a report that will subsequently be confirmed, refuted or modified by other investigators. It is difficult for any individual to keep abreast of the exponential growth in reports describing tumour-associated changes. The fact that the majority of these changes will be of minor biological interest and no clinical relevance acts as a further disincentive. It might be more rewarding to focus research activities upon tumour cell attributes that are thought to be of particular importance in determining malignant behaviour. These include activation of oncogenes leading to uncontrolled growth, breakdown of the normal mechanisms of cell to cell interaction as determined by the altered expression of cell surface glycoconjugates, avoidance of recognition and destruction by the host's immune system (EBERT et al. 1987) and abnormal invasiveness due to the secretion of proteolytic enzymes such as urokinase (GELISTER et al. 1987). Some of the more recent advances in these areas will be reviewed.

5.1 Immunohistochemical Studies

Despite the investment of considerable research activity into the immunohistochemical study of differentiation antigens such as blood group substances and class I and II histocompatibility antigens, the findings have been disappointing up to now. Some differentiation antigens are lost pari passu with structural dedifferentiation. An example is the IgA carrier molecule, secretory component (ISAACSON 1982; ROGNUM et al. 1982). The expression of this molecule is associated with an improved survival, but is not independent of more traditional pathological variables (ARENDS et al. 1984a). Loss of HLA class I antigens might be expected to be related to prognosis since immune T cell attack depends on the co-expression of these as well as non-self antigens (SANDERSON and BEVERLEY 1983). However, CSIBA et al. (1984) failed to show a correlation between the expression of class I antigens and the extent and type of mononuclear cell infiltrate in colorectal tumours. On the other hand loss of class I antigens has been described in mucinous carcinomas of the colorectum (VAN DEN INGH et al. 1987) and this may be related to the scant mononuclear cell infiltrate associated with these tumours (SASAKI et al. 1987). HLA class II antigens are detected on cells whose function is to present antigen to T cells. The anomalous expression of HLA-D subregion products by colorectal cancer epithelium shows no correlation with either Dukes stage or differentiation (GHOSH et al. 1986). It should be appreciated, however, that the focal expression of HLA-DR by normal colorectal epithelium appears to be a physiological event, particularly with respect to lymphoepithelial complexes (SPENCER et al. 1986) or in inflammatory conditions (SELBY et al. 1983). Thus it could be argued that the *failure* of colorectal cancer to express HLA-DR in the presence of lymphokines (γ interferon) might be abnormal.

Another feature of malignant epithelium which lends itself to immunohistochemical study is the expression of so-called oncodevelopmental antigens. This phenomenon may be explained by the derepression of genes that are normally active during embryonic or fetal life and allows one to speculate on possible parallels between the rapid growth and migratory activities of embryonic tissues and the behaviour of malignant cells. However, it would appear that many of the oncodevelopmental antigens, including carcinoembryonic antigen, gastrointestinal cancer-associated antigen (sialylated Lewis^a), stage-specific embryonic antigen (Lewis^x) and other blood group antigens are expressed by adult tissues also. Furthermore the increased expression of these antigens has not been shown to have an independent influence upon survival (ARENDS et al. 1984b; HAMADA et al. 1985; SCHOENTAG et al. 1987).

The glycoprotein laminin is an important component of the basement membrane. It is now appreciated that invasion of the basement membrane is not a prerequisite for the diagnosis of malignancy and that the presence of this structure depends on whether its integrity has been maintained through the secretory activity of the tumour cell. Absence of laminin correlates with distant spread and poor survival rates (FORSTER et al. 1984).

5.2 Oncogenes and Molecular Biology

Interest in the activation and control of growth has been stimulated in the last few years by the discovery of oncogenes. These are genes which have a physiological role in the control of growth and differentiation. Point mutations, translocations or gene amplification may account for the abnormal activities of these genes in tumours. The end-point will be increased growth which may be mediated by such mechanisms as uncontrolled synthesis of growth factors leading to autostimulation by tumour cells (SPORN and TODARO 1980), to the abnormal functioning of growth factor receptors or to the switching on of DNA synthesis. Over 30 oncogenes have now been described, but only a few have been implicated in the pathogenesis of colorectal cancer. This review will consider only c-*myc* and the c-*ras* family.

The c-*myc* oncogene codes for a nuclear protein which plays a role in the control and switching on of the cell cycle. Increased expression of this oncogene has been demonstrated in colorectal neoplasms by RNA measurement (Northern blotting) (CALABRETTA et al. 1985) and by means of a monoclonal antobody raised against the protein product of the oncogene (STEWART et al. 1986). The increased expression is not explained by either amplification or rearrangement of the gene (ERISMAN et al. 1985). It has been reported that well differentiated adenocarcinomas contain more of the gene product ($p62^{c\text{-}myc}$) than poorly differentiated tumours (STEWART et al. 1986). It would appear that more c-*myc* oncogene expression occurs in cancers of the rectum and left colon than in those of the right colon (ROTHBERG et al. 1985). The level of c-*myc* oncogene expression has not been shown to be of prognostic significance. However, when messenger RNA levels of the c-*myc*, c-*fos*, c-Ha-*ras* and c-Ki-*ras* (see below) genes were studied in a small series of colon cancers, high levels of one or more correlated with a poor outcome (MONNAT et al. 1987).

Protein products of the c-*ras* family ($p21^{ras}$) are thought to transduce signals from growth factor receptors by activating the nucleotide guanosine triphosphate (GTP). Mutated forms of the *ras* protein may be associated with a continuous GTPase activity which would lead to overpromotion of the mitogenic pathway. The c-*ras* oncogenes have been studied by different methods. Monoclonal antibodies have been raised against sections of the protein product which have then been demonstrated immunohistochemically. This approach fails to distinguish between the mutated and non-mutated forms of the gene and the results have generally been disappointing (KERR et al. 1985). Although raised levels of the protein may be detected in tumours, this shows no correlation with the stage of the disease. Indeed metastatic deposits may contain decreased levels of $p21^{ras}$ (GALLILCK et al. 1985). The relation of *ras* oncogene expression to stage has been studied by messenger RNA blotting techniques (KERR et al. 1986). Again there was no correlation between level of mRNA and stage of the disease. It would appear that $p21^{ras}$ plays a role in the early stages of neoplastic transformation (SPANDIDOS and KERR 1984), but is not essential for tumour progression and spread. Recently it has been shown that a proportion of colorectal cancers have a point mutation at codon 12 of the c-Ki-*ras* oncogene (BOS et al. 1987; FORRESTER et al. 1987). The prognostic significance of this finding is unknown at present.

Single somatic mutations that lead to an observable alteration are of course dominant for that condition. It is a relatively easy matter to observe the effects of a dominant oncogene by, for example, transfecting the cloned mutant oncogene into a well characterised cell line. It is very much more difficult to identify recessive oncogenes. However, there is now evidence to suggest that recessive genes (usually deletions of genes that control growth) are important in the aetiology of colorectal cancer. Recessive genes are known to be implicated in the pathogenesis of inherited tumours such as retinoblastoma. Loss of the homologous gene is required to terminate synthesis of the gene product and lead to malignancy. This is usually due to complete loss of the normal chromosome through non-disjunction, but could also be due to a partial deletion or to a point mutation. This loss can be demonstrated by means of a molecular probe that is heterozygous for the affected individual. Homo- or hemizygosity within tumour DNA when normal DNA from the same individual is heterozygous for the particular probe will thereby indicate loss (or partial loss) of the normal chromosome. KNUDSON (1971) suggested that the initial inherited mutation within familial neoplasms might be acquired in sporadic forms of the same disease. In familial adenomatous polyposis (FAP) there is an inherited deletion on the long arm of chromosome 5 (BODMER et al. 1987). Hemizygosity is rarely observed within adenomatous DNA, but occurs in up to 40% of sporadic colorectal cancers (SOLOMON et al. 1987). The implication of the latter finding, therefore, is that the first somatic mutation is equivalent to the inherited mutation of FAP and gives rise to an adenoma. However, since the gene is recessive for cancer, loss of the second normal chromosome, leading to hemizygosity, is a prerequisite for malignant transformation. Interestingly, similar mechanisms may implicate growth controlling or suppressor genes on other chromosomes also. Cytogenetic studies have demonstrated consistent deficiences of chromosome 18 and the short arm of chromosome 17 (MULERIS et al. 1985). Utilising molecular biological techniques, others have shown somatic loss of chromosome 17p sequences in 76% of colorectal cancers but in only 1/30 adenomas (FEARON et al. 1987). It is not yet known whether there are any prognostic implications for cancers that have become hemizygous for chromosome 5, 17 or 18 sequences.

5.3 DNA Flow Cytometry

Flow cytometry provides a simple method for measuring tumour DNA content. In a series of colorectal cancers the DNA content will follow a clear bimodal distribution. Thus about 40% of cancers are near-diploid and the remaining 60% are aneuploid (TRIBUKAIT et al. 1983; GOH et al. 1987). The fact that the technique is unable to resolve the relatively minor changes of karyotype which characterise the near-diploid group is unimportant for the purposes of this discussion. There is a high level of agreement on the pattern of DNA distribution that is found in a series of large bowel cancers. It is also agreed that there is no relationship between DNA ploidy and tumour differentiation. However, it is unclear whether a relationship exists between ploidy and stage. Some studies report a trend between increasing stage and aneuploidy (BANNER et al. 1985; KOKAL et al. 1986; SCOTT et al. 1987b) whereas others do not (WOLLEY et al. 1982; TRIBUKAIT et al. 1983; ROGNUM et al. 1983; ARMITAGE et al. 1985; MELAMED et al. 1986; QUIRKE et al. 1987). There are no reports of a negative trend. It should be appreciated that most of these studies have been relatively small and when the data are stratified by stage and ploidy, small differences may not be detected. A summation of the published data would probably indicate a weighting of DNA aneuploidy amongst tumours at a more advanced stage. Indeed it would be difficult to explain the survival advantage of near-diploid tumours if there were no such relationship. In our own series of 203 rectal adenocarcinomas, there was a borderline relationship with Dukes stage ($\chi^2 = 3.77$; $P = 0.077$) and a significant relationship with extent of direct spread in continuity ($\chi^2 = 6.12$; $P = 0.014$) (GOH et al. 1987). However, the most significant association was with the stromal reaction at the advancing edge of the tumour. A cellular stroma that included a prominent lymphocytic infiltrate predicted near-diploidy whereas a dense fibrotic stroma predicted aneuploidy (GOH et al. 1987). The latter somewhat unexpected finding has been recorded by others (SCOTT et al. 1987 b).

The survival curves for near-diploid and aneuploid cancers are gratifyingly similar in most large series, with diploid tumours having a clear survival advantage. However, the magnitude of the independent predictive value of DNA ploidy varies enormously. In our own study, ploidy was dwarfed into near insignificance by Dukes stage (GOH et al. 1987). Others have found ploidy to be as important (SCOTT et al. 1987 b) or even more important (KOKAL et al. 1986) than Dukes stage. Since the survival curves for cancers stratified by DNA ploidy are similar in the majority of reports, it would seem that the quality of pathological reporting is the variable factor. One contribution stands apart from all the others in reporting a cure rate for near-diploid tumours of 100% (KOKAL et al. 1986). However, this was a small and highly selected series with only three aneuploid Dukes C cancers.

The predictive value of DNA flow cytometry might be increased by removing cases having either a very poor prognosis or a very good prognosis. Once cancers have spread to distant sites, ploidy status becomes immaterial (FINAN et al. 1986) and the same would presumably apply to incompletely removed cancers. Similarly cancers with no positive lymph nodes and little or no direct extension beyond the bowel wall will have an excellent prognosis regardless of ploidy status. It is in patients undergoing curative surgery and subsequently placed within prognostic group III (see above) that flow cytometry might prove to be of particular value.

It is possible that near-diploid tumours are heterogeneous. For example, there might be a subgroup with a near normal chromosomal constitution and characterised by a low biological aggressiveness. There is some evidence that near-diploid cancers with a low proliferative index (as indicated by a low proportion of cells in the S and G_2 phases) fare better than those with a high proliferative index (QUIRKE et al. 1987). Such a subgroup would account for the overall better prognosis of near-diploid tumours. The artificial selection of the same subgroup might account for the findings of KOKAL et al. (1986). This possibility warrants further study.

It has been suggested that aneuploidy predicts local recurrence in rectal tumours (SCOTT et al. 1987b), but this report did not heed the extent of radial spread or clearance at the deep excision margin. These factors would provide more direct guidance on the adequacy of surgical excision.

In conclusion, DNA flow cytometry may have a small part to play in the assessment of surgical specimens of large bowel cancer. However, this would probably apply only to cases that could not otherwise be placed within excellent or poor prognostic categories.

6 Conclusion

Although there have been new and interesting insights into the biological nature of colorectal cancer, these have made little clinical impact so far. Cancerous and non-cancerous cells have been shown to differ in innumerable ways. However, most of these differences are qualitative and most are lacking in clinical significance. This will change in the next few years and it seems likely that colorectal malignancy will be understood to result from a small number of key somatic mutations. These exciting developments will not take place unless there is close liaison between clinician, diagnostic pathologist and experimentalist. It is essential that basic research is coupled to a standardised and meticulous system for recording clinical and pathological variables which are known to be of prognostic importance. New prognostic variables should not be studied in isolation. Their clinical value may be demonstrated by identifying an important and independent contribution in the presence of a sound and comprehensive set of pathological variables.

References

Alexander P (1983) Dormant metastases – studies in experimental animals. J Pathol 141: 379–383

Arends JW, Wiggers T, Thijs CT, Verstijnen C, Swaen GJV, Bosman FT (1984a) The value of secretory component (SC) immunoreactivity in diagnosis and prognosis of colorectal carcinomas. Am J Clin Pathol 82:267–274

Arends JW, Wiggers T, Verstijnen C, Hilgers J, Bosman FT (1984b) Gastrointestinal cancer-associated antigen (GICA) immunoreactivity in colorectal carcinoma in relation to patient survival. Int J Cancer 34:193–196

Arends JW, Bosman FT, Hilgers J (1985) Tissue antigens in large bowel carcinoma. Biochim Biophys Acta 780:1–19

Armitage NC, Robins RA, Evans DF, Turner DR, Baldwin RW, Hardcastle JD (1985) The influence of tumour cell DNA abnormalities on survival in colorectal cancer. Br J Surg 72:828–830

Banner BG, Tomas-De La Vega JE, Roseman DL, Coon JS (1985) Should flow cytometric DNA analysis precede definitive surgery for colon carcinoma? Ann Surg 202:740–744

Bodmer WF, Bailey CJ, Bodmer J et al. (1987) Localization of the gene for familial adenomatous polyposis on chromosome 5. Nature 328:614–616
Bos JL, Fearon ER, Hamilton SR, Verlaan-de Vries M, Boom JH van, Eb AJ van der, Vogelstein B (1987) Prevalence of *ras* gene mutation in human colorectal cancers. Nature 327:293–297
Calabretta B, Kaczmarek L, Ming P-ML, Au F, Ming S-C (1985) Expression of c-*myc* and other cell cycle-dependent genes in human colon neoplasia. Cancer Res 45:6000–6004
Carlon CA, Fabris G, Arslan-Pagnini C, Pluchinotta AM (1984) Prognostic correlations of operable carcinoma of the rectum. Dis Colon Rectum 28:47–50
Chan KW, Boey J, Wong SKC (1985) A method of reporting radial invasion and surgical clearance of rectal carcinoma. Histopathology 9:1319–1327
Cox DR (1972) Regression models and life tables (with discussion). J R Stat Soc B 34:187–200
Csiba A, Whitwell HL, Moore M (1984) Distribution of histocompatibility and leucocyte differentiation antigens in normal human colon and in benign and malignant colonic neoplasms. Br J Cancer 50:699–709
Dukes CE, Bussey HJR (1958) The spread of rectal cancer and its effect on prognosis. Br J Cancer 12:309–320
Ebert EC, Roberts AI, O'Connell SM, Robertson FM, Nagase H (1987) Characterization of an immunosuppressive factor derived from colon cancer cells. J Immunol 138:2161–2168
Erisman MD, Rothberg PG, Diehl RE, Morse CC, Spandorfer JM, Astrin SM (1985) Deregulation of c-*myc* gene expression in human colon carcinoma is not accompanied by amplification or rearrangement of the gene. Mol Cell Biol 5:1969–1976
Fearon ER, Hamilton SR, Vogelstein B (1987) Clonal analysis of human colorectal tumors. Science 238:193–196
Finan PJ, Quirke P, Dixon MF, Dyson DED, Giles GR, Bird CC (1986) Is DNA aneuploidy a good prognostic indicator in patients with advanced colorectal cancer? Br J Cancer 54:327–330
Finlay IG, McArdle CS (1986) Occult hepatic metastases in colorectal carcinoma. Br J Surg 73:732–735
Forrester K, Almoguera C, Han K, Grizzle WE, Perucho M (1987) Detection of high incidence of K-*ras* oncogenes during human colon tumorigenesis. Nature 327:298–303
Forster SJ, Talbot IC, Critchley DR (1984) Laminin and fibronectin in rectal adenocarcinoma: relationship to tumour grade, stage and metastasis. Br J Cancer 50:51–61
Gallick GE, Kurzrock R, Kloetzer WS, Arlinhaus RB, Guttermann JU (1985) Expression of p21 *ras* in fresh primary and metastatic human colorectal tumours. Proc Natl Acad Sci 82:1795–1798
Gelister JSK, Jass JR, Mahmoud M, Gaffney PJ, Boulos PB (1987) Role of urokinase in colorectal neoplasia. Br J Surg 74:460–463
Ghosh AK, Moore M, Street AJ, Howat JMT, Schofield PF (1986) Expression of HLA-D subregion products on human colorectal carcinoma. Int J Cancer 38:459–464
Goh HS, Jass JR, Atkin WS, Cuzick J, Northover JMA (1987) Value of flow cytometric determination of ploidy as a guide to prognosis in operable rectal cancer: a multivariate analysis. Int J Colorect Dis 2:17–21
Hamada Y, Yamamura M, Hioki K, Yamamoto M, Nagura H, Watanabe K (1985) Immunohistochemical study of carcinomabryonic antigen in patients with colorectal cancer. Correlation with plasma carcinoembryonic antigen levels. Cancer 55:136–141
Hart IR, Fidler IJ (1981) The implications of tumor heterogeneity for studies on the biology and therapy of cancer metastases. Biochim Biophys Acta 651:37–50
Isaacson P (1982) Immunoperoxidase study of the secretory immunoglobulin system in colonic neoplasia. J Clin Pathol 35:14–25
Jass JR (1986) Lymphocytic infiltration and survival in rectal cancer. J Clin Pathol 39:585–589
Jass JR, Atkin WS, Cuzick J, Bussey HJR, Morson BC, Northover JMA, Todd IP (1986) The grading of rectal cancer: historical perspectives and a multivariate analysis of 447 cases. Histopathology 10:437–59

Jass JR, Love SB, Northover JMA (1987) A new prognostic classification of rectal cancer. Lancet I:1303–1306

Kerr IB, Lee FD, Quintanilla M, Balmain A (1985) Immunocytochemical demonstration of p21 *ras* family product in normal mucosa and in premalignant and malignant tumours of the colorectum. Br J Cancer 52:695–700

Kerr IB, Spandidos DA, Finlay IG, Lee FD, McArdle CS (1986) The relation of the *ras* family oncogene expression to conventional staging criteria and clinical outcome in colorectal carcinoma. Br J Cancer 53:231–235

Knudsen JB, Nilsson T, Sprechler M, Johansen A, Christensen N (1983) Venous and nerve invasion as prognostic factors in postoperative survival of patients with resectable cancer of the rectum. Dis Colon Rectum 26:613–617

Knudson AG (1971) Mutation and cancer: statistical study of retinoblastoma. Proc Natl Acad Sci USA 68:820–823

Kokal W, Sheibani K, Terz J, Harada R (1986) Tumor DNA content in the prognosis of colorectal carcinoma. JAMA 255:3123–3127

Kronborg O, Hage E, Fenger C, Deichgraeber E (1986) Do synchronous adenomas influence prognosis after radical surgery for colorectal cancer? A prospective study. Int J Colorect Dis 1:99–103

Melamed MR, Enker WE, Banner P, Janov AJ, Kessler G, Darzynkiewicz Z (1986) Flow cytometry of colorectal carcinoma with three-year follow-up. Dis Colon Rectum 29:184–186

Monnat M, Tardy S, Saraga P, Diggelmann H, Costa J (1987) Prognostic implications of expresion of the cellular genes *myc*, *fos*, Ha-*ras* and Ki-*ras* in colon carcinoma. Int J Cancer 40:293–299

Morson BC (1966) Factors influencing the prognosis of early cancer of the rectum. Proc R Soc Med 59:607–608

Muleris M, Salmon RJ, Zafrani B, Girodet J, Dutrillaux B (1985) Consistent deficiences of chromosome 18 and of the short arm of chromosome 17 in eleven cases of human large bowel cancer: a possible recessive determinism. Ann Genet 28:206–213

Quirke P, Durdey P, Dixon MF, Williams NS (1986) Local recurrence of rectal adenocarcinoma due to inadequate surgical resection. Histopathological study of lateral tumour spread and surgical excision. Lancet II:996–999

Quirke P, Dixon MF, Clayden AD, Durdey P, Dyson JED, Williams NS, Bird CC (1987) Prognostic significance of DNA aneuploidy and cell proliferation in rectal adenocarcinomas. J Pathol 151:285–291

Redman BG, Pazdur R (1987) Colonic small cell undifferentiated carcinoma: a distinct pathological diagnosis with therapeutic implications. Am J Gastroenterol 82:382–385

Rognum TO, Elgjo K, Brandtzaeg P, Ørjasaeter H, Bergan A (1982) Plasma carcinoembryonic antigen concentrations and immunohistochemical patterns of epithelial marker antigens in patients with large bowel carcinoma. J Clin Pathol 35:922–933

Rognum TO, Brandtzaeg P, Thorud E (1983) Is heterogeneous expression of HLA-DR antigens and CEA along with DNA-profile variations evidence of phenotypic instability and clonal proliferation in human large bowel carcinomas? Br J Cancer 48:543–551

Rothberg PG, Spandorfer JM, Erisman MD, Staroscik RN, Sears HF, Petersen RO, Astrin SM (1985) Evidence that *c-myc* expression defines two genetically distinct forms of colorectal adenocarcinoma. Br J Cancer 52:629–632

Sanderson AR, Beverley PCL (1983) Interferon, β2 microglobulin and immunoselection in the pathway to malignancy. Immunol Today 4:211–213

Sasaki O, Atkin WS, Jass JR (1987) Mucinous carcinoma of the rectum. Histopathology 11:259–272

Schoentag R, Primus FJ, Kuhns W (1987) ABH and Lewis blood group expression in colorectal carcinoma. Cancer Res 47:1695–1700

Scott NA, Grande JP, Weiland LH, Pemberton JH, Beart RW, Lieber MM (1987 a) Flow cytometric DNA patterns from colorectal cancers – how reproducible are they? Mayo Clin Proc 62:331–337

Scott NA, Rainwater LM, Wieand HS, Weiland LH, Pemberton JH, Beart RW, Liebner MM (1987b) The relative prognostic value of flow cytometric DNA analysis and conventional clinicopathologic criteria in patients with operable rectal carcinoma. Dis Colon Rectum 30:513–520

Selby WS, Janossy G, Mason DY, Jewell DP (1983) Expression of HLA-DR antigens by colonic epithelium in inflammatory bowel disease. Clin Exp 53:614–618

Solomon E, Voss R, Hall V et al. (1987) Chromosome 5 allele loss in human colorectal carcinomas. Nature 328:616–619

Spandidos DA, Kerr IB (1984) Elevated expression of the human *ras* oncogene family in premalignant and malignant tumours of the colorectum. Br J Cancer 49:681–688

Spencer J, Finn T, Isaacson PG (1986) Expression of HLA-DR antigens on epithelium associated with lymphoid tissue in the human gastrointestinal tract. Gut 27:153–157

Sporn MB, Todaro GJ (1980) Autocrine secretion and malignant transformation of cells. N Engl J Med 303:878–880

Stewart J, Evan G, Watson J, Sikora K (1986) Detection of the c-*myc* oncogene product in colonic polyps and carcinomas. Br J Cancer 53:1–6

Svennevig JL, Lunde OC, Holter J, Bjorgsvik D (1984) Lymphoid infiltration and prognosis in colorectal carcinoma. Br J Cancer 49:375–377

Thomas GDH, Dixon MF, Smeeton NC, Williams NS (1983) Observation variation in the histological grading of rectal carcinoma. J Clin Pathol 36:385–91

Tribukait B, Hammarberg C, Rubio C (1983) Ploidy and proliferation patterns in colorectal adenocarcinomas related to Dukes' classification and to histopathological differentiation: a flow cytometric DNA study. Acta Pathol Microbiol Scand [A]91:89–95

van den Ingh HF, Ruiter DJ, Griffioen G, Muijen GNP van, Ferrone S (1987) HLA antigens in colorectal tumours – low expression of HLA class I antigens in mucinous colorectal carcinomas. Br J Cancer 55:125–130

Weiss J, Holmes JC, Ward PM (1983) Do metastases arise from pre-existing subpopulations of cancer cells? Br J Cancer 47:81–89

Whiteway J, Nicholls RJ, Morson BC (1985) The role of surgical local excision in the treatment of rectal cancer. Br J Surg 72:694–687

Wolley RC, Screiber K, Koss LG, Karas LG, Sherman A (1982) DNA distribution in human colon carcinomas and its relationship to clinical behavior. J Natl Cancer Inst 69:15–22

Wood WQ, Wilkie DPD (1933) Carcinoma of the rectum. An anatomico-pathological study. Ed Med J 40:321–43

Zhou X-G, Yu B-M, Shen Y-X (1983) Surgical treatment and late results in 1226 cases of colorectal cancer. Dis Colon Rectum 26:250–256

Polyposis Syndromes – An Update

N. A. SHEPHERD and H. J. R. BUSSEY

1 Introduction

The term polyposis encompasses a heterogeneous group of gastrointestinal conditions which includes relatively well defined inherited syndromes, less well defined syndromes characterised by multiple polyps in the gut and acquired conditions such as inflammatory and lymphoid polyposis. There are three major inherited gastrointestinal polyposis syndromes which are, in order of prevalence, familial adenomatous polyposis (FAP, formerly called familial polyposis coli), Peutz-Jeghers polyposis (PJP) and juvenile polyposis (JP). It should be emphasised that, while the colon is the predominant site of involvement in FAP and JP, no part of the alimentary tract is immune from pathology in these syndromes: significant morbidity and mortality result from lesions both in the upper alimentary tract and outside the gut in all three conditions.

A similar mode of inheritance is shared by FAP, PJP and JP, all three conditions being inherited on an autosomal dominant basis. However, although JP is often familial, sporadic cases make up a large proportion. FAP is undoubtedly the commonest of the three syndromes, with an incidence rate of approximately 1 in 10000. This rate is remarkably consistent throughout the Western world and Japan (BULOW 1986). It is less easy to assess accurately the incidence and prevalence of PJP and JP as they are clearly much rarer and, in the case of JP, less well defined both clinically and genetically.

In this chapter it is intended to concentrate on recent advances in the inherited polyposis syndromes. In FAP recent molecular biological techniques which have localised the gene of FAP to chromosome 5 and have assessed the clonality of FAP adenomas, methodologies which attempt to find abnormality in the 'normal' colorectal mucosa of FAP, and the extracolonic manifestations of FAP are discussed. In PJP and JP we have concentrated on the risk of gastrointestinal malignancy and on the extracolonic manifestations of the syndromes. Finally other rarer polyposis syndromes are briefly reviewed. Some of these may simulate the commoner types of polyposis syndrome, particularly FAP, and unnecessary surgery may be performed if biopsies are not taken.

2 Familial Adenomatous Polyposis

2.1 Genetic and Clonality Studies

A major recent finding in FAP is the localisation of the FAP gene to chromosome 5. The clue to this localisation was provided by a single case report describing a patient with multiple congenital abnormalities who developed colonic carcinoma (HERRERA et al. 1986). Subsequent examination of the colon revealed FAP and cytogenetic studies showed deletion of part of chromosome 5. Molecular biological techniques using DNA probes closely linked to the region of chromosome 5 that contain the putative gene have clearly demonstrated that the gene was indeed on chromosome 5 and that it was probably in the q 21–22 region (BODMER et al. 1987). Further studies are in progress to characterise the gene. DNA probes closely linked to the FAP gene are now being used at St. Mark's Hospital for the screening of FAP families and they show great potential for the genetic counselling of affected families.

Further studies from the ICRF (SOLOMON et al. 1987) have shown that more than 20% of sporadic carcinomas of the colorectum lose one of the alleles of chromosome 5 which are present in normal matched tissues. They have further suggested that loss of one normal allele giving rise to an active recessive gene may be a critical step for the progression of many

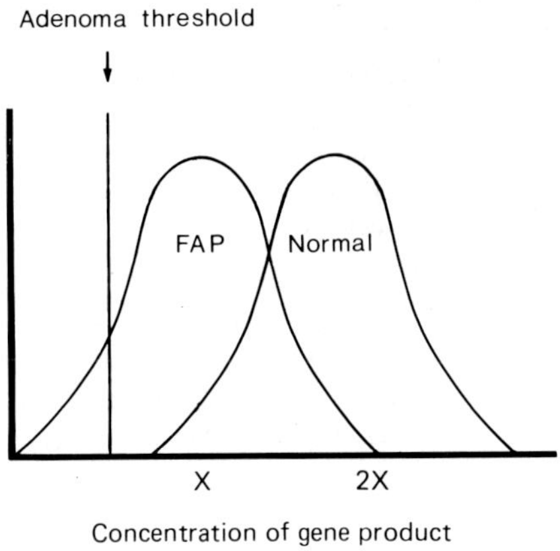

Fig. 1. Suggested mechanism for adenoma formation in FAP patients due to reduction in the FAP gene product, a growth factor repressor, below a threshold

sporadic colorectal cancers. This recessivity is not seen in the preceding adenomas and it is suggested that the heterozygosity for the deficiency may give rise to localised growth abnormalities by a threshold effect which involves negative control over the production of growth factors. Thus the FAP gene product may fluctuate in the deficient heterozygote and focally there may be a reduction such that the gene product falls below a threshold (Fig. 1). When this occurs a localised area of growth abnormality (i.e. the adenoma) occurs.

It is at present uncertain whether the adenoma in FAP arises as a result of clonal proliferation of epithelial cells. HSU et al. (1983) studied three patients who were heterozygous for the enzyme glucose-6-phosphate dehydrogenase (G6PD). All three patients' polyps displayed the AB phenotype, suggesting that the polyps were multiclonal in origin. However, more recently, workers from the same group have demonstrated by use of DNA probes that adenomas in FAP are probably monoclonal (FEARON et al. 1987). They have suggested that their initial demonstration of polyclonality using G6PD assays was due to inclusion of stromal tissues in the analysed material which obscured the monoclonality of the adenomatous epithelium.

2.2 The 'Normal' Colorectal Mucosa in FAP

Presently the diagnosis of FAP in patients at risk depends on the demonstration of adenomatous polyps in the colon and rectum but these polyps are not usually present until late childhood or early adulthood (BUSSEY 1975). There have been many attempts to improve the early identification of patients who have inherited the genotype of FAP. The localisation of the FAP gene to chromosome 5 (BODMER et al. 1987) and the use of probes to genes closely linked to this region will allow the early identification of patients but only in those families whose pedigree is informative.

The latter property depends not only on information gathering of the whole family but also on the distribution of the polymorphic genes which are being probed in order to detect the presence or absence of the abnormal gene for FAP. The detection of a phenotypic abnormality in the histologically normal colonic mucosa would be of use, not only in 'non-informative' families but also to confirm the genetic analysis.

Approaches that have been used in an attempt to demonstrate abnormalities in the morphologically normal colonic mucosa of FAP patients have included proliferative activity as assessed by tritiated thymidine incorporation, mucin histochemistry, biochemical assays for the proliferation-associated enzyme ornithine decarboxylase and immunohistochemical methods using monoclonal antibodies.

2.2.1 Epithelial Proliferative Activity

In the normal colonic mucosa, cell renewal takes place in the lower third of the crypt (COLE and MCKALEN 1961). The work of several groups suggests that, in FAP, there is a shift of this proliferative compartment from the lower third of the crypt towards the surface (DESCHNER et al. 1963; BLEIBERG et al. 1972; IWAMA et al. 1977; LIPKIN et al. 1984). The proliferative activity in these studies has been assessed by incubation of rectal mucosal biopsy specimens with tritiated thymidine followed by autoradiography. In this way those cells undergoing DNA synthesis are visualised. About 15%–20% of cells in the proliferative compartment are engaged in DNA synthesis and the number of cells diminishes as the cells mature up the crypt (LIPKIN 1980). Once the surface epithelium is reached, DNA synthesis has ceased. In FAP a focal abnormality has been described in which DNA synthesis continues up the crypt and the surface epithelium may show proliferative abnormality. This change occurs in the normal appearing colonic epithelial cells before the mucosa develops the cytological features associated with adenoma. The abnormal activity has been observed in about 80% of random biopsy specimens (LIPKIN 1978). LIPKIN has suggested that abnormal proliferation is due to failure of repression of DNA synthesis. These findings are in keeping with the postulates of BODMER et al. (1987), who have suggested that the FAP gene encodes for a growth inhibiting protein and that the level of this protein has to reach a certain low threshold before a focal abnormality (i.e. an adenoma) is produced.

We have recently studied the morphologically normal mucosa of FAP patients using the monoclonal antibody Ki-67 (GERDES et al. 1983), which detects proliferating cells. We have been unable to demonstrate convincingly differences between FAP patients and age/sex-matched controls (Fig. 2). These studies have used, as controls, colorectal mucosal samples from patients with idiopathic constipation and Crohn's disease and it may be that these are not entirely suitable controls. We are attempting further

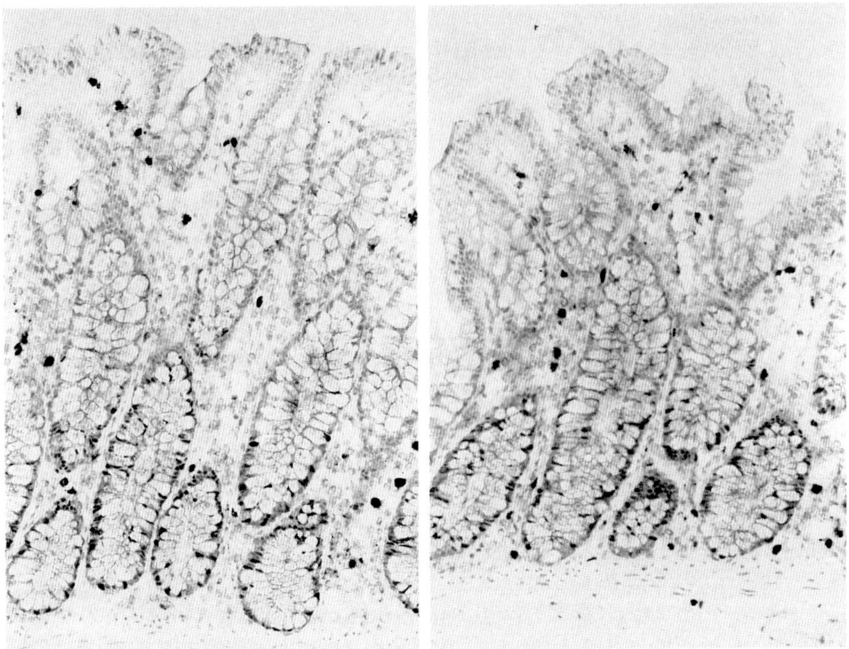

a b

Fig. 2a, b. A comparison of Ki-67 derived proliferative activity in the flat mucosa of age-, sex- and site-matched patients with idiopathic constipation (**a**) and FAP (**b**). Proliferative activity, as determined by nuclear staining in epithelial cells, is restricted to the lower third of the crypts in both biopsies. Stromal staining is due to endogenous peroxidase in mononuclear cells. Ki-67 immunoperoxidase, × 200

prospective studies using rectal mucosal biopsies taken from untreated FAP patients and age/sex-matched control patients with no evidence of gastrointestinal disease to corroborate our earlier findings. To date we have been unable to demonstrate any proliferative abnormality in the mucosa of FAP other than in micro-adenomas. We believe that further studies are necessary before proliferative studies can be used as a diagnostic test in FAP.

2.2.2 Mucin Histochemistry

Several investigators have reported abnormalities in the mucin histochemistry of the morphologically normal colonic mucosal goblet cells in FAP. Filipe et al. (1980) have suggested that there is an increased sialomucin expression in the flat mucosa of FAP patients. It has also been suggested that the flat mucosa of the left colon of FAP patients shows increased expression of the lectin Ulex europaeus agglutinin 1 (UEA-1) (Yonezawa et al. 1983) compared with the goblet cell mucin of normal left colonic mucosa (Yonezawa et al. 1982). Sugihara and Jass (1987) were, however, unable to confirm these findings and they found no difference in UEA-1 binding between patients with FAP and site-matched controls. They did note a pronounced regional difference in UEA-1 binding in both FAP patients and controls.

MUTO et al. (1985) have used the periodic acid thionin Schiff/potassium hydroxide:periodic acid-Schiff method which differentiates *N*-acetyl sialomucin and neutral mucins (a blue colour) from *O*-acetyl sialomucins (a red colour). In their study the flat mucosa of FAP patients produced a blue product with this stain in 83% of patients whereas only 36% of normal controls showed this reaction. They have suggested that sialomucin properties of the flat mucosa in FAP are different from those of normal colon and that this simple histochemical technique may be of use in the early detection of at-risk patients (MUTO et al. 1987). However, SUGIHARA and JASS (1987) were unable to confirm these findings in a much larger series of patients and suggested that the lack of specificity of the method for sialic acid combined with a failure to appreciate the existence of regional variation would account for the differential expression described by MUTO and his colleagues. Apart from a possible reduction in the expression of neutral sugars in the right colon of patients with FAP, SUGIHARA and JASS (1987) could find no mucin or lectin histochemical differences in the normal mucosa of FAP patients and matched controls. These results would suggest that mucin histochemistry has little part to play in the early detection of patients at risk of FAP.

2.2.3 Ornithine Decarboxylase Activity

Ornithine decarboxylase is the rate-limiting enzyme in the polyamine synthesis pathway. The enzyme is intimately involved in epithelial proliferation (HEBY 1981). Biochemical analysis of mucosal biopsy specimens from patients with FAP has shown significantly higher levels of the enzyme in these patients compared with controls (LUK and BAYLIN 1984). It has been suggested that colonic mucosal ornithine decarboxylase may be a sensitive biological marker for FAP. However, there are problems: the level of ornithine decarboxylase is unequivocally raised in both adenomas and carcinomas of the colon (LAMURAGLIA et al. 1985) and the studies of LUK and BAYLIN do not conclusively rule out the possibility that small adenomas and micro-adenomas were present in the tissues that they used for their analysis. Further studies are required to test the sensitivity and specificity of mucosal ornithine decarboxylase in much younger patients at risk from FAP. The mucosa of these patients is less likely to be contaminated by numerous adenomas and micro-adenomas.

2.2.4 *Monoclonal Antibodies*

Two recent studies have suggested that monoclonal antibodies which recognise two very different antigens may be useful in the early identification of FAP patients. In a wide-ranging study using the antibodies AE1 and AE3, which are directed against cytokeratin determinants, CHESA et al. (1986) studied five cases of FAP and noted that the epithelial cells showed uniformly strong immunoreactivity with the monoclonal antibody AE1 throughout the crypt. In the control tissues only the cells of the proliferative compartment stained with the antibody. A similar immunoreactivity pattern was noted by HARA et al. (1987) using a monoclonal antibody to the carbohydrate stage-specific embryonic antigen 1 (SSEA-1). Following these reports, we stained mucosal biopsies from five FAP patients and five age-, sex- and site-matched controls with AE1 and a monoclonal antibody directed against SSEA-1 (SOLTER and KNOWLES 1978) but could find no differences between the FAP mucosal specimens and the controls (JASS and SHEPHERD 1988, unpublished observations). In conclusion, despite numerous descriptions of various functional differences between the morphologically normal mucosa of FAP patients and controls, critical study casts doubt on many of these reports and at present we have no clinically useful method, excepting the genetic analyses, of diagnosing the disease before adenomas are demonstrated by sigmoidoscopy.

2.3 Extracolonic Manifestations of FAP

Until GARDNER (1951) described the syndrome which now bears his name, FAP was thought to be an entirely colorectal condition. It is now realised that the disease is a multisystem disorder. Adenoma proneness extends throughout the gastrointestinal tract and the adenoma-carcinoma sequence that is so readily observed in the colon in FAP can also occur in the remaining gastrointestinal tract. There is also a propensity to skin, soft tissue and bony lesions in FAP, some of which are included under the term Gardner's syndrome.

GARDNER (1951) originally described a patient group in whom FAP coexisted with osteomas of the skull and jaw and numerous epidermal cysts of the skin. On subsequent review of the kindred, further dental abnormalities were identified and osteomas were also found throughout the entire skeleton (GARDNER and RICHARDS 1953; GARDNER 1962). There is now much debate as to whether Gardner's syndrome and classical FAP are different conditions or merely differing expressions of the same genetic defect. Many have regarded any extracolonic disease associated with FAP as a manifestation of Gardner's syndrome. However, it has been shown that more than 90% of FAP patients have occult osteomas of the jaw, one of the cardinal signs of Gardner's syndrome (UTSUNOMIYA and NAKAMURA 1975). Also there are kindreds with Gardner's syndrome in which some of the patients do not have extracolonic manifestations of FAP and further families with classical FAP are known in whom some members show features of Gardner's syndrome. Many would now regard FAP and Gardner's syndrome to be differing manifestations of the same genetic abnormality rather than the expression of two abnormal genes at different loci and doubt whether the term Gardner's syndrome should continue to be used.

Many of the extracolonic conditions present in FAP, such as epidermal cysts and bony osteomas, are trivial and do not cause significant morbidity. Similarly congenital hypertrophy of the retinal pigment epithelium has been associated with FAP (BLAINE and TREMPE 1980; LLOPIS and MENEZO 1987). This is probably not of clinical importance but may be of significance as a diagnostic sign of FAP. Nevertheless there are extracolonic conditions which are clinically more important and may give rise to significant morbidity and mortality.

2.3.1 Desmoid Disease

The association of desmoid tumours and FAP was first described by MILLER and SWEET (1937). Between 5% and 10% of patients with FAP have clinically significant desmoid disease (SMITH 1959; BUSSEY 1975; KLEMMER

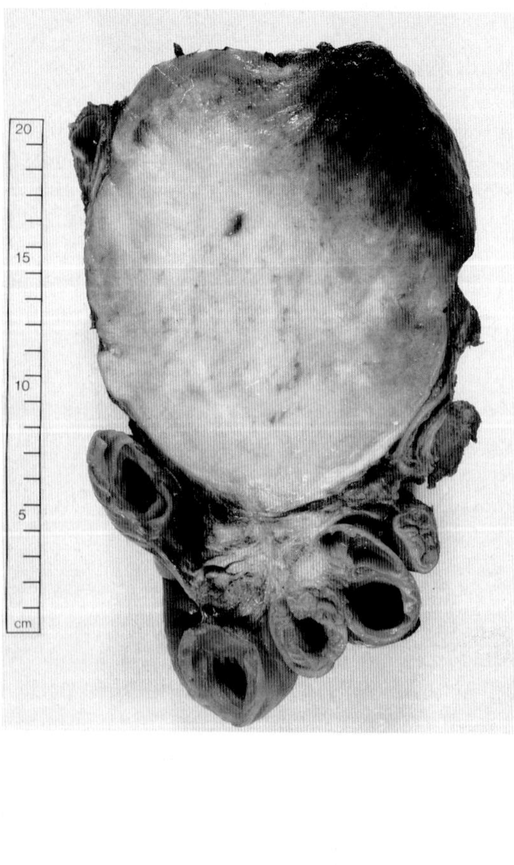

Fig. 3. A mesenteric desmoid tumour in a 32-year-old female FAP patient who presented with small bowel obstruction. The tumour has involved loops of small bowel and there is a large area of intratumoral haemorrhage

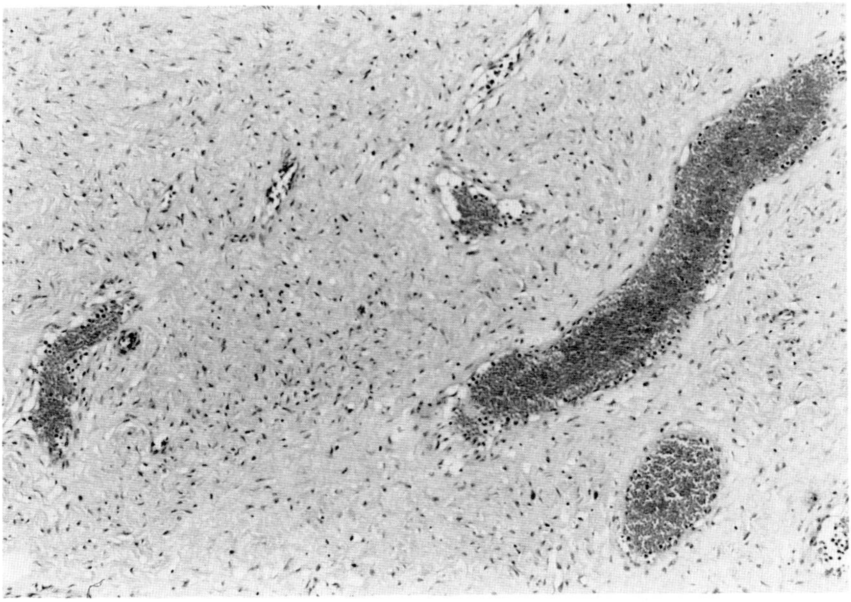

Fig. 4. Histology of the desmoid shown in Fig. 3. There are numerous fibroblasts in a myxoid stroma with relatively little collagen. Note the widely ectatic blood vessels which account for the high rate of peri-operative haemorrhage. HE, × 100

et al. 1987). The tumour occurs in young patients and in particular women are affected, a ratio of 3:1 being recorded by the Cleveland Clinic Group (JONES et al. 1986). Most tumours present after previous surgery, the onset usually being 1–2 years after colectomy. Although fibromatoses may be found in musculo-aponeurotic sites outside the abdomen in FAP patients, the clinically important desmoids are most commonly found within the abdomen, especially in the retroperitoneum and mesentery (Fig. 3). The tumours may occur in the scar on the anterior abdominal wall. Clinical presentation is with a mass and/or small intestinal obstruction (Fig. 3). Unlike extra-abdominal fibromatosis, desmoids associated with FAP may show rapid growth, particularly after surgery, and are a cause of significant mortality in FAP patients (HERRERA-ORNELAS et al. 1987).

Histologically desmoids associated with FAP are indistinguishable from fibromatosis elsewhere (ENZINGER and WEISS 1983). However, the histological appearances are variable and there is a tendency for FAP desmoids to be more cellular with a myxoid stroma and numerous small blood vessels (Fig. 4). The blood vessels that characterise desmoid tumours are of capillary size but lack a well-defined wall, the pericytes appearing to merge with the tumour cells. The vessels are often widely ectatic and this presumably accounts for the haemorrhage that may occur during surgery and may be life threatening. Stromal haemorrhage is often a prominent feature on both macroscopic examination and histological study of intra-abdominal desmoid tumours (Fig. 3).

The treatment of desmoids has been predominantly surgical although many surgeons with a wide experience of FAP are very reluctant to undertake surgery for asymptomatic desmoids even in the presence of a large mass because of problems associated with haemorrhage and rapid regrowth after surgery. Radiotherapy has in the past been attempted but fibromatoses are relatively insensitive to radiotherapy and doses in excess of 5000 rads are likely to be required: such doses are likely to cause significant radiation enteritis. Successful outcome has been reported with chemotherapy (HUTCHINSON et al. 1979) but generally results with chemotherapy have been disappointing. Some response to non-steroidal anti-inflammatory agents, particularly indomethacin and sulindac, has occurred in isolated cases (WADDELL and GERNER 1980; BELLIVEAU and GRAHAM 1984; PROCTER et al. 1987; KLEIN et al. 1987). It has been suggested that prostaglandin inhibition produced by these agents causes T cell and killer cell induction and hence tumour regression (BELLIVEAU and GRAHAM 1984). Alternatively these agents may act by blocking ornithine decarboxylase activity, thus reducing cell proliferation (WADDELL et al. 1983).

Desmoid tumours as a whole, and in particular in FAP, are more common in women and are known to enlarge during pregnancy (MCADAM and GOLIGHER 1970) and after taking oral contraceptives (JONES et al. 1986). Therefore it has been intimated that these tumours are under hormonal influence, in particular by oestrogens. Oestrogen receptor activity has been demonstrated in some desmoid tumours (REITAMO et al. 1986) although more recently we have been unable to demonstrate oestrogen or progesterone receptors by biochemical assay in seven intra-abdominal desmoids in patients with FAP (SHEPHERD and PUDDEFOOT 1987, unpublished observations). Nevertheless response to anti-oestrogen compounds such as tamoxifen has been described in FAP-associated desmoids (WADDELL et al. 1983; KINZBRUNNER et al. 1983) and in multicentric desmoid tumours (PROCTER et al. 1987). Whatever the mechanism of action of non-steroidal anti-inflammatory agents and tamoxifen, the reports of response are encouraging and worthy of a full prospective multicentre trial.

2.3.2 Upper Gastrointestinal Tract Neoplasia

Duodenal lesions in FAP patients were considered very unusual until recently. HOFFMANN and GOLIGHER (1971) reviewed the world literature and could only find ten cases of FAP associated with duodenal polyps. The precise frequency of neoplastic change in the duodenum in patients with FAP is to this day uncertain but there are now reports which indicate that about 50% of FAP patients will have duodenal adenomas (BULOW 1986; JARVINEN and SIPPONEN 1986) whilst about 30% of patients were found to

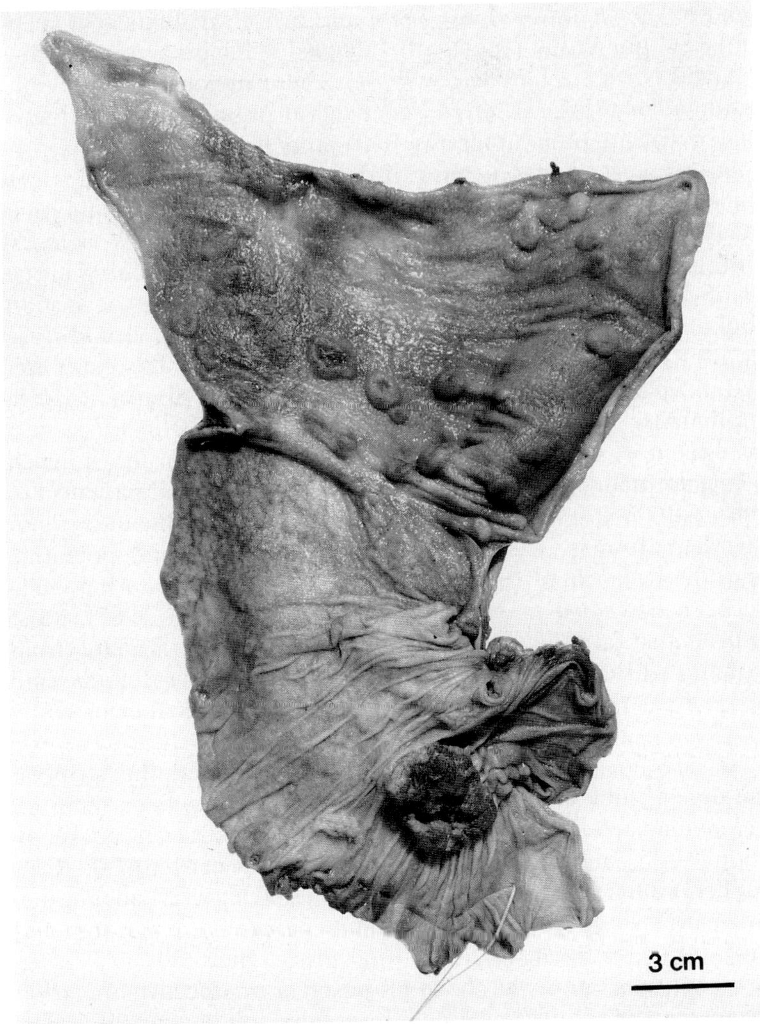

Fig. 5. Whipple's operation specimen from an FAP patient (gastric antrum *above* and duodenum *below*). A large protuberant carcinoma is present at the ampulla. There is an adenomatous polyp adjacent to the carcinoma. The gastric antral polyps are non-neoplastic hyperplastic polyps

have duodenal adenomas on a single endoscopic screen (KURTZ et al. 1987; SARRE et al. 1987). Many FAP patients with endoscopically normal duodenum have adenomas on histological examination of random peri-ampullary biopsies (ALEXANDER et al. 1987; SPIGELMAN et al. 1988). The increased neoplastic potential in this area is not confined to the duodenal mucosa. There are reports of adenomatosis and carcinoma arising in the extrahepatic bile ducts, the gall-bladder and the pancreatic ducts in FAP patients (LEES and HERMAN 1981; JARVINEN et al. 1983; KOMOROWSKI et al. 1986).

The high prevalence of duodenal adenomas in FAP patients is in keeping with the now numerous reports of duodenal carcinoma complicating FAP (JONES and NANCE 1977; BULOW 1987). These tumours are predominantly peri-ampullary (Fig. 5), often advanced at presentation and therefore associated with a poor prognosis. Peri-ampullary carcinoma is probably the second most common cause of death in FAP patients after colorectal cancer (JAGELMAN 1987). SUGIHARA et al. (1982) found that duodenal carcinomas occur at a mean age of 45 and that 40% were associated with synchronous adenomas. The risk of carcinoma arising in the duodenum of FAP patients appears to be sufficiently high to warrant prophylactic screening by upper gastrointestinal endoscopy. Studies are now under way in many countries in order to determine the exact frequency of duodenal neoplasia and malignancy to enable routine surveillance programmes to be formulated.

The assessment of the frequency of neoplastic change in the stomach is difficult because many of the polyps in the stomach of FAP patients are fundic gland cysts (WATANABE et al. 1978). These lesions, which are considered to be hamartomas, have little or no added malignant potential. Adenomas of the stomach, a particularly unusual lesion in Western populations, have been described in 4%–13% of patients (BULOW 1987). Most of the reports associating gastric carcinoma with FAP originate from Japan, a country with a high incidence of sporadic gastric carcinoma, and the incidence of gastric carcinoma in Western FAP patients appears to be very low (DESIGAN et al. 1986; KURTZ et al. 1987).

Adenomas are not infrequently seen in the mucosa of the terminal ileum at the time of total colectomy for FAP and cases have been reported in which adenomas are found in the ileum by intra-operative endoscopy (OHSATO et al. 1977) and after colectomy (HAMILTON et al. 1979). ROSS and MARA (1974) described the occurrence of jejunal and ileal adenocarcinoma in two patients but the risk of malignant change in the jejunum and ileum appears to be minimal. Recently total proctocolectomy, ileal reservoir and ileo-anal anastomosis has been proposed as an effective operation for FAP. However, both in ileo-anal ileal reservoirs and in continent ileostomy reservoirs, a form of colonic metaplasia appears to take place (PHILLIPS 1985; SHEPHERD et al. 1987a) and it may be that the creation of an ileal reservoir which subsequently undergoes a form of colonic metaplasia provides an environment in which adenomas and possibly carcinomas may arise. Adenomas have been noted both in FAP patients with continent ileostomy reservoirs and in those with ileo-anal ileal reservoirs (BEART et al. 1982; SHEPHERD et al. 1987a; STRYKER et al. 1987).

2.3.3 *Extra-gastrointestinal Neoplasia*

Associations have been reported between FAP and several extra-gastrointestinal tumours. Perhaps the strongest association is with papillary carcinoma of the thyroid gland. PLAIL et al. (1987) reviewed the St. Mark's Hospital Polyposis Register and found seven women with a history of thyroid carcinoma out of a total of 465. There were no cases of thyroid carcinoma amongst males. These authors suggested that the risk of women with FAP under the age of 35 developing thyroid cancer was increased 160-fold and that all patients with FAP should have regular thyroid examinations. There is strong evidence that there is also an increased incidence of childhood hepatoblastoma in FAP families (KINGSTON et al. 1983; LI et al. 1987). There is a suggestion of an increased incidence of non-thyroid endocrine tumours in FAP. These include multiple endocrine adenomatosis type II b, pituitary adenomas, islet cell tumours and tumours of the adrenal cortex (NAYLOR and GARDNER 1981; SCHNEIDER et al. 1983; PAINTER and JAGELMAN 1985; PERKINS et al. 1985).

The association between polyposis coli and malignant tumours of the central nervous system has been termed Turcot's syndrome. TURCOT and his colleagues (1959) described two siblings in whom multiple colonic polyps were associated with astrocytoma and medulloblastoma. There are controversies about the syndrome, particularly its suggested autosomal recessive inheritance (ROTHMAN et al. 1975; ITOH et al. 1979; LEWIS et al. 1983) and the fact that the adenomas in the colon are relatively few in number compared with classical FAP (BAUGHMAN et al. 1969). Therefore, like Gardner's syndrome, the separate identity and specificity of Turcot's syndrome is still in doubt.

3 Peutz-Jeghers Polyposis

The association of gastrointestinal polyposis and mucocutaneous pigmentation was first described from Holland by PEUTZ (1921). JEGHERS et al. (1949) reviewed the features of ten patients, producing what is now regarded as a classic description of the syndrome. Peutz-Jeghers polyposis (PJP) shows an autosomal dominant inheritance. The polyps are found throughout the gastrointestinal tract but are most prevalent in the small intestine (MORSON 1962). Polyps have been described in the urinary tract as part of the syndrome (SOMMERHAUG and MASON 1970), although in some cases these polyps are not hamartomatous but merely oedematous mucosal folds (HAGGITT and REID 1986). It is doubtful, therefore, whether true hamartomatous polyps occur in the urinary tract as part of the Peutz-Jeghers syndrome.

Although Peutz-Jeghers polyps are classified as hamartomas, they show a very orderly architecture. The core of the polyp is composed of tree-like branching bundles of smooth muscle covered by mucosa of the type native to that part of the bowel in which the polyp arises. The mucosa of the polyp, which appears morphologically normal, contains all specialised cells present in that part of the gastrointestinal tract. Peutz-

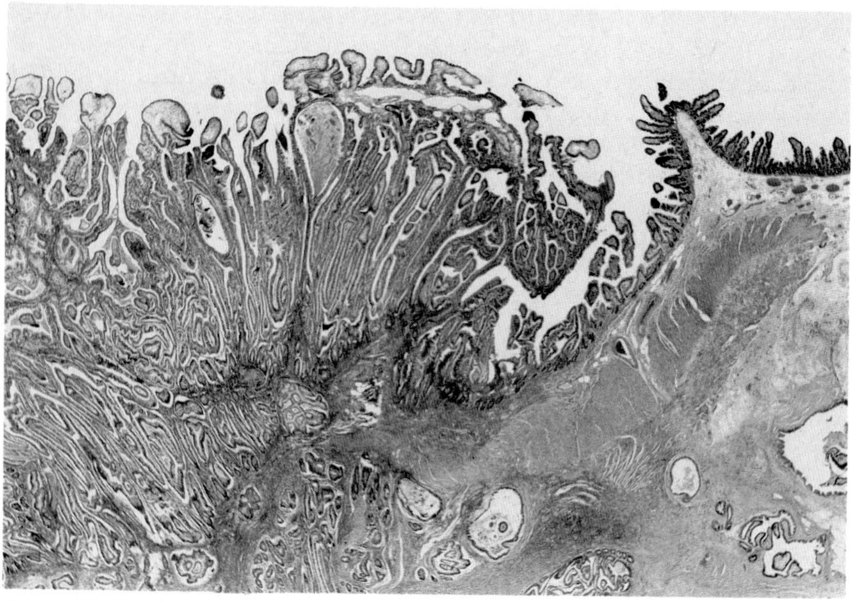

Fig. 6. Epithelial misplacement in the jejunal Peutz-Jeghers polyp in an 18-year-old female. The presence of glandular epithelium and mucinous cysts within the muscularis propria and serosa mimics invasive carcinoma. Normal small intestinal mucosa is present at *right*. HE, × 25

Jeghers polyps are especially prone to intussusception, particularly in the small intestine, and may also cause bowel obstruction. It is these mechanisms which probably account for the epithelial misplacement that may be seen in small intestinal polyps. In a review of 40 patients with PJP, it was shown that epithelial misplacement is a not uncommon accompaniment of small intestinal PJP, occurring in approximately 10% of polyps (SHEPHERD et al. 1987 b). It is important to recognise this complication of PJP, which has previously been referred to as enteritis cystica profunda (KYRIAKOS and CONDON 1978), as the epithelial misplacement, which may extend into the muscularis propria and into serosal tissues, closely mimics invasive carcinoma (Fig. 6). This epithelial misplacement has resulted in an appreciable number of cases, especially in the early literature, being misdiagnosed as invasive malignancy.

3.1 Risk of Gastrointestinal Malignancy

There is still controversy about the magnitude of risk of gastrointestinal malignancy in PJP. Reviews of the early literature give incidences of gastrointestinal malignancy which vary from 0% (BARTHOLOMEW et al. 1957; DORMANDY 1957) to 24% (BAILEY 1957). DOZOIS et al. (1969) reviewed the world literature but could only find 11 cases of bona fide malignancy

Table 1. Frequency of gastrointestinal (GI) cancer in PJP

Series	Patients with PJP	Patients with GI carcinoma
Dozois et al. (1969)	326	11
Utsunomiya et al. (1975)	102	13
Linos et al. (1981)	48	1
Giardiello et al. (1987)	31	4
St. Mark's Hospital PJP patients (unpublished data)	28	3
	535	32

in Peutz-Jeghers polyps whilst Utsunomiya et al. (1975) found a 13% incidence of gastrointestinal carcinoma in a review of 102 patients with PJP. Reid (1974) reviewed the world literature and concluded that the estimated lifetime risk of gastrointestinal carcinoma in PJP was 2% and that gastric and duodenal malignancies were most common. In Japan, the colorectum appears to be the site with the highest incidence of carcinoma in PJP (Utsunomiya et al. 1975; Konishi et al. 1987) although in this country some of these cases (Konishi et al. 1987; Narita et al. 1987) would be diagnosed as severe dysplasia in view of the apparent absence of invasion across the muscularis mucosae. Differences in histological interpretation of what is clearly a rare finding only add to the difficulties in assessing the risk of malignancy in PJP.

In the Mayo Clinic series of 48 PJP patients observed in a 45-year period, only one patient has developed gastrointestinal carcinoma (Linos et al. 1981). There are 68 PJP patients registered at St. Mark's Hospital and of these, 28 have been seen at the hospital. Of these 28 patients, three men, aged 38, 39 ad 34, have died of adenocarcinoma of the stomach, caecum and pancreas respectively. In the cases of gastric and caecal carcinoma it could not be convincingly demonstrated that the carcinomas actually arose in Peutz-Jeghers polyps. Recently we have reviewed the histology of all Peutz-Jeghers polyps held in the St. Mark's Polyposis Registry (Shepherd et al. 1987 b) and the absence of epithelial dysplasia in any of the 491 polyps examined suggests that neoplastic change in Peutz-Jeghers polyps is a very rare occurrence. Nevertheless there are at least 40 convincing case reports of gastrointestinal cancer in PJP. Most of these cancers have arisen in the stomach and upper small bowel. Table 1 documents the frequency of gastrointestinal cancer in five of the largest series of PJP. It should be emphasised that many of these cancers have arisen in patients under the age of 40. From the data available, we conclude that, whilst PJP is generally considered to be a relatively benign condition, there is a small but definite increased propensity to gastrointestinal carcinoma in the syndrome. We would, however, agree with the conclusion of Linos et al. (1981) that surgical conservatism should be practiced in the management of PJP due to the small risk of malignancy and the high risk of complications of radical surgery.

3.2 Extra-gastrointestinal Neoplasia

Extra-gastrointestinal associations are being increasingly recognised in PJP, as they are in FAP and juvenile polyposis. The association between PJP and an unusual ovarian tumour, 'sex cord tumour with annular tubules' (SCTAT) was first described by SCULLY (1970). The tumour is thought to arise from granulosa cells but has a morphological pattern more like that of Sertoli cells. The tumour may have oestrogenic effects, leading to endometrial hyperplasia. It is probable that most female patients with PJP have small SCTAT tumours if the ovaries are diligently examined. There appears to be an association between PJP, SCTAT and low grade adenocarcinoma of the endocervix, so-called adenoma malignum (YOUNG et al. 1982). More recently YOUNG et al. (1983) have described a functioning ovarian sex cord tumour which is apparently unique to PJP.

The increased frequency of extra-gastrointestinal malignancy has been highlighted by GIARDIELLO et al. (1987). In their series of 31 patients, 15 patients developed malignant tumours, only four of which arose in the gastrointestinal tract. The majority of these tumours were adenocarcinomas, four in the pancreas and two in the breast. An apparently increased incidence of breast cancer in female PJP patients is manifest in reports describing the association of PJP with bilateral breast cancer (RILEY and SWIFT 1980; TRAU et al. 1982; LEHUR et al. 1984). The four patients with pancreatic carcinoma in the Johns Hopkins series of 31 patients represent a 100-fold increase in the disease over that expected in a normal population. One patient in the St. Mark's Hospital Registry died of pancreatic carcinoma at the age of 34 and a 19-year-old patient with PJP and pancreatic carcinoma has been described (BOWLBY 1986). Although many types of tumour have been associated with PJP, there does seem to be a markedly increased incidence of certain tumours in the syndrome and these undoubtedly include ovarian tumours, breast cancer and pancreatic cancer.

4 Juvenile Polyposis

The third of the triumvirate of hereditary polyposis syndromes, juvenile polyposis (JP), was not fully defined until 1964 (MCCOLL et al. 1964), although several groups had previously described polyposis syndromes in children which, although originally called adenomatous polyposis, in retrospect probably represented JP (KERR 1948; GORDON et al. 1957; HINES et al. 1959). The confusion that abounds in the literature regarding JP is hardly surprising considering the difficulties in defining the disease, its rarity and the plethora of clinical presentations.

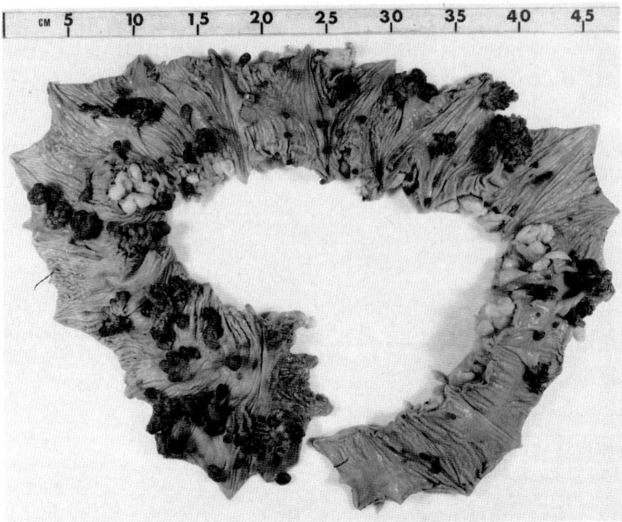

Fig. 7. Colectomy specimen from a 17-year-old boy with JP. Note the relative paucity of polyps compared with FAP and the large, papillary 'atypical' juvenile polyps

The sporadic juvenile polyp is a relatively common polyp amongst children and adolescents and occasionally occurs in adults. In countries where adenomas are rare, the juvenile polyp is one of the commoner clinically significant polyps. It usually presents with bleeding per rectum and there is no family history. Sporadic juvenile polyps may be multiple; up to five juvenile polyps in the rectum is not an unusual finding. Dysplasia is extremely uncommon in isolated juvenile polyps. There is only a single report of dysplasia in a sporadic juvenile polyp (FRIEDMAN and FECHNER 1982) and only two cases of carcinoma arising in solitary juvenile polyps (LIU et al. 1978, JONES et al. 1987). Clearly the risk of dysplasia and carcinoma in isolated juvenile polyps is very low indeed.

Whereas FAP and PJP are now well-defined syndromes, JP is less clearly defined. A working definition of the syndrome should include one of the following (a) more than ten juvenile polyps, (b) juvenile polyps throughout the gastrointestinal tract, or (c) any number of juvenile polyps with family history of JP (SACHATELLO et al. 1974). Patients who meet these requirements fall into three major clinical groups:

1. JP of infancy
2. Generalised JP (throughout the gastrointestinal tract) with or without a family history
3. JP of the colon (juvenile polyposis coli) with or without a family history (Fig. 7).

Data from the St. Mark's Polyposis Registry indicate that juvenile polyposis coli is much commoner than generalised JP. The sporadic form of generalised JP is commoner than the familial form. Congenital defects are more likely to occur in sporadic JP and approximately 20% of these patients will show such congenital abnormalities as malrotation of the bowel, Meckel's diverticulum, mesenteric lymphangioma, congenital heart disease, hypertelorism and hydrocephalus (VEALE et al. 1966; BUSSEY 1975). Familial JP appears to be an autosomal dominant condition; this is suggested by its occurrence in three generations (SMILOW et al. 1966). JP of infancy has a very poor prognosis. Infants present with bleeding, diarrhoea, rectal prolapse, malnutrition, dehydration and large numbers of typical juvenile polyps in the colon. Death usually occurs at an early age (SACHATELLO et al. 1974). Such cases of infantile JP are very rare. Non-infantile cases of JP usually present with rectal bleeding or the symptoms and signs of anaemia.

4.1 Risk of Gastrointestinal Malignancy

The magnitude of risk of malignant change in JP is at present uncertain. The condition is undoubtedly rare and currently there are only seven reported cases of unequivocal colorectal carcinoma in association with histologically confirmed JP (Table 2). STEMPER et al. (1975) reported a large kindred in which ten patients had single or multiple juvenile polyps and 11 had carcinoma of the gastrointestinal tract. Of the patients with colorectal cancer, only one had definite JP. The rarity of reported cases of gastrointestinal malignancy arising in JP led authors to conclude that regular follow-up of patients with JP is probably not warranted because the risk of malignancy appears to be low, carcinoma in JP families is (allegedly) more common in those family members who do not have juvenile polyps and carcinoma in patients with JP can arise anywhere in the gastrointestinal tract and not necessarily within juvenile polyps themselves.

Table 2. Reports of concurrent colorectal carcinoma and JP

Reference	Age[a]	No of polyps of colorectum	Dysplasia	FH of juvenile polyps	FH of GIT cancer
1	59	15	?	Yes	No
2	30	?	Yes	Yes	Yes
3	40	Many	Yes	No	No
4	23	Numerous	Yes	No	No
5	25	Multiple	Yes	No	Yes
6	58	Numerous	Yes	Yes	No
7	49	3 + gastric	Yes	Yes	Yes

[a] Age at diagnosis of carcinoma; FH, family history; GIT, gastrointestinal tract.
References: 1, SMILOW et al. 1966; 2, STEMPER et al. 1975; 3, RESTREPO et al. 1978; 4, GOODMAN et al. 1979; 5, GRIGIONI et al. 1981; 6, ROZEN and BARATZ 1982; 7, JARVINEN and FRANSSILA 1984.

Table 3. A classification of polyps in the St. Mark's series of JP patients (JASS et al. 1987)

	Dysplasia				
	None	Mild	Moderate	Severe	Total
Typical juvenile	758	70	6	0	834
Atypical juvenile	90	50	25	3	168[a]
Adenomas					21[b]
Metaplastic polyps					2
					1025

[a] One atypical polyp contained a focus of carcinoma.
[b] One adenoma contained a focus of carcinoma.

There are now grounds for questioning this assessment of the risk of malignant change. The St. Mark's Polyposis Registry holds records of 87 JP patients, ascertained through 64 index cases. Seventeen patients have developed colorectal cancer. Seven of the index patients had colorectal cancer at the time of referral but two of these cancers were only discovered at histological examination at St. Mark's Hospital. Consequently five patients have been removed from the analysis to avoid bias. In the remaining patients, the incidence of carcinoma is 14.6%. The median age of patients with cancer was 32 years (range 16–58) and the majority of these cancers occurred in patients under the age of 35. Although this is a small series of a rare disease and there is inevitably some bias towards recording of JP patients with colorectal cancer, there is little doubt that these data represent a greatly increased risk of colorectal cancer in JP, especially considering the young age of the patients concerned (JASS et al. 1988). The increased risk clearly justifies clinical surveillance of affected individuals and their families by regular endoscopy and prophylactic removal of polyps.

The intimation that carcinoma in JP patients can arise anywhere in the gastrointestinal tract and not necessarily within juvenile polyps can be countered by the increasing evidence to suggest that cancer does indeed arise within juvenile polyps. Dysplasia has been described in two forms in patients with JP. It may occur within juvenile polyps, producing so-called mixed polyps (HAGGITT and PITCOCK 1970; STEMPER et al. 1975; RESTREPO et al. 1978; GOODMAN et al. 1979; GRIGIONI et al. 1981; JARVINEN and FRANSSILA 1984). Secondly, dysplasia may be seen in an adenoma which shows no residual features of the juvenile polyp (RESTREPO et al. 1978; RABIN et al. 1979). It is uncertain whether such adenomas arise de novo or through neoplastic change within pre-existing juvenile polyps. The absence of small adenomas in these cases argues against a de novo origin (GOODMAN et al. 1979).

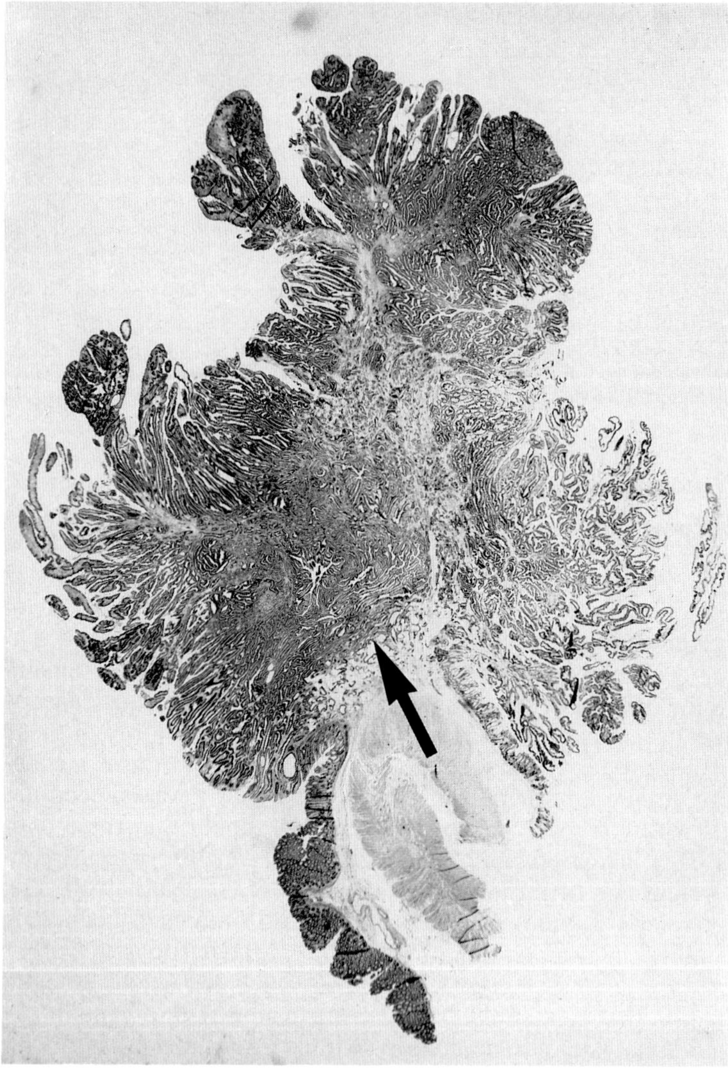

Fig. 8. A polyp from a 16-year-old boy with JP. The papillary configuration and the relative paucity of lamina propria and cystic crypts are characteristic of 'atypical juvenile polyps'. In addition there is focal invasive adenocarcinoma (*arrowed*). HE, × 10

Examination of the large series of multiple juvenile polyps at St. Mark's Hospital supports the suggestion that dysplasia arises in juvenile polyps (Table 3; JASS et al. 1987). This study has shown that dysplasia is more likely to occur in a subtype of juvenile polyp that is defined by certain morphological features. Two types of juvenile polyp are recognised. One type is the classical juvenile polyp with its well-known histological features. The second type of polyp is usually multilobated, lacks surface ulceration and often shows a papillary configuration (Figs. 7, 8). These polyps lack the abundant lamina propria that is so characteristic of classical juvenile polyps. They have been called atypical juvenile polyps. The demonstration of various grades of dysplasia and a focus of carcinoma (Fig. 8) within the St. Mark's series of juvenile polyps provides indirect but important evidence for the origin of carcinoma within the juvenile polyp itself (Table 3; JASS et al. 1987).

In conclusion, there is an undoubted increased risk of gastrointestinal cancer, particularly colorectal cancer, in JP. The demonstration of all grades of dysplasia within a series of JP polyps suggests that cancer probably arises within the polyp itself. Further research is required from other centres to corroborate these findings in an attempt to define adequate surveillance programmes and management of affected families and individuals.

5 Other Polyposis Syndromes

5.1 Inflammatory and Lymphoid Polyposis

Inflammatory polyposis is the commonest form of polyposis to affect the colon and rectum. It is usually the sequel of inflammatory bowel disease, particularly ulcerative colitis, but is also seen in Crohn's disease, diverticular disease, schistosomiasis and amoebiasis. Because of the association with inflammatory bowel disease, it is unlikely to be confused with other forms of polyposis. Lymphoid polyposis, on the other hand, clinically simulates the polyposis syndromes, especially FAP. Multiple lymphoid polyps, which histologically are hyperplastic lymphoid follicles, may mimic small adenomas of FAP and are especially common in the defunctioned rectum (Fig. 9). Benign lymphoid polyposis is rare and characteristically occurs in children, probably the result of viral infection. It is also seen in the immunodeficient (SHAW and HENNIGAR 1974).

Malignant lymphomatous polyposis (MLP) (see p. 157), which has also been given the tautologous title of multiple lymphomatous polyposis, is a primary gastrointestinal malignant lymphoma of diffuse centrocytic type (BLACKSHAW 1980; ISAACSON et al. 1984). Although any part of the bowel may be affected in MLP, the colon and rectum are most usually involved and a recent review suggests that MLP is a relatively common subtype of primary malignant lymphoma of the colon and rectum, comprising one-quarter of the 45 cases (SHEPHERD et al. 1988). Clinically MLP may closely mimic FAP although it is most often a disease of the middle-aged and elderly.

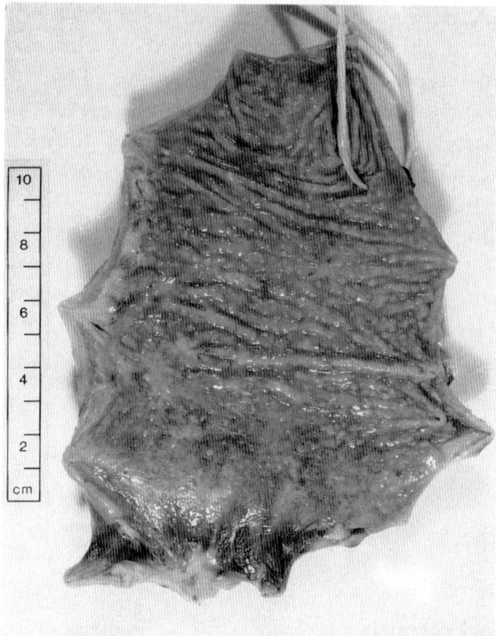

Fig. 9. The defunctioned rectum of a 33-year-old female patient with FAP. The polyps, which could easily be mistaken for adenomas, are in fact lymphoid polyps

5.2 Metaplastic Polyposis

Metaplastic polyps are the commonest polyps of the colorectum in the elderly and are usually multiple. However, cases of metaplastic polyposis have been described in younger, predominantly male, patients (WILLIAMS et al. 1980; BENGOECHEA et al. 1987). In these cases typical though relatively large metaplastic polyps, mostly in excess of 50 in number, have been present and in the case of BENGOECHEA et al. (1987) were associated with a carcinoma at the age of 28. In the records of the Pathology department of St. Mark's Hospital are several cases of adenocarcinoma of the colon and rectum associated with multiple metaplastic polyps (at least 50) in young and middle-aged adults. Although it may be that the metaplastic polyps are a secondary or independent phenomenon, it is possible that there is a syndrome of metaplastic polyposis which is associated with an increased risk of colorectal malignancy. Further research into metaplastic polyposis is warranted.

5.3 Other Rare Polyposis Syndromes

Cowden's disease is an inherited syndrome in which multiple hamartomas of the skin are associated with polyps of the gastrointestinal tract. The polyps, which are probably only present in about 35% of cases (SALEM

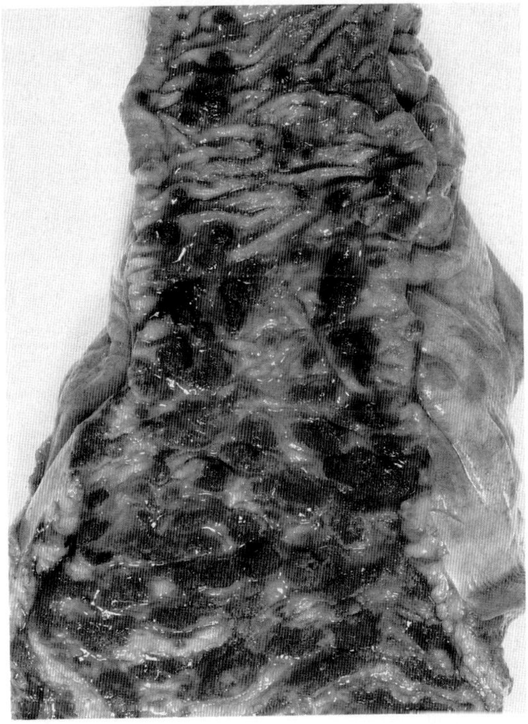

Fig. 10. The sigmoid colon of a 35-year-old male patient with inflammatory cap polyposis. The polyps are particularly located on the mucosal folds, best seen at the *top*, and appear dark and granular

and STECK 1983), are varied histologically and have features of juvenile polyps, lymphoid polyps, inflammatory polyps and ganglioneuromas (HAGGITT and REID 1986). There does not appear to be any increased risk of gastrointestinal malignancy although patients with the syndrome have very high rates of breast and thyroid carcinoma (SALEM and STECK 1983). In the Ruvalcaba-Myhre-Smith (RMS) syndrome, first described in 1980 (RUVALCABA et al. 1980), ileal and colonic polyps are associated with severe mental deficiency, macro-encephaly and penile pigmentary lesions. The polyps appear to be histologically similar to juvenile polyps (HAGGITT and REID 1986). As extra-gastrointestinal congenital abnormalities are common in sporadic JP, it is probable that the RMS syndrome is a variant of JP.

Inflammatory 'cap' polyposis is a rare syndrome which affects the sigmoid colon and rectum of adults who present with rectal bleeding and mucous diarrhoea (WILLIAMS et al. 1985). The polyps are red, granular and sessile and concentrate on the apices of the mucosal folds (Fig. 10). Histologically there is elongation and dilatation of the crypt epithelium with fibromuscular obliteration of the lamina propria and a cap of inflammatory granulation tissue covering the luminal surface. The histological features are similar to those of the solitary ulcer (mucosal prolapse) syndrome; mucosal prolapse is probably a major aetiological factor. Other conditions such as multiple lipomas (YATTO 1982), multiple ganglioneuromas (CARNEY et al. 1976), multiple inflammatory fibroid polyps (ANTHONY et al. 1984), pneumatosis coli (PIETERSE et al. 1985) and the Cronkhite-Canada syndrome (DANIEL et al. 1982) may present clinically as polyposis. Only in the Cronkhite-Canada syndrome is there a suggestion of an increased risk of gastrointestinal malignancy (DANIEL et al. 1982)

References

Alexander JR, Becker JM, Buchi KN, Burt RW (1987) The frequency of adenomatous polyps of the duodenal papilla in familial polyposis coli. Gastroenterology 92:1293 A

Anthony PP, Morris DS, Vowles KDJ (1984) Multiple and recurrent inflammatory fibroid polyps in three generations of a Devon family: a new syndrome. Gut 25:854–862

Bailey D (1957) Polyposis of gastrointestinal tract: the Peutz syndrome. Br J Med I:433–439

Bartholomew LG, Dahlin DC, Waugh JM (1957) Intestinal polyposis associated with mucocutaneous melanin pigmentation (Peutz-Jeghers syndrome). Gastroenterology 32:434–451

Baughman FA, List CF, Williams JR, Muldoon JP, Segarra JM, Volkel JS (1969) The glioma-polyposis syndrome. N Engl J Med 281:1345–1346

Beart RW, Fleming CR, Banks PM (1982) Tubulovillous adenomas in a continent ileostomy after protocolectomy for familial polyposis. Dig Dis Sci 27:553–556

Belliveau P, Graham AM (1984) Mesenteric desmoid tumor in Gardner's syndrome treated with sulindac. Dis Colon Rectum 27:53–54

Bengoechea O, Martinez-Penuela JM, Larrinaga B, Valerdi J, Borda F (1987) Hyperplastic polyposis of the colorectum and adenocarcinoma in a 24-year-old man. Am J Surg Pathol 11:323–327

Blackshaw AJ (1980) Non-Hodgkin's lymphoma of the gut. In: Wright R (ed) Recent advances in gastrointestinal pathology. WB Saunders, London, pp 213–240

Blaine NP, Trempe DL (1980) Hypertrophy of the retinal pigment epithelium associated with Gardner's syndrome. Am J Ophthalmol 90:661–667

Bleiberg H, Mainguet P, Galand P (1972) Cell renewal in familial polyposis coli. Comparison between polyps and adjacent healthy mucosa. Gastroenterology 63:240–245

Bodmer WF, Bailey CJ, Bodmer J et al. (1987) Localization of the gene for familial adenomatous polyposis on chromosome 5. Nature 328:614–616

Bowlby LS (1986) Pancreatic adenocarcinoma in an adolescent male with Peutz-Jeghers syndrome. Hum Pathol 17:97–99

Bulow S (1986) Familial polyposis coli. A clinical and epidemiological study. Laegeforeningens, Copenhagen

Bulow S (1987) Incidence of associated diseases in familial polyposis coli. Sem in Surg Oncol 3:84–87

Bussey HJR (1975) Familial polyposis coli. The Johns Hopkins University Press, Baltimore

Carney JA, Go VLW, Sizemore GW, Hayles AB (1976) Alimentary tract ganglioneuromatosis. N Engl J Med 295:1287–1291

Chesa PG, Rettig WJ, Melamed MR (1986) Expression of cytokeratins in normal and neoplastic colonic epithelial cells. Implications for cellular differentiation and carcinogenesis. Am J Surg Pathol 10:829–835

Cole JW, McKalen A (1961) Observations of cell renewal in human rectal mucosa in vivo with thymidine-H^3. Gastroenterology 41:122–125

Daniel ES, Ludwig SL, Lewin KJ, Ruprecht RM, Rajacich GM, Schwabe AD (1982) The Cronkhite-Canada syndrome. An analysis of clinical and pathologic features and therapy in 55 patients. Medicine 61:293–309

Deschner EE, Lewis CM, Lipkin M (1963) In vitro study of human rectal epithelial cells. J Clin Invest 42:1922–1928

Desigan G, Wang M, Dewey Dunn G, Halter S, Vaughan S (1986) Intramucosal gastric carcinoma in a patient with familial polyposis coli. Am J Gastroenterol 81:19–22

Dormandy TL (1957) Gastrointestinal polyposis with mucocutaneous pigmentation (Peutz-Jeghers syndrome). N Engl J Med 256:1093–1102, 1141–1146, 1186–1190

Dozois RR, Judd ES, Dahlin DC, Bartholomew L (1969) The Peutz-Jeghers syndrome. Is there a predisposition to the development of intestinal malignancy? Arch Surg 98:509–517

Enzinger FM, Weiss SW (1983) Soft tissue tumors. CV Mosby, St. Louis, pp 45–70

Fearon ER, Hamilton SR, Vogelstein B (1987) Clonal analysis of human colorectal tumours. Science 238:193–196

Filipe MI, Mughal S, Bussey HJR (1980) Patterns of mucus secretion in the colonic epithelium in familial polyposis. Invest Cell Pathol 3:329–343

Friedman CJ, Fechner RE (1982) A solitary juvenile polyp with hyperplastic and adenomatous glands. Dig Dis Sci 27:946–948

Gardner EJ (1951) A genetic and clinical study of intestinal polyposis, a predisposing factor for carcinoma of the colon and rectum. Am J Hum Genet 3:167–176

Gardner EJ (1962) Follow-up study of a family group exhibiting dominant inheritance of a syndrome including intestinal polyps, osteomas, fibromas and epidermal cysts. Am J Hum Genet 14:376–390

Gardner EJ, Richards RC (1953) Multiple cutaneous and subcutaneous lesions occurring simultaneously with hereditary polyposis and osteomatosis. Am J Hum Genet 5:139–147

Gerdes J, Schwab U, Lemke H, Stein H (1983) Production of a mouse monoclonal antibody reactive with a human nuclear antigen associated with cell proliferation. Int J Cancer 31:13–20

Giardiello FM, Welsh SB, Hamilton SR et al. (1987) Increased risk of cancer in Peutz-Jeghers syndrome. N Engl J Med 316:1511–1514

Goodman ZD, Yardley JH, Milligan FD (1979) Pathogenesis of colonic polyps in multiple juvenile polyposis. Report of a case associated with gastric polyps and carcinoma of the rectum. Cancer 43:1906–1913

Gordon DL, Hallenbeck GA, Dockerty MB, Kennedy RLJ, Jackman RJ (1957) Polyps of the colon in children. Arch Surg 75:90–95

Grigioni WF, Alampi G, Martinelli G, Piccaluga A (1981) Atypical juvenile polyposis. Histopathology 5:361–376

Haggitt RC, Pitcock JA (1970) Familial juvenile polyposis of the colon. Cancer 26:1232–1238

Haggitt RC, Reid PJ (1986) Hereditary gastrointestinal polyposis syndromes. Am J Surg Pathol 10:871–887

Hamilton SR, Bussey HJR, Mendelsohn G et al. (1979) Ileal adenomas after colectomy in nine patients with adenomatous polyposis coli/Gardner's syndrome. Gastroenterology 77:1252–1257

Hara A, Watanabe M, Kodaira S et al. (1987) The expression of stage-specific embryonic antigen-1 in the non-cancerous colorectal epithelia of familial polyposis coli. Dis Colon Rectum 30:440–443

Heby O (1981) Role of polyamines in the control of cell proliferation and differentiation. Differentiation 19:1–20

Herrera L, Kakati S, Gibas L, Pietrzak E, Sandberg AA (1986) Gardner syndrome in a man with an interstitial deletion of 5q. Am J Med Genet 25:473–476

Herrera-Ornelas L, Elsiah S, Petrelli N, Mittelman A (1987) Causes of death in patients with familial polyposis coli (FPC). Sem in Surg Oncol 3:109–117

Hines MO, Hawley PH, Ray JE, Rush BM (1959) Polyps of the colon and rectum in children: experience with 27 cases. Dis Colon Rectum 2:161–165

Hoffmann DC, Goligher (1971) Polyposis of the stomach and small intestine in association with familial polyposis coli. Br J Surg 58:126–128

Hsu SH, Luk GD, Krush AJ, Hamilton SR, Hoover HH (1983) Multiclonal origin of polyps in Gardner syndrome. Science 221:951–953

Hutchinson RJ, Norris DG, Schnaufer L (1979) Chemotherapy: a successful application in abdominal fibromatosis. Pediatrics 63:157–159

Isaacson PG, Maclennan KA, Subbuswamy SG (1984) Multiple lymphomatous polyposis of the gastrointestinal tract. Histopathology 8:641–656

Itoh H, Obsato K, Yao T, Iida M, Watanabe H (1979) Turcot's syndrome and its mode of inheritance. Gut 20:414–419

Iwama T, Utsunomiya J, Sasaki J (1977) Epithelial cell kinetics in the crypts of familial polyposis of the colon. Jpn J Surg 7:230–234

Jagelman DG (1987) Extracolonic manifestations of familial polyposis coli. Cancer Genet Cytogenet 27:319–325

Jarvinen H, Franssila KO (1984) Familial juvenile polyposis coli: increased risk of colorectal cancer. Gut 25:792–800

Jarvinen HJ, Sipponen P (1986) Gastroduodenal polyps in familial adenomatous and juvenile polyposis. Endoscopy 18:230–234

Jarvinen HJ, Nyberg M, Peltokallio P (1983) Biliary involvement in familial adenomatosis coli. Dis Colon Rectum 26:525–528

Jass JR, Bussey HJR, Williams CB, Morson BC (1987) Juvenile polyposis: a precancerous condition. Gut 28:1367 A

Jass JR, Williams CB, Bussey HJR, Morson BC (1988) Juvenile polyposis: a precancerous condition. Histopathology 13:619–630

Jeghers H, McKusick VA, Katz KH (1949) Generalised intestinal polyposis and melanin spots of the oral mucosa, lips and digits. A syndrome of diagnostic significance. N Engl J Med 241:993–1005, 1031–1036

Jones IT, Jagelman DG, Fazio VW, Lavery IC, Weakley SL, McGannon E (1986) Desmoid tumors in familial polyposis coli. Ann Surg 204:94–97

Jones MA, Hebert JC, Trainer TD (1987) Juvenile polyp with intramucosal carcinoma. Arch Pathol Lab Med 111:200–201

Jones TR, Nance FC (1977) Periampullary malignancy in Gardner's syndrome. Ann Surg 185:565–573

Kerr JG (1948) Polyposis of the colon in children. Am J Surg 76:667–671

Kingston JE, Herbert A, Draper GJ, Mann JR (1983) Association between hepatoblastoma and polyposis coli. Arch Dis Child 58:959–962

Kinzbrunner B, Ritter S, Domingo J, Rosenthal CJ (1983) Remission of rapidly growing desmoid tumours after tamoxifen therapy. Cancer 52:2201–2204

Klein WA, Miller HH, Anderson M, DeCosse JJ (1987) The use of indomethacin, sulindac and tamoxifen for the treatment of desmoid tumours associated with familial polyposis. Cancer 60:2863–2868

Klemmer S, Pascoe L, DeCosse J (1987) Occurrence of desmoids in patients with familial adenomatous polyposis of the colon. Am J Med Genet 28:385–392

Komorowski RA, Tresp MG, Wilson SD (1986) Pancreaticobiliary involvement in familial polyposis coli/Gardner's syndrome. Dis Colon Rectum 29:55–58

Konishi F, Wyse NE, Muto T, Sawada T, Morioka Y, Sugimara H, Yamaguchi K (1987) Peutz-Jeghers polyposis associated with carcinoma of the digestive organs. Dis Colon Rectum 30:790–799

Kurtz RC, Sternberg SS, Miller HH, DeCosse JJ (1987) Upper gastrointestinal neoplasia in familial polyposis. Dig Dis Sci 32:459–465

Kyriakos M, Condon SC (1978) Enteritis cystica profunda. Am J Clin Pathol 69:77–85

Lamuraglia GM, Lacaine F, Malt RA (1986) High ornithine decarboxylase activity and polyamine levels in human colorectal neoplasia. Ann Surg 204:89–93

Lees CD, Herman RE (1981) Familial polyposis coli associated with bile duct cancer. Am J Surg 145:378–380

Lehur PA, Madarnas P, Devroede G, Perey BJ, Menard DB, Hamade N (1984) Peutz-Jeghers syndrome: association of duodenal and bilateral breast cancers in the same patient. Dig Dis Sci 29:178–182

Lewis JH, Ginsberg AL, Toomey KE (1983) Turcot's syndrome: evidence for autosomal dominant inheritance. Cancer 51:524–528

Li FP, Thurber WA, Seddon J, Holmes GE (1987) Hepatoblastoma in families with polyposis coli. JAMA 257:2475–2477
Linos DA, Dozois RR, Dahlin DC, Bartholomew LG (1981) Does Peutz-Jeghers syndrome predispose to gastrointestinal malignancy? A later look. Arch Surg 116:1182–1184
Lipkin M (1978) Susceptibility of human population groups to colon cancer. Adv Cancer Res 27:281
Lipkin M (1980) The prevention of colon cancer. Am J Med 68:917–931
Lipkin M, Blattner WA, Gardner EJ et al. (1984) Classification and risk assessment of individuals with familial polyposis, Gardner's syndrome and familial non-polyposis colon cancer from [^{3}H] thymidine labelling patterns in colonic epithelial cells. Cancer Res 44:4201–4207
Liu TH, Chen M-C, Tseng H-C (1978) Malignant change of juvenile polyp of colon. A case report. Chin Med J (Engl) 4:434–439
Llopis MD, Menezo JL (1987) Congenital hypertrophy of the retinal pigment epithelium and familial polyposis of the colon. Am J Ophthalmol 103:235–236
Luk GD, Baylin SB (1984) Ornithine decarboxylase as a biological marker in familial colonic polyposis. N Eng J Med 311:80–83
McAdam WAS, Goligher JC (1970) The occurrence of desmoids in patients with familial polyposis coli. Br J Surg 57:618–631
McColl I, Bussey HJR, Veale AMC, Morson BC (1964) Juvenile polyposis coli. Proc R Soc Med 57:896–897
Miller RH, Sweet RH (1937) Multiple polyposis of the colon. Ann Surg 105:511–515
Morson BC (1962) Some peculiarities in the histology of intestinal polyps. Dis Colon Rectum 5:337–344
Muto T, Kamiya J, Sawada T, Agawa S, Morioka Y, Utsunomiya J (1985) Mucin abnormality of colonic mucosa in patients with familial polyposis coli. A new tool for early detection of the carrier? Dis Colon Rectum 28:147–148
Muto T, Agawa S, Ooya M, Morioka Y (1987) Mucin abnormality in colonic mucosa in patients with familial polyposis coli. Semin Surg Oncol 3:179–182
Narita T, Eto T, Ito T (1987) Peutz-Jeghers syndrome with adenomas and adenocarcinomas in colonic polyps. Am J Surg Pathol 11:76–81
Naylor EW, Gardner EJ (1981) Adrenal adenomas in a patient with Gardner's syndrome. Clin Genet 20:67–73
Ohsato K, Yao T, Watanabe H, Iida M, Itoh H (1977) Small intestinal involvement in familial polyposis diagnosed by operative intestinal fiberscopy. Dis Colon Rectum 20:414–420
Painter TA, Jagelman DG (1985) Adrenal adenomas and adrenal carcinoma in association with hereditary adenomatosis of the colon and rectum. Cancer 55:2001–2004
Perkins JT, Blackstone MO, Riddell RH (1985) Adenomatous polyposis coli and multiple endocrine neoplasia type 2b. A pathogenetic relationship. Cancer 55:375–381
Peutz JLA (1921) 'Very remarkable case of familial polyposis of mucous membrane of intestinal tract and nasopharynx accompanied by peculiar pigmentations of skin and mucous membrane.' Ned Maandschr Geneesk 1:134–146
Phillips SF (1985) Altered physiology. In: Dozois RR (ed) Alternatives to conventional ileostomy. Year Book Medical, Chicago, pp 146–159
Pieterse AS, Leong ASY, Rowland R (1985) The mucosal changes and pathogenesis of pneumatosis cystoides intestinalis. Hum Pathol 16:683–688
Plail RO, Bussey HJR, Glazer G, Thomson JPS (1987) Adenomatous polyposis: an association with carcinoma of the thyroid. Br J Surg 74:377–380
Procter H, Singh L, Baum M, Brinkley D (1987) Response of multicentric desmoid tumours to tamoxifen. Br J Surg 74:401
Rabin ER, Patel T, Chen F-H, Gunalp S, Brown HW (1979) Juvenile colonic polyposis coli with villous adenoma and retroperitoneal fibrosis: report of a case. Dis Colon Rectum 22:63–67
Reid JD (1974) Intestinal carcinoma in the Peutz-Jeghers syndrome. JAMA 229:833–834
Reitamo JJ, Scheinin TM, Hayry P (1986) The desmoid syndrome: new aspects in cause, pathogenesis and treatment of the desmoid tumor. Am J Surg 151:230–237

Restrepo C, Moreno J, Duque E, Cuello C, Amsel J, Corren P (1978) Juvenile colonic polyposis in Colombia. Dis Colon Rectum 21:600–612
Riley E, Swift M (1980) A family with Peutz-Jeghers syndrome and bilateral breast cancer. Cancer 46:815–817
Ross JE, Mara JE (1974) Small bowel polyps and carcinoma in multiple intestinal polyposis. Arch Surg 108:736–738
Rothman D, Su CP, Kendall AB (1975) Dilemma in a case of Turcot's (glioma-polyposis) syndrome: report of a case. Dis Colon Rectum 18:514–515
Rozen P, Baratz M (1982) Familial juvenile colonic polyposis with associated colon cancer. Cancer 49:1500–1503
Ruvalcaba RHA, Myhre S, Smith DW (1980) Sotos syndrome with intestinal polyposis and pigmentary changes of the genitalia. Clin Genet 18:413–416
Sachatello CR, Hahn IS, Carrington CB (1974) Juvenile gastrointestinal polyposis in a female infant. Report of a case and a review of the literature of a recently recognised syndrome. Surgery 75:107–113
Salem OS, Steck WD (1983) Cowden's disease (multiple hamartoma and neoplasia syndrome). J Am Acad Dermatol 8:686–696
Sarre RG, Frost AG, Jagelman DG, Petras RE, Sivak MV, McGannon E (1987) Gastric and duodenal polyps in familial adenomatous polyposis: a prospective study of the nature and prevalence of upper gastrointestinal polyps. Gut 28:306–314
Schneider NR, Cubilla AL, Chaganti RSK (1983) Association of endocrine neoplasia with multiple polyposis of the colon. Cancer 51:1171–1175
Scully RE (1970) Sex cord tumour with annular tubules. A distinctive ovarian tumour of the Peutz-Jeghers syndrome. Cancer 25:1107–1121
Shaw EB, Hennigar GR (1974) Intestinal lymphoid polyposis. Am J Clin Pathol 61:417–422
Shepherd NA, Jass JR, Duval I, Moskowitz RL, Nicholls RJ, Morson BC (1987 a) Restorative proctocolectomy with ileal reservoir: pathological and histochemical study of mucosal biopsy specimens. J Clin Pathol 40:601–607
Shepherd NA, Bussey HJR Jass JR (1987 b) Epithelial misplacement in Peutz-Jeghers polyps: a diagnostic pitfall. Am J Surg Pathol 11:743–749
Shepherd NA, Hall PA, Coates PJ, Levison DA (1988) Primary malignant lymphoma of the colon and rectum: a histopathological and immunohistochemical study of 45 cases with clinicopathological correlations. Histopathology 12:235–252
Smilow PC, Pryor CA, Swinton NW (1966) Juvenile polyposis coli. A report of three patients in three generations of one family. Dis Colon Rectum 9:248–254
Smith WG (1959) Desmoid tumors in familial multiple polyposis. Mayo Clin Proc 34:31–38
Solomon E, Voss R, Hall V et al. (1987) Chromosome 5 allele loss in human colorectal carcinomas. Nature 328:616–619
Solter D, Knowles BB (1978) Monoclonal antibody defining a stage-specific mouse embryonic antigen (SSEA-1). Proc Natl Acad Sci USA 75:5565–5569
Sommerhaug RG, Mason T (1970) Peutz-Jeghers syndrome and ureteral polyposis. JAMA 211:120–122
Spigelman AD, Phillips RKS, Williams CB, Bussey HJR (1988) Foregut screening in familial adenomatous polyposis (FAP). Gut 29:A 1445
Stemper TJ, Kent TH, Summers RW (1975) Juvenile polyposis and gastrointestinal carcinoma. Ann Intern Med 83:639–646
Stryker SJ, Carney JA, Dozois RR (1987) Multiple adenomatous polyps arising in a continent reservoir ileostomy. Int J Colorectal Dis 2:43–45
Sugihara K, Jass JR (1986) Colorectal goblet cell mucin heterogeneity and its relation to malignant disease. J Clin Pathol 39:1088–1095
Sugihara K, Jass JR (1987) Colorectal goblet cell mucin in familial adenomatous polyposis. J Clin Pathol 40:608–611
Sugihara K, Muto T, Kamiya J, Konishi F, Sawada T, Morioka Y (1982) Gardner's syndrome associated with periampullary carcinoma, duodenal and gastric adenomatosis. Dis Colon Rectum 25:766–771

Trau H, Schewach-Millet M, Fisher BK, Tsur H (1982) Peutz-Jeghers syndrome and bilateral breast carcinoma. Cancer 50:788–792

Turcot J, Despres JP, St. Pierre F (1959) Malignant tumors of the central nervous system associated with familial polyposis of the colon: report of two cases. Dis Colon Rectum 2:465–468

Utsunomiya J, Nakamura T (1975) The occult osteomatous changes in the mandible in patients with familial polyposis coli. Br J Surg 62:45–51

Utsunomiya J, Gocho H, Miyanga T, Hamaguchi E, Kashimure A, Aoki N, Komatsu I (1975) Peutz-Jeghers syndrome: its natural course and management. Johns Hopkins Med J 136:71–82

Veale AMO, McColl I, Bussey HJR, Morson BC (1966) Juvenile polyposis coli. J Med Genet 3:5–16

Waddell WR, Gerner RE (1980) Indomethacin and ascorbate inhibit desmoid tumours. J Surg Oncol 15:84–90

Waddell WR, Gerner RE, Reich MP (1983) Non-steroidal anti-inflammatory drugs and tamoxifen for desmoid tumours and carcinoma of the stomach. J Surg Oncol 22:197–211

Watanabe H, Enjoji M, Yao T, Ohsato K (1978) Gastric lesions in familial adenomatosis coli. Hum Pathol 9:269–283

Williams GT, Arthur JF, Bussey HJR, Morson BC (1980) Metaplastic polyps and polyposis of the large intestine. Histopathology 4:155–170

Williams GT, Bussey HJR, Morson BC (1985) Inflammatory 'cap' polyps of the large intestine. Br J Surg 72 [Suppl]:S 133

Yatto RP (1982) Colonic lipomatosis. Am J Gastroenterol 77:436–437

Yonezawa S, Nakamura T, Tanaka S, Sato E (1982) Glycoconjugate with Ulex europaeus agglutinin-1 binding sites in normal mucosa, adenoma and carcinoma of the human large bowel. JNCI 69:777–785

Yonezawa S, Nakamura T, Tanaka S, Maruta K, Nishi M, Sato E (1983) Binding of Ulex europaeus agglutinin-1 in polyposis coli: comparative study with solitary adenomas in the sigmoid colon and rectum. JNCI 71:19–24

Young RH, Welch WR, Dickersin GR, Scully RE (1982) Ovarian sex cord tumour with annular tubules. Review of 74 cases including 27 with Peutz-Jeghers syndrome and four with adenoma malignum of the cervix. Cancer 50:1384–1402

Young RH, Dickersin GR, Scully RE (1983) A distinctive ovarian sex cord tumor causing sexual precocity in the Peutz-Jeghers syndrome. Am J Surg Pathol 7:233–243

Subject Index

The numbers set in *italics* refer to those pages on which the respective catch-word is discussed in detail

Index of Volumes 77–80 Current Topics in Pathology

Volume 77: Morphological Tumor Markers. Edited by G. SEIFERT

G. L. WRIGHT JR., A. D. COX, Monoclonal Antibodies to Human Tumor Antigens

T. M. CHU, Immunohistochemical Markers for Human Cancer

H. DENK, Immunohistochemical Methods for the Demonstration of Tumor Markers

R. MOLL, Epithelial Tumor Markers: Cytokeratins and Tissue Polypeptide Antigen (TPA)

G. KLÖPPEL, J. CASELITZ, Epithelial Tumor Markers: Oncofetal Antigens (Carcinoembryonic Antigen, Alpha Fetoprotein) and Epithelial Membrane Antigen

T. O. ROGNUM, P. S. THRANE, F. R. KORSRUD, P. BRANDTZAEG, Epithelial Tumor Markers: Special Markers of Glandular Differentiation

W. ALTMANNSBERGER, M. OSBORN, Mesenchymal Tumor Markers: Intermediate Filaments

H. F. OTTO, R. BERNDT, K. SCHWECHHEIMER, P. MÖLLER, Mesenchymal Tumor Markers: Special Proteins and Enzymes

R. V. IOZZO, Proteoglycans and the Intercellular Tumor Matrix

J. CASELITZ, Basal Membrane Antigen as Tumor Markers

J. CASELITZ, Lectins and Blood Group Substances as "Tumor Markers"

PH. U. HEITZ, Neuroendocrine Tumor Markers

P. KLEIHUES, M. KIESSLING, R. C. JANZER, Morphological Markers in Neuro-Oncology

TH. LÖNING, K. MILDE, Viral Tumor Markers

I. DAMJANOV, Cell, Tissue and Organ Specific Tumor Markers: An Overview

Volume 78: Ovarian Pathology. Edited by F. NOGALES

I. DAMJANOV, Ovarian Tumours in Laboratory and Domestic Animals

H.-E. STEGNER, Hormonally Related Non-Neoplastic Conditions of the Ovary

L. L. ADCOCK, L. P. DEHNER, Surgical Staging of Ovarian Tumours: The Individual and Integrative Roles of the Oncologist and Pathologist

C. NUÑEZ, Cytopathology and Fine-Needle Aspiration in Ovarian Tumours: Its Utility in Diagnosis and Management

S. G. SILVERBERG, Prognostic Significance of Pathologic Features of Ovarian Carcinoma

H. FOX, The Concept of Borderline Malignancy in Ovarian Tumours: A Reappraisal

E. SAKSELA, Advances in Immunohistochemistry of Ovarian Tumours

Volume 79: Cell Kinetics of the Inflammatory Reaction.
Edited by O. IVERSEN

O. H. IVERSEN, The Cell Kinetics of the Inflammatory Reaction. Introduction and Overview

H. B. BENESTAD, O. D. LAERUM, The Neutrophilic Granulocyte

I. C. M. MACLENNAN, S. Oldfield, Y.-J. LIU, P. J. L. LANE, Regulation of B-Cell Populations

G. JANOSSY, D. CAMPANA, A. AKBAR, Kinetics of T Lymphocyte Development

S. FOSSUM, The Life History of Dendritic Leucocytes (DL)

R. VAN FURTH Origin and Turnover of Monocytes and Macrophages

D. O. ADAMS, T. A. HAMILTON, The Activated Macrophage and Granulomatous Inflammation

L. ENERBÄCK, K NORRBY, The Mast Cells

J. L. VAN LANCKER, Molecular Events in Liver Regeneration and Repair

Volume 80: Biological Characterization of Bone Tumors.
Edited by A. ROESSNER

G. C. STEINER, Neuroectodermal Tumor Versus Ewing's Sarcoma – Immunohistochemical and Electron Microscopic Observations

A. SCHULZ, G. JUNDT, Immunohistological Demonstration of Osteonectin in Normal Bone Tissue and in Bone Tumors

J. ALTHOFF, P. QUINT, H. J. HÖHLING, A. ROESSNER, E. GRUNDMANN, Tumor Bone Formation in Different Osteosarcomas: Topological, Biochemical, and Histochemical Analyses

E. VOLLMER, A. ROESSNER, P. WUISMAN, A. HÄRLE, E. GRUNDMANN, The Proliferation Behavior of Bone Tumors Investigated with the Monoclonal Antibody Ki-67

W. MELLIN, W. DIERSCHAUER, W. HIDDEMANN, A. ROESSNER, G. EDEL, P. WUISMAN, A. HÄRLE, E. GRUNDMANN, Flow Cytometric DNA Analysis of Bone Tumors

L. E. WOLD, T. SPELSBERG, N. JIANG, F. SIM, Steroid Receptors and Giant Cell Tumor of Bone

J. J. BROOKS, J. Q. TROJANOWSKI, V. A. LIVOLSI, Chondroid Chordoma: A Low-Grade Chondrosarcoma and Its Differential Diagnosis

V. BOUROPOULOU, A. BOSSE, A. ROESSNER, E. VOLLMER, G. EDEL, P. WUISMAN, A. HÄRLE, Immunohistochemical Investigation of Chordomas: Histogenetic and Differential Diagnostic Aspects

A. ROESSNER, E. VOLLMER G. ZWADLO, C. SORG, M. KOLVE, D. B. v. BASSEWITZ, P. WUISMAN, A. HÄRLE, E. GRUNDMANN, The Cytogenesis of Macrophages and Osteoclast-like Giant Cells in Bone Tumors with Special Emphasis on the So-Called Fibrohistocytic Tumors